THE NIGERIAN HEALTH SYSTEM'S DEBACLE AND FAILURE!

THE NIGERIAN HEALTH SYSTEM'S DEBACLE AND FAILURE!

DANIEL M. N. McDIKKOH, MD, PhD

LIBRARY OF CONGRESS CONTROL NUMBER:		2009914135
ISBN:	HARDCOVER	978-1-4500-2105-0
	SOFTCOVER	978-1-4500-2104-3
	EBOOK	978-1-4500-2106-7

To order additional copies of this book, contact:
Xlibris Corporation
1-888-795-4274
www.Xlibris.com
Orders@Xlibris.com
72276

CONTENTS

DEDICATION

First, to my late mother, Gimbiya Markus N. McDikkoh (Gyi Jeb Sawntong), who rested in the Lord on July 15, 2001. Mom, you made sacrifices and dedicated your entire life for our upbringing—dead and alive—while we still miss you. You now reside in the bosom of our heavenly Father in eternal bliss, where you really belong! You most definitely were one of those whom this " . . . world was not worthy of . . . them" (Hebrews 11:38).

Second, to my uncle, Lt. Col. John Ngan Jeb Sawntong (Rtd.), a one-of-a-kind uncle whose love and dedication toward my progress was second to none in the early years of my life. There's no way that an ordinary words of "thank you" can or will ever adequately express my deep gratitude for your kindness! However, some deeds are best left for the expression of those simple words of "T-h-a-n-k-y-o-u"!

Finally, to a very special friend, a bosom pal at that, one aptly referred to in the divine definition and the biblical lingo in Psalms of David, "a friend closer than a brother," Chief Dr. Steven B. Manya, the Shatima of Adara, who through the years has been a dear friend, confidant, an immense source of strength and hope to all those who know him. Our friendship, to my belief, is not a happenstance or coincidental by human design, but clearly divinely predestined. There's no way that our friendship could, in any way, have been by chance or by human arrangement. All the years that we've been friends, you have touched my life, brought meaning to it in more ways than one or imagine. For this, I remain eternally grateful to Almighty God for His providence of and in this wise or arrangement! And this I sincerely mean with all my heart and with every fiber of my being!

My prayer and hope in all this is that during our affiliation over the years, I would hope that you too have experienced a similar satisfaction, at least at some point, in some small way, even if it's a smidgen of satisfaction as I have over the years of friendship. Should that be the case, then my joy would, indeed, be complete!

Finally, I wish you every blessing available in the Almighty's abundant storehouse of blessings!

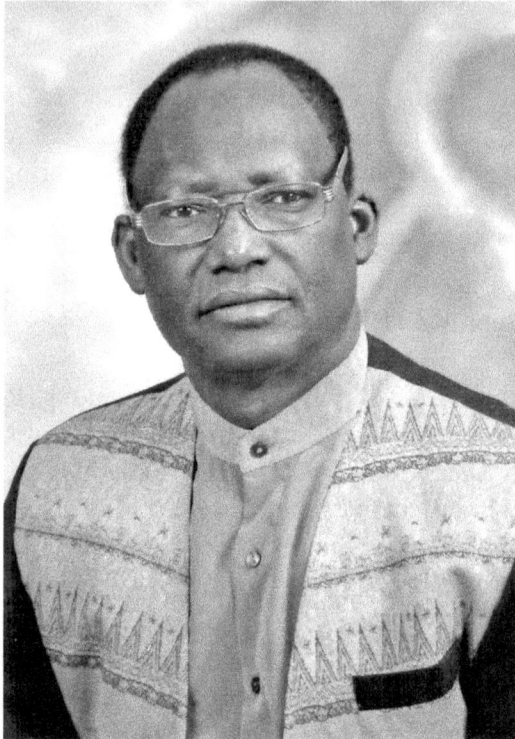

FOREWORD

There is a well-known health adage in Nigeria that is also a universally recognized dictum that goes something like this: "Health is wealth!" I stand corrected, but doesn't every known human group has a word for good health—what it means—and how to describe it to people who may not be from the same group? The literal meaning of the adage "Health is wealth" in Nigeria simply refers to the fact that it is when people are well that they can entertain any idea including work, seek wealth or accumulate it. Even self-defense, in certain poor health situations, is sometimes neglected. This simple explanation—I hope if I might venture to add, say, if I might add—is generally accepted as pretty accurate.

Then based on that premise, I would venture to make a categorically bold statement, but also claim as also universally accepted that a healthy nation comprises of healthy citizens. Therefore, a healthy nation is not only a nation of healthy citizens but one also of high productivity!

The definition of this concept, *health*, and to paraphrase the United Nations' definition, is complete fitness or freedom from any physical sickness or mental illness and/or social restraints or constraints. With this broad definition, it is therefore fair to conclude that the sum total of the citizens' health of a nation should reflect positively on the sum total of the nation's productivity. It is arguable that since this is not the case in the Nigeria's situation as we know it today, i.e., that a great number of Nigerians do not enjoy "good" or optimum health, that is all because of the poor state of the health system in the country, which has fallen woefully into a very bad disrepair state. Ironically, though, Nigeria happens to be one of the richest countries in Africa because it is one of those African economic "giants" that produces and exports oil (sells) to the greatest superpower (United States) in the world with the best health care system and prosperity that the world has ever known.

A cursory look at these raised issues, there is, or so it appears, as it seems as if there is a disconnect here, or somewhere, somehow, between the ideal and the actual, given the superlatives used in describing these two countries—Nigeria and the United States. However, there just might be a very simple explanation that seems to lie in the simple fact that one of the two () seems to care "more" about the health of its citizens while the other (Nigeria) does not seem even to be bothered. At least, at this juncture anyway, it shows only token concern (lip service) to the health concerns of its people. But how can that be in this day and age?

The answer to this question lies in the following pages of this book's edition. Dr. McDikkoh's perspective and his hypothesis that the problem of Nigeria's health system and their causes do, however, offer a clearer and more concise description and explanation as to the nature of contemporary social issues, which seem to galvanize and so presided over a stupendous slippery a slope in descending into such a degree of moral decay. These changes, if handled properly, can arrest the rate of decadence and perhaps reverse the course of events, not just in health system alone but also in all other social institutions in the country.

Furthermore, this book also delves into other issues and areas far beyond its purview and limited pages. These issues and or areas are also implied, by extension, even if they are distantly associated with the conventional meaning of health, but still within the concept and scope of a health as a system, at least to the limited in understanding of people who are uninformed. It is very obvious that education: politics; economics; culture; some aspects of the public health and its services (i.e., electricity, available and good water sources, etc.); transportation; and other related areas are all issues that, by extension, affect any health system directly and indirectly. However, it is remarkable that the author has not left any area out, but seems to find each and every area of the Nigerian lifestyle linked, affected or somehow directly influenced by the Nigerian health system. Moreover, his vast experience based on his vast travel experience here in Nigeria, other parts of Africa, Europe, Continental America (USA, Canada, and the Caribbean Islands) and parts of the Middle East have given him great exposure to different cultures, religions, lifestyles, and health systems of the world.

The author was himself a product, perhaps by happenstance, but he was probably a "victim" of the defunct British colonial legacy and rule in the then Northern Nigeria (or was he?). He started his education from a very humble beginning in elementary education system in the defunct Sudan Interior Mission (SIM) school system. He camped out (almost literally) for four long years in class one (first grade) in his native town of Kurmin Musa in Kachiya District of then Zaria Province. He was admitted to the nursing training at the VOM Christian Hospital, in Plateau, by sheer divine providence and determination. When he graduated in December of 1968 by passing the Nigerian Registered Nurse (NRN) that same year, he merely worked just four short years before proceeding to the United States to earn his BS Nursing, MA, MEd also in nursing and eventually PhD in Health Care Facility Administration. To top it all, he graduated as a doctor of medicine from a medical school in St. Lucia in 1994. Therefore, because of these qualifications and experience, to my mind, he is qualified to deal with this subject squarely. Thus he is able to compare and contrast as well as give appropriate commentary on the subject at hand.

He is of the belief, first and foremost, that the problems embedded in the health system in Nigeria must need thorough examination, if the correct diagnosis and effective cure are to come about. He believes not only in identifying the problem(s) as he sees it or them, but also he has a vehement aversion to the concept of a "band-aid or patchwork—policy—the so-called "make-do" or passing the buck—nor by the same token does he believe in "palliative" approach or "nipping" at the edges of a problem either. The failure to do what needs to be done is tantamount to dressing up a pig with an expensive dress and jewelry, which, at the tail of it, the expensive garb and ornaments that adorn the outside do not change the monster within. The dressed pig so adorn is still a pig, even with lipstick, ornaments, and all!

For me at this juncture, this edition is solid—a solid critique of not just the health system in Nigeria but also of the entire social order of the Nigerian society in general. In his considered opinion, the health system is completely broken down as it has failed all those for whom it was created and meant to serve. Therefore, it needs a complete overhaul. This is why the author laments the deplorable attitude and lack of professionalism of all health care professionals who have failed to live up to the Hippocratic Oath, the code of conduct that governs the behavior of all workers in the health care professions, a noble field for serving humanity. As a group, they seem to have abandoned all ethical scruples that circumscribe the profession as a noble one, but sadly been in favor of materialism and whims of wanton greed. These, according to the author, is little wonder that the health system, with most of the care facilities within its domain, has fallen prey and is in the shape that is being witnessed now!

To the keen reader, this book presents some challenges at least on two fronts. The first area of challenge attempts to provide insights to issues that affect the lives of ordinary Nigerians and the role of one in the society, to say the least. This area of challenge presents two fronts with the social ills and their causes as the first front and the second comprising of the solution or possible solutions. One is then challenged to take a look at our societal problems as identified afresh with some suggested solutions and to explore other ways that can better affect the type of change in the health system in which you would like to see take place.

The second area of challenge, after all, is not so much of a challenge per se, as commonly understood, rather, it is a point that the reader can grasped, or at least to ponder. For those who are satisfied with the health system in Nigeria or are not sure of what to think about it, for whatever reason, the issue at this point is rather a mute point at this juncture as they are, either blind, an axe to grind, or just downright intellectually dishonest by preferring to "sit on the fence," as all the clamor in this book or any where else is not nothing more than absolute balderdash—a well-managed complete exercise in futility, one incapable of rousing them from their intellectual stupor.

Simply and plainly put another way, it is like putting a wonderful world-class orchestral display of wonderful, angelic music composed by a world-renown composer for an audience that is both deaf and dumb, with none blessed with neither the sense of hearing nor speech to express appreciation. However, every single one in that unfortunate audience is blessed with sight, but visual ability without the complementing auditory sense of hearing is similar to viewing paradise through a very thick glass wall. This is worse than being in hell, even though the "hell" might be imaginary! If that be the case, then of course, this is a complete waste of your so-called precious time.

However, at the other end of the spectrum, there are those that the issues raised in this issue have provided them a juicy fodder that can spark nervous conversation, if not altogether reasonable and meaningful discussion. This is where the concept of synergy becomes handy.

Synergism is a more powerful effect that a group of parts can exert by working in unity harmoniously, or call it what you want, than what individual part can do alone. Working can and will explore both feelings and avenues of finding solutions and not just venting frustrations; it may even place you on the plane that enables to both view and scan the horizons of reality for frank assessment of direction to head to or to avoid.

Those that do see nothing wrong with health system in the country, sad to say, are capable of a frank assessment of the health situation or any situation in the country for that matter, much less to take any action that could lead to change.

So, by the author's candid assessment, now is no time for frolicking. We own our country and not the other way around, as some would have us believe. Just as the destruction of a society starts from within, one person at a time, slowly, but surely, so is building it or its restoration. It is time for action, and yes, it is now time for a united front, as only the wise with foresight are capable of positive thinking and looking ahead—looking for ways that will help affect change. Positive thinking leads to action that helps galvanize those agitated by what they see; and only the agitated are able to move, yes, move even mountains on some occasions, in the quest to change status quo when they finally concertedly determine to act. The choice is not only clear but also available and, I dare say, also solidly for the taking by those who are willing to get involved. To this I wholeheartedly concur. It's now totally all up you!

Dr. Steven B. Manya, Shattima of Adara, and Commissioner of Electoral Commission of the Federal Republic of Nigeria.

DISCLAIMER

Necessary steps and precautions have been employed to correct most, if not all, the mistakes that were contained in the first editorially unedited edition that was published by the Ahmadu Bello University Printing Press, Limited in Samaru Zaria, Nigeria in 2005. However, this does not guarantee or even warrant any assumption of total accuracy of the content and all quoted information within the context of this book, as typographical errors and, or some omissions, might still exist. Since its text is not claimed as absolutely complete, no any illicit activity based on any of the ideas expressed within its pages, either in application or its misapplication, for that matter, expressed or implied, is supported or sanctioned.

Furthermore, certain aspects of quoted information or material and, in some cases, information about some of the authors may be incomplete. In view of all the above, therefore, the reader's discretion in applying of any of the information in its text, whether in general or in particular, is strongly encouraged; this continues to remain under the sole volitional control and the domain of the reader.

Lastly, I do cherish and will continue to cherish all encouragement and, I might add, your constructive criticisms, also, of all who will read this book; that means every single one of all of you!

PREFACE

Before writing this book, I had contemplated writing about the health system in Nigeria for years. However, it was in mid November, 1994 that I actually started jotting ideas about the book down in earnest. Many titles for the book at the time came to mind, but I finally settled on this one: Nigerian Health System: Efficient as Designed or Debacle, in Shambles and Taters? All of the research notes and the entire first draft of the manuscript were handwritten and later typed out by my late brother, Mr. Dawuda Markus N. McDikkoh, who passed away in early May 1999.

From the time period between the early (or when first draft was began, on November 14, 1994,) and the final copy in June 2005, which was then submitted to the Ahmadu Bello, University Printing Press, Samaru, Zaria, in Nigeria, is about ten and a half years. There were many alterations, as you might have imagined, a result of the following:

1. Typographical errors (typos) either

   a. due to misreading (intentional or otherwise) of handwritten words or letters, leading to alterations in word meaning, as well as a sentence or paragraph, and
   b. due to changes in the political climate of the country of the time period, or the rampant shortages of essentials, but especially of gasoline (petrol), food, services—i.e., electricity, telephone, transportation, et cetera, in a country so blessed with all of the above and more.

2. Rate and tone of politics, political flux (which had started with the coming to power of General Ibrahim Babangida in 1983):

    a. Turmoil in an unstable country, like Nigeria, caught up in too fast a speed in development.

    b. Such a situation culminated in the election of a former head of state, General Olusegun Obasanjo, in 1997 before the final copy was printed in mid-August 2005.

3. All the changes, in both the political atmosphere and social institutions services in the country, made revision or changes inevitably necessary and regular, if not constant, of the research material.

The alterations referred to in the preceding paragraph did, as a matter of fact, continue in spite and despite all attempts and every precautionary measures that were available in my arsenals to prevent them from recurring again. They persisted even when the very last copy was taken to press as we had given up the correction as they simply were just too many. My fears had been confirmed after proofreading the previous copies as mistakes reoccur time and again. To my shock and surprise, as my fears and dismay were all confirmed, this particular press was hell-bent in producing junk work out of this book, so I gave up trying and permitted the print work to continue. My only regret and absolute chagrin was that I had to pay, and handsomely too, for it!

It was abundantly clear to me at that point that there was little or no professional editorial oversight during the printing process of the book as should have been. The Ahmadu Bello University Printing Press did such a poor job in the process that the degree of unprofessionalism, so clearly displayed in the final product, is just numbingly mind-boggling that it defies every reason or explanation.

All printing presses, good and professional ones that is, have set criteria for publishing all book materials from manuscripts. To add more insult to injury, the charges for this piece of sorry mess were so exorbitant, which I still paid. Finally and in addition to all that I have just described, the management of the press abrogated on the agreement agreed—terms and conditions governing payment.

First, one-third of the total charges agreed would be paid before the printing process started and the balance only after completion of the total work was done. I fulfilled my part of that obligation as part of the prearranged agreement. However, before the printing process had even started, I was approached by the management to give more money for the down payment of about fifty percent (50%). The excuse given for this attempted breach of contract was the unforeseen increase in the cost of materials. After a protracted period of time with no progress made in printing, I authorized upping the payment to 50 percent (which proved to be a mistake after all), yet shortly after this episode, I was again asked to make more payment to enable management meet staff payroll. My insistence that the publisher should keep its part of the agreement, as I had no way of gauging progress, fell on deaf ears. Only later did my representative assured me that the work was "making some progress" since I was away in the United States.

Let me spare you all the details. This work that was supposed to be done in two to three months was finally done in one year and two months plus, and only after I had permitted increasing the down payment to 75 percent as the work was not going to advance any further without further payment. I absolutely refused to give anything over the 75 percent as the demand had been that all the money had to be paid for the work to be completed.

The publisher sent two representatives for the launching of the book in August 2005, and to confirm that it was free of any modicum of professionalism or professional shame, its representative brought with them some individuals claiming to represent some bookstores that can or will help me market the sales of my book. This to me, ladies and gentlemen, epitomizes the zenith of shamelessness by a business enterprise that has no business whatsoever being in noble profession of publishing! If this so-called university press were anywhere near a developed society where contracts laws are respected and enforced, today I would be sitting pretty. Yes, you guess it, on a heap of doe!

FIRST EDITION: LAUNCH AND REVIEW

During the launching of the book in at the Prison Staff College compound, Barnawa, Kaduna, in August 2005, one Alhaji Yakubu Aliyu, director of the Kaduna State Library Board, sent a representative—perhaps one of his lieutenants—who did a pretty good job in pointing out areas of deficiencies and errors based on his observation in several areas. He was, in all fairness, kinder in his critique than I would have been had I been the one who evaluated this piece of work—as a matter of fact, any piece of work with such level of errors. These included typographical, grammar, and syntax errors. He also advanced some recommendations that he felt needed to be addressed in future for the next edition. The following points were some of the several that he stressed in his critique:

1. "Too many mistakes, including typographical, grammatical, as well as syntactical mistakes".
2. "A lot of unnecessary spelling mistakes."
3. "Copious opinions but dirge [shortage or scant—addition and emphasis mine] of facts backing presented opinions."
4. Addressing "wrong issues with a fixation and deliberation centering on a very few areas, but to the exclusion of some of the more serious ones."
5. A deliberate attempt to "ignore palpable achievement and progress made in several social fronts, i.e., a fixation on only the negatives as the main thrust or approach the book."

These points were very well taken then, as I also do now, as I promised to "keep them in mind" and would review them whenever revision or a new edition were ever to be contemplated in future. However, the only revision that is necessary and the only one that should be made here, basically, has two facets: correcting the typographical errors—which is a must, yet one that could easily have been corrected or done by the publisher had the publisher so chose. Instead, the publisher, for lack of professional ethical values, chose to botch publishing the book even as it was paid handsomely!

While I do not wish to shirk from my responsibility, nor do I want to give the impression that I nurse a grudge and so quoting, "Pass the buck," yet it was abundantly clear to me then, based on all that was taking place, that there was some effort exerted by the publisher to sabotage the book because of the issues raised in the book. For some unexplained reason, there was this insistence, if not zeal, at constantly changing the spelling of words that I would correct and correct time after time, yet when the next copy is delivered for proofreading, there would always be repeated each time. The new version always seemed to reflect a British spelling and writing style, a version quite different from the style (American) that I had used or intended. On the surface, this may appear to be a harmless oversight; however, the net result, like it or not, was alteration of the meaning the words were meant to portray. These alterations did more than change the meaning of the words, they also changed the sentences and/or paragraphs in which they appeared, also ultimately the meaning they were meant to define or clarify.

Last but not the least, the other aspect of change that is necessary, and so of necessity called for here, is to change the publisher, period! It will, indeed, be foolhardy for me to make the same mistake twice (as the saying "Once bitten, twice shy" is aptly applicable here) with a full knowledge of all that has transpired between me and an enterprise that has no savvy in professional publishing, nor does it have even the minutest of inkling proper business etiquettes or professional manners. The Ahmadu Bello University Printing Press displayed a total sense of depravity by abdication with reckless abandon of ethical any standards, as it relates to professional standards of book publication and a complete absence professionalism. If I or anyone who reads this sorry account of this type of professional misconduct should choose to go to this so-called publisher in future, then they deserve all that the ABU Printing Press can dish out and more!

THIS EDITION

The main reason for writing this book is, principally, to describe the deplorable state of the health system of Nigeria and the poor services delivered within its care facilities and to look at some possible solutions to the problems. In addition to this deplorable state of affairs, which essentially is a failure to accomplish the noble mission of effectively delivering health services as mandated by law[*] to the citizens of Nigeria. And attendant to the abject failure of the health system are a host of other problems that have made the state of affairs in health sector bitterly unpalatable, i.e., the unprofessional attitude of health care workers with

---

[*]   Note that no specific Nigerian law is cited in support of this assertion, but for the fact that each year the legislatures at federal, states, and local government levels budget or include in their budgets funds specifically targeted for the running of health programs at their various levels of jurisdictions. Were this not the case, then why they bother in the first place? However, though, argument can be posited with ample evidence to back the claim that budgeting funds for failed social programs in Nigeria, all too often, have become legitimate avenues of misspending (through the misappropriation) of public funds.

the attendant and the deep-seated corruption of some of these health care workers—professional and paraprofessional alike.

SOCIETY: TOTAL SUM OF ALL ITS INDIVIDUAL PARTS

Nigeria has been in the doldrums of a moral morass for quite some time now, and that is putting it mildly. Changes first started occurring in the moral fiber and value system of Nigerians, then and only then did changes in all other areas started following suit. These changes did not happen overnight, but were rather very gradual when they started. Nigerians did not just wake up one day and find out that a lot of areas in their social lives have changed inalterably, thus causing changes in most social institutions as well as the services these social institutions provide, which no longer meet the needs of those whom they are supposed to serve in the first instance. When this slippery slope started, but no remedial measures were instituted, the natural outcome was the gathering of momentum, which has now reached "critical mass," and therefore, there is no stopping in it, or so it seems.

CHANGES THAT RESULT DUE TO CHANGE IN MORAL AND VALUE SYSTEM

Changes in one's value system—positive or negative—are brought about by a change here and there in an individual's value system that is dismissed as harmless. In time, these small alterations have cumulative effects that do tally up, and the result, a major shift in value system. After this then comes a similar shift in one's moral value system. It always starts with one individual or a group; change of beliefs or world views (value system) which inevitably begin to affect others or some within the community (local and/or societal) and the established norms. But it is also coupled with inadequate sanctions that are severe enough to forestall the spread of such aberrant behavior. Failure to nip the problem in time in the butt encourages its spread and so a shift in societal social values.

To summarize the system theory of organization by paraphrasing Rakich et al, (1977), an organization is only the sum of all of its individual parts.[*][2]

---

*   "A system consists of parts organized in a manner that produces a unified whole" from Jonathan S. Rakich et al., *Managing Health Care Organization* (Philadelphia, PA: W. B. Saunders Co., 1977), 157.

THE VERY FIRST SIGNS

When enough individuals in a society have experienced similar change or alteration, the nation is then bound to drift morally and, consequently, a shift in direction. In this particular case which I will tag the "Nigerian case," the effects have been so negative that services in the country are at the poorest level that they have ever been in, in all the history of the country. The health system, as do other social services in the country, did not just wake up one morning and noted to have gone south or bad all of a sudden. These changes did not sauntered in, but rather, they crept up slowly and to the surprise of only the naive, who happened to be in cahoots with materially minded, by either playing the ostrich or thinking that they really could eat their cake and also have it all at the same time.

The dangerous trail all began early in the 1980's although, frankly speaking, the seeds of corruption had been planted very much earlier and were evident as far back as early 1970s or even in the late 1960s during the military regime of General (Rtd) and Dr.—doctor of philosophy—Yakubu Gowon. Some may discount this as a litigate argument, but you may also remember a general attitude that was pervasive with vendors of food and other essential commodities in the era of the early to mid 1980's and the emergence of the diabolic vice, which some then and perhaps now would deliberately discount as inconsequential, but one that began to be witnessed when hawkers would not sell their commodities to anyone that wanted to buy them, but without the exact change. For sure, there were some of these vendors who legitimately did not have the change or had run out of it and unable to give back to the buyer their due change. However, many just used the "no change" available argument statement or a means used to defraud unsuspecting patrons/customers who needed to buy merchandise and were forced to forgive or ignore the spare change of their money. The vendor then walked away with the spare cash as a "dash" (gift), a superficial "tank-u, sa" with a huge and a gulf-like wide smile on his/her face, having successfully pulled off another fraudulent scheme for the day!

CONTINUATION OF THE SLIDE

Another clear example that indicated that the Nigerian nation was heading into moral and value abyss of depravity and degeneration was the paradigms of instances that also started showing up back in the 1980s. At this juncture, I will use some such instances to demonstrate the signs of erosion as the beginning of decay of moral values in the country.

During that era, government contracts had three pronged venues or approaches for procurement:

1. Knowing someone in "higher places" who could serve either as the one to award the contract or having a link to someone who could,
2. Having an agreement or a promise on the part of the person soon to procure the contract to pay 10 percent (10%) or more of the contract to be awarded prior to securing the contract.
3. Then selling the contract to someone else who might be in better financial position to execute the contract, and
4. Going to this stage that is part of step c above. Whoever the contract is allocated would collect the so-called mobilization funds meant for the purchase of material with which to start or complete the contract; but at this stage, the secured contract is then sold yet to someone else who is able to execute the contract, but he may or may not carry the contract to completion.

MORE EXAMPLES

Another and more alarming instance of the moral decay, at least to some of us anyway, involved corruption by the police force personnel who were charged with public and property safety protection—by a supposed honest law enforcement arm of the federal government. It turned out that the Nigerian police personnel started accepting bribe to the point that they grossly bastardized the graft process. For instance, assume that two vehicles were involved in a traffic accident and the police were involved, as the police was in charge for determining who of the two drivers was in breach of the traffic rules. Well, then as now, even though the situation is far worse today than way back then, according to the Nigerian police, the driver with more money and/or influence to give to the police is the driver at no fault even if he was the one at fault to cause the accident. The person who caused the accident and clearly at fault, but is a "big man"—meaning he/she is either a highly placed government official and/or has money—ended up being the victim in the traffic accident situation! Go figure!

HEAVENS HELP THE POLICE IN CHARGE!

By mid-1980s, the police behavior had become such a byword that police report commonly became derisively regarded as "erasable" or "rubutun yan sanda" in the Hausa language (police writing), meaning, a written report that can easily be erased, if the right amount of bribe money is advanced! At the very beginning, when such police misconduct started surfacing, people dismissed it or blamed it on the poor police pay/salary, which could easily be corrected by pay raises, or increase in salary was the argument. This was after the fact that the police personnel pay, on the average, was by far better than the salary structures of most ordinary Nigerians who worked in factories teachers or worked the farm. By comparison, the police pay was similar to the pay that blue-collar workers or that of the middle class in other western societies in the West. At the tail end of it, we have now come to realize that no matter what amount of the increase in salary or pay raise for the Nigerian police force, it is never enough as the police conduct only continues to worsen—their appetite for money and material goods is never satiated!

The examples cited above are only a few out of many more others. Some of the prominent ones which held sway at the very early stages of this moral decline, a herald that not very many Nigerians remember either because they are too young or were not even around when these events started surfacing. Others, especially oldsters—people fifty years and over—would remember, but they prefer to forget these events, in which case it could then be surmised that this is either because they were complicit or enablers to this mess of a national shame.

COLONIAL WHITE RULE VERSUS BLACK COLONIAL RULE

WHITE COLONIALS IN CHARGE

The following sayings: "Look before you leap" and "You cannot eat your cake and have it too" and other similar adages are axiomatic or essentially true statements. While these statements may be overused, yet they convey some essential truths about given situations, and in this instance, it is the black African and, specifically, Nigerian situation. On the first several paragraphs, we have discussed the moral and value system decay in

Nigeria. Now let us look back just some few decades back when, if you will recall, some self-righteous elite (from some of Nigeria's institutions of higher learning) were harping on the constant refrain of the white man doing all kinds of things to us: he "enslaved," "ruled," and "pillaged" us, this, that, and million other unsavory "things" as this list continues ad infinitum. The so-called mean, unkind, and rotten "white man" has done all that and more to us poor black people, not only here in continental Africa but also elsewhere around the globe.

And yet when the so-called evil white man was in charged, the health system worked very well! The health care facilities functioned well, the pharmacies were well supplied with every drug imaginable available to all that plied the corridors of every hospital. Electricity was available twenty-four hours a day and seven days a week; where pipe-borne water was available, it was supplied to every home that could afford to pay—both to Muslims and the Kafirs or kafirai all alike. I can go on and on as the list is inexhaustible, but I believe you get my drift!

To be perfectly honest with you, I have traveled far and wide in Europe and the Americas and have never met or come across any such creature called "white man" with all these horrible attributes or characteristics as described in the preceding lines in my thirty-six years of sojourn in United States or anywhere else in the world. Never! But let me describe the white man that I constantly meet in my constant travels: I constantly meet a kind and compassionate white man, one who is both willing and has repeatedly demonstrated this in taking all kinds of risks (the like of David Livingstone, Mungo Park, and many others) to help people of all races. I constantly meet compassionate white people who believe all people everywhere to be virtually equal, thus the sharing of information of every discovery in all fields, but especially in science, to help improve the lives of people everywhere. This definitely cannot be said of black people in Africa, who were responsible of selling their fellow black Africans into slavery and especially certain tribes of black people in Nigeria who are so heartless as to deny fellow black Nigerians electricity, medical care, pipe-borne water because of tribalism and religious beliefs!

Even more ridiculously ridiculous is the zany idea perpetrated by these so-called enlightened dons or elites—take your pick—that all the social problems in Nigeria (and therefore by extension all blacks' problems in the world) are caused by this unknown white man! This game or blame game or hate of white people, if you will, however, of the white man (or nasarathe Hausa word for a white person), that is, conveniently omits, wittingly or otherwise, some geographical areas of the world that white people come from. This blame or accusation is leveled at whites from certain regions of the world, while the "white man" from others is conveniently exempt, excluded, or "excused" from this implied so-called global blame. You see, this selective, yet at the same time supposedly "global" blame applies only to white people from the West, i.e., from the United States, Europe, Canada and Australia. It, however, does not apply to the white man from the Middle East (Arab countries) communist countries or the Latin Americas! This is astounding!

Before going any further, let me first at this point deal with this business of the "hate-of-the-white-man" façade of these hypocrites once and for all! For a start, I will like to posit that this so-called hate is not even a dislike, much less a hate. As a matter of fact, I believe that the so-called hate is in fact a very strong self-dislike. In other words, this is what Freudian psychology refers to as a defense mechanism of "projection" where the person with the strong feeling of hate toward someone or an object turns and accuses the object their hate as the one who hates them!

BLACK "COLONIAL" RULE (BLACK POWER)
BLACKS (AFRICANS) NOW IN CHARGE

Black people claim that white people do all of the things mentioned above, yet we take every opportunity that presents and, many at times, even invent the opportunities to imitate white people. We imitate the way the white people cook and eat, we dress like them, we live like they do as we have abandoned a good amount of our cultural, traditional heritage and still muster the visceral effrontery to claim or accuse white people of treating us badly, when we are guilty of treating our fellow blacks worse than the white man could never ever dream of doing. We dare to point any fingers at the white people! This is beyond amazing! This defies any imagination!

I am, however, not naïve as to want to give the impression that the white man gets a pass for his past mistakes. Not at all! White people have made more than their fair share of mistakes in dealings with black people in general, but especially with their Nigerian subjects during the British colonial presence and rule (from the mid-1850s to 1960) in Nigeria. When the colonial whites ruled in South Africa, all African politicians with clout and who wanted to matter in African politics in unison riled and lambasted white South Africans as racist negrophobes (fear of the black people or the black color), and perhaps rightly so.

Now, in referring to the "white man," I am not speaking exclusively about geography of the West or the predominantly Christian religion of the Western European countries that most white people from that circumscribed geography of that area—the so-called "West", as others conveniently choose to either forget or omit to include. I am referring to the universal white man in the west, east, north, south, or any other areas of our human-inhabited globe, period. That means a white person from every region of the globe, including the Arabs regions and all Arab countries, none is exempt here. A white person from any of the Arab countries is as guilty as the next one that happens to hail from elsewhere. Some, however, may argue that Arabs are not a white race. Well, that is a topic for debate another day, but not for right now, they are—they will serve the purpose here just fine.

Let us take a look at the behavior of some white people. Generally, as this is common knowledge, some white people see the white race as innately better and so a superior human race than the black race. This kind of feeling or belief, as claimed by psychologists, is a psychological disorder called "superiority complex." Unfortunately, white folks are not the only ones suffering from this aberration or mutant disorder, as black folks also suffer from its nasty variant called "tribalism" or "ethno-centricism."

The issue here, though, is not that white people believe themselves to be superior to black people, a false belief by the way, with no cogent basis whatsoever. If, for example, the physical features of white people (Caucasoid)—color (white) and straight hair (primates also have straight hair)—were the sole basis that serve as proof of superiority and/or the grounds of judging intelligence, then the question that naturally confronts such a postulate then is, "How come some white societies seem more intelligent than others?" For instance, why are the Caucasoid race group—i.e., Anglos and Germanic (Arian)—seem more intelligent than others,* say for example, Araboids (meaning from the Arabian stock, this neogilistic concoction is totally my creation) or Mongoloids? Please note the word *seem* because as they say and as far I am concerned, "beauty is in the eye of the beholder."

I will again further posit that the ability to dominate does not necessarily prove a superior intelligence. Actually, it all depends on the circumstances under which the domination occurs, since any variety of variables or factors can affect such a circumstance and so alter the outcome. A clear example is the use of guns. When white people came into contact with the black people in Africa, such primary or first contacts were exploratory in nature, subsequent to the initial ones that followed trading contacts aimed at further inland adventures into the hinterlands. Having firmly been established firm control following the initial contacts, subsequent but continuous contacts that followed were deliberately and systematically established trading posts, which were also aimed at disarming the so-called African "brutes."

Some argument could be made that it might have been for self-defense—i.e., the fear of self harm or the so-called "self" preservation, if you will—that drove these explorers into disarming the natives. However, there is very little evidence or facts, if there were ever any, that support the notion that the white missionaries, explorers or any other races that were not were threatened or attacked by the natives to cause such level of proactive change in behavior. There is, however, ample or perhaps an avalanche of evidence to suggest that there might have been fewer attacks (that resulted in either injury or death or both) to either explorers or the Christian missionaries in the jungles of Africa than the great numbers of deaths and at times massacres in the South Americas and/or the islands of the Pacific Ocean during the late 17th, 18th, and 19th centuries. In fact, if anything, the natives in continental Africa were less hostile and, I might add, very helpful to white explorers, as they went with these newcomers, showing them ways to move from place to place, to adapt and survive the harsh elements of climatic changes unfamiliar to these missionaries-explorers and wild animals, etcetera.

---

*   "Carl C. Brigham (1923), arguing for the exclusion of southern and eastern European immigrants who had scored poorly on supposed tests of innate intelligence" from Stephen J. Gould, *The Mis-measure of Man* (New York: W. W. Norton & Co., 1981) 20.

While the white man was neither naïve nor stupid, he was brave as this level of brevity had seen him all over and then known the world by looking for hidden treasures. While his smart abilities, at this time, allowed and enabled him to be familiar with all types of cues that indicated where to look for as well as how to get the hidden riches, of course, his level of astuteness cued him in and on areas of, real or hidden, dangers in attitude and behaviors of strange peoples he is in the midst of—people of different background and with customs unfamiliar to him. Finally, he was also very subtle because while he knew exactly what he was looking, he did not betray this desire in the process.

But with all that having been said about the white man, this can also equally be said on just about any race, for that matter, because the foregoing description does not require some superior intellect or very high level of intelligence to accomplish. Come to think of it, there is nothing to it really, other than ordinary intelligence, cunningness, and a lot of courage to adequately execute. The other necessary components to complete the drama are for the prey (victim in this instant) to be unarmed, or in possession of an ineffective weapon, and be oblivious or unsuspecting to the dangers of what is about to take place. Besides, this style of cunning behavior is always effective especially in situations where the so-called smart person is prepared, as this is almost always the case because the perpetrators would have had plenty of time to prepare and in possession of powerful weaponry, which, inevitably, they are always ready to use.

Another well-known saying "Duplicity is a vice and not a virtue" is so apt in its application, especially in this particular instance. This type of behavior is constantly in use by armed robbers or in such other situations, which those employing the deceptive behavior have nothing but ill will for their victims. At any rate, talk of a mismatch! In any given war or conflict, when one side is not appropriately equipped, for whatever reason, it is definitely not a match for its opponent because, of such a mismatch, the end result is bound to be disastrous, except and only if there is some divine miraculous intervention.

Therefore, it would be laughable if, for instance, an unsuspecting group armed with machetes would be expected to prevail in a conflict with a group that was armed with pistols and other sophisticated gadgets of war with a hidden agenda. No match, as was the expected outcome goes naturally, as any rational mind would rightly conclude and rightly so! A machete against a pistol is a joke and a bad joke at that, as anyone involved in that kind of arrangement, but belong to the group armed with machete, is either crazy or else he has secretly prearranged his funeral!

Here again, let me posit the point that had the black people in Africa—who found themselves at the receiving end of this bad deal which ultimately ended in white domination for several decades, had even locally made guns, in addition to bows and arrows—the white colonizers would have had to think twice, maybe trice, before attempting to go on with this inhuman crusades and carnage, which led to the subjugation of the so-called African brutes. But, alas! This was not the case! Africans were subjugated and treated terribly by these wealth-seeking colonialists who found it rather necessary, when on the contrary this was not so at all, to complete their domination, ravished the pristine resources of these countries by pillaging their resources' wealth bare. Finally, to show how totally deprived racists they were, the poor natives were treated to lives of slavery in their own countries.

What was the motive behind the actions of these white colonial rulers? Well, the answer lies in the first position that I posited earlier, which is, some white people feel that their race is a superior to the rest of the other human races, but especially the black race. This racist position has no explanation as there is no other way to adequately or appropriately explain it, at least to my satisfaction anyway! The result of this unfortunate racist behavior led to the near total destruction of natural resources of the dominated domains, which were carted off in order to develop the colonialists' countries of origins in the Europe. At the same time, they neglected the countries from where their newfound riches were taken.

However, whatever precious little development might have been done in these areas of their wealth's acquisition (the territories of domination) were not done as tokens of appreciation, but rather they were for the purpose to provide comfort to the brigands, the so-called superiors, as they ravished the natural resources of these countries. This facilitated in order to enable by furthering their complete parasitic decimation of these resources as they were intent in exploring for more. They were going to make sure every stone had been turned, with every diamond, gold, or any other precious stone extracted! And yes, this is only a very small part of the story that the white racist colonialists on the poor, defenseless Africans, as there are more and abundant horror stories of the awful acts, perpetrated on the African continent and its black natives that are absolutely and unpalatably gut-wrenching in literature in the history books!

Now let us turn our attention on black people's misdeeds perpetrated against fellow blacks. It is necessary to be even-handed—if we discussed some of the faults of the white colonialists, then it is only fair that evil deeds of black Africans are also equally partially portrayed and discussed as well.

The fact that white race is not superior to any other race is, without equivocation, and absolutely outside the realm of any dispute or debate. The white colonialists, or any white person for that matter, who that may harbor such a zany thought is inane and beyond help and plain dangerous! But what if I were to suggest that white racism pales in comparison to tribalism, what would be your reaction? While I do not know how you would react to this hypothesis, one thing I do know is that some black folks—including black Africans and especially some of the black ruling groups (ethnic tribes or tribal groups)—in Nigeria are, plain and simple, worse than the white racist colonialists.

Let me explain this carefully so as to make it to easy to grasp. The white colonial conquerors that invaded black Africa had, at least, "some" excuses for their racist attitude and reaction to black Africans. This is because, for some of them anyway, they had never seen the African creature who, to their utter surprise, looked very much like them and yet very different and all at the same time! While these Africans looked, talked like them and indeed were human beings, they wore black (actually dark) skin, while theirs—the white people—was very, very fair (not the common description of *white* as no skin of any race in the entire globe is white) skin; straight hair; long, narrow, and towering nose; and thin lips (some of the features characteristics of a Caucasoid). For them, this was a true paradox of nature. These apparent differences created, at least in the mind of some of the, the so-called real differences that warranted the intense and irrational racist belief which led to their racist activities.

On the other hand, the features or physical characteristics which seem to differentiate blacks (Negroid) from most other races are typically dark, skin, kinky hair, flat or broad nose, and thick lips. Most black people in continental Africa, but especially in the sub-Saharan desert including the southern aspects of the Sudan, share these common features that some wish they could change (refer to my previous insinuations of black people imitate white people and yet claim an intense hate for them).

Now let us go back to my assertion that some black people are intensely racist by way of tribalism (simply means an intense hate for your own kind or race), which is the worst kind of racism there is because this is exactly premise the assertion that "white racism pales in comparison to tribalism." Apologists for every misbehavior of black people invariably constantly go back to the same tired and old argument of the long wicked era of rule by the white man, who left the countries that they ruled, in quote "such deplorable states" and employed the "divide and conquer" as well as "divide and rule" arguments as sources of separation and disunity of the black folk. These approaches made governance easier for the colonial masters, but have proven elusive, if not difficult, even impossible for African politicians from the time we were granted independence, as it continues to be so even to the present day. Apartheid was roundly and soundly condemned by all African leaders—and rightly so, I might add, because it was the white man then in power. However, the same apartheid soon reared its ugly tentacles, under the governance of these same leaders, as soon as some of these leaders had secured power and total control. More will be said about this in subsequent chapters. Of course and conveniently, no one speaks about it either by default or by design, no one seems to care. This argument, however, conveniently and deliberately ignores the fact that the avenue toward achieving unity and easy governance resides only by way, perhaps the highway of freedom, and that is by treating the governed humanely and with dignity. Again more will be said about this topic later on.

Let me see if I can properly paraphrase the argument against the white man so as to better understand its premise: black mistreatment of other blacks is because of the white's long rule and mistreatment of the black people in Africa. I am now confused, really confused, and can understand if you are just as flummoxed! Let me get this right: the white person that we suppose so much dislike, even hate, is the same one that has taught our black leaders how to mistreat us, their very own black brothers and sisters, right? Hmm, this is interesting! Very interesting! In other words, blacks mistreat blacks because they were not only shown how to mistreat fellow blacks, but also taught or directed them as to how to mistreat their fellow blacks! Were this be the case, then these black leaders are not, after all, all that bright as they would like to have us all believe! As a matter of fact, they are both dumb and stupid—won't you say? If all they had to do was follow and carry out dumb directives foolishly without questions, then to my mind they are not smart at all!

I have never, as I am yet, read anywhere in history books, commentaries, or anywhere else that the colonial rulers left instructional manuals or blueprints for succeeding African nationals, who later assumed power, on how to mistreat other Africans. Nor I am yet to see blueprint left behind by white colonialists on how to be selfish and continue to stay in power perpetually and invent new ways to exercise dictatorial authority! But even if this were so, and any such "blueprints" of instruction on how to prey on your ilk and kind are found, why would anyone accept instructions from someone that they claim they hate so much anyway? And if anyone were to accept such instructions, does the person accepting such directives take any responsibility for his/her action? Does he or she have a mind, a conscience? Maybe, just maybe, answers to all the above questions are negative, thus the resort to the scapegoat game! To ask that objective be employed here to these people is far-fetched, but then, to rely on their subjectivity is definitely a mistake it is so wrapped in—damaged beyond retrieve. This is because nowhere in the world is such blatant disregard for human life and rights as is done in Africa, but particularly in the present-day Nigeria. A large section of population wallows in abject poverty and neglect by its own government as these people are denied the most basics essentials for a descent living. No good drinking water, no good roads to access in medical emergencies and electricity, simply because of tribal or ethnic group and/or religious affiliation. Amazing!

Some Nigerians, as are some blacks and whites everywhere, do want to eat their cakes and have them all at the same time too, yet these apologists and these dictators in Nigeria do not seem to appreciate the degree of impossibility of this situation! The white colonial powers handed power to the nationals of African countries, including those in Nigeria. There were no Martians within this group of would-be leaders, all 100 percent of them—tangible and palpably human Africans.

The handing of power to them was tantamount to giving them self-rule or governance, but to this group of new "rulers," it was a symbol of "black power" colloquially translated to mean the misuse or misapplication of power (seen in the conduct of bullies or misrule). Granted some white folks are also negrophobes or have a condition of that can be described as "negrophobia" (fear of black people) and, to some degree, this is understandable on the basis of previous discussion on this issue, an interracial phenomenon which continues to defy both explanation and common sense!

But enough has already been said about this topic in this section with some scattered commentary now and then throughout the entire of this new edition. Attention now needs to shift onto the organization of this edition and what new approach is used in dealing with the health system of the Nigerian society.

This edition is divided into four sections. The first section is comprised of chapters one and two1, with chapter 1 dealing with the historical development of the country as a nation and chapter 2 attempting to trace the development of the health system of the country right from the very first contacts of coastal dwellers of the country with the Western explorers and finally to the organization of the health system to its current state.

The second section comprises of chapters 3 and 4 with chapter 3 dealing with the definition of a health system and its general divisions, setups, its various professions, professionals, and the general preparations of these self same professions. Chapter 4 addresses the processes involved in the health system, the distribution of health care facilities, and the manner in which health care is delivered to clients who patronize these health care facilities.

Section 3 comprises of chapters 5, 6, 7, and 8. Chapter 5 attempts to describe the different types of health care facilities, their distribution and availability, while chapter 6 attempts to delve into the general administrative principles and theories. Chapter 7 describes the current state of health care services in Nigeria's health care facilities as it is compared and contrasted with health care services as obtained in other societies. Chapter 8 analyses the differences in the Nigerian health care services from those in Western societies, like that of the United States and especially that of the Great Britain, since it is the archetype after which the Nigerian health system and the delivery of health care were fashion after. This particular chapter, chapter 8, serves as the concluding chapter where opinions and commentary are made, as these help the reader to judge for him/herself and reach some conclusion as to what the information presented and discussed mean—that is, if they amount to anything, or what the portends are for Nigeria.

ACKNOWLEDGMENT

In writing this edition, I have incurred a debt of thanks to the following: my late brother, Dawuda Markus McDikkoh, who typed the very first handwritten and the second corrected version.

Chief, Dr. Steven B. Manya, the Shattima of Adara who also, worked assiduously to provide some innovative ideas for both the first edition as well as this one. Mr. Samuel D. Maida, who served as representative during the printing process of the first edition, without which there was no telling of how our dealings with the Ahmadu Bello Printing Press experience could have ended. As a matter of fact, it is the result of that experience that this particular issue has finally come about.

My late brother-in-law Saidu Gajere, who helped immensely, with the initial contacts and arrangements for the publication of the first edition at the Ahmadu Bello University Campus complex, without which it would be all the more difficult. Also to Mr. Yohanna Yahmen Yerima, who assisted Samuel D. Maida in running important errands during that crucial period.

To Mrs. Magdalene Olivas in ISC office of El Pas Community College-Rio Grande Campus, El Paso, Texas, for typing the corrected manuscripts of this very edition.

And finally, a profound thanks to Gabriela F. Carlos and Espie Cepeda, in charge of the Business Laboratory in the fourth floor of the B building of Rio Grande Campus, both of whom were of tremendous assistance. Because the propinquity of my office to the Business Laboratory made it convenient for me to call for the help of these two noble ladies each time during the proofreading phase of the manuscripts. When I ran into any "computer trouble," each time that I would call for assistance, I would expect a rebuke, yet each time, they would respond without any complaints.

CHAPTER ONE

GENERAL BACKGROUND AND DEFINITION OF HEALTH SERVICES

INTRODUCTION

The World Health Organization's preamble, according to John M. Last, 1987 contains a certain idea, that at some level seems to convey the state of health. This I have tried to paraphrase to mean the state of total physical, mental, and social well-being, which allows individuals to function within the normal confines of their communities. In other words, it is a state of balance, if you will, that allows the individual to live a happy life in pursuit of personal goal or goals that are consonant with those of his/her aspirations and community, within context of the society's norms.

Health and *good health* are usually synonymous terms that are commonly used interchangeably[1] to describe elusive entity or phenomenon that is valued greatly in every known human society. Edward F. Lehman's statement implied this truth when he stated that

> ". . . all known human societies have had people who diagnose sickness as well as those who provide methods for managing it."[2]

The acts of diagnosis and managing sickness are avenues of pursuing "health" or "good health," if you will, by people with the objective of health in mind, who are not performing at their very best. Levey and

1

Loomba expressed a similar thought in a slightly different way and yet capture the most essential aspect that concerns health in all societies:

> The domain of the term 'health' is as large and complex as the entire scope of human activities. Each and every human being is concerned with the concept of health—directly or indirectly, individually or collectively, consciously or unconsciously. A state of good health is the most basic prerequisite for performing the tasks and duties associated with the diverse roles that individuals assume at different stages in their lives.[3]

Health or good health—take your pick—indeed, is the goal of all normal people who aspire to go through life, from birth to death. Each one wants to be free of any and all ailments, physically, mentally, psychologically, or otherwise. However, very few people, if any, ever lived without ever getting sick! Most people—regardless of race, color, creed, or lifestyle—live and die with countless disease encounters, and "pain" is usually a common denominator that heralds the presence of most diseases. This is true with most disease states, which may range from a headache (which, often than not, is a symptom of something more serious) to cancer: same difference, that is, the result or effect is the same: discomfort.

However, there are stories and speculations in this day and age of claims of people living healthy lives with some of these human antiques as old as 120 years or more. This may indeed be the case, I don't know for sure. All I do know is that none of these breathing antiques can claim that they never had pain of any sort. Even Enoch in Genesis did not die, as indicated in the holy scriptures, as well as a very selected few others, many of whom lived an average of range of 150 to 960 years.[*4]

Before written history, ancients were known to practice certain fundamentals of hygiene at both the personal and communal levels.

---

*   Genesis 5:21 through24: "And Enoch lived sixty and five years and begat Methuselah. And Enoch walked with God after he begat Methuselah three hundred years and begat Sons and daughters." Also refer to the rest of chapter 5, chapters 6 through 9, and chapter 25:7 for more information on the years of the very "selected few" group mentioned in previous paragraphs.

For instance, taking a bath after the performing of a dirty job, for all intent and purpose, was and still is considered a normal behavior. This behavior has been in practice in most, if not all, human societies from time immemorial.

Isolation of people with such infectious skin diseases as leprosy and smallpox is also another area that shows a common human behavior that relates to hygiene in the effort to stay well or healthy. The Hebrews or Jews especially and Egyptians, as recorded in the Old Testament section of the Holy Bible, were known to have practiced isolation as an effort keep infectious diseases like leprosy from spreading to others in their communities. Also, millennia before written history, most human societies buried their dead, while even in some more advance ones, burying such human wastes as feces, urine, vomitus, or even spittle in holes and pits were also practiced.

Furthermore, for most human communities, no matter how civilized or uncivilized, the source of drinking water is almost always kept clean, clear from dirt and every possible source of contamination, like excrement or fecal matters. Finally, the practice of fumigation, burning, and/or abandonment of contaminated belongings of one who might have died of smallpox or some other infectious diseases, which has been in practice[5, 6] as far back to prehistoric times. These efforts all constitute health activities by people seeking to remain or in order to achieve good health.

Archeological evidence[*7] abounds, which reveals that ancients suffered from leprosy, gum or other dental maladies, nutritional problems, arthritis, tuberculosis, and many other forms of chronic diseases.[8] While the progenitors of the human race, Adam and Eve, according to the Bible,[9] lived during as well as in the post-Eden period, several hundred years on the average, with no mention of anyone of them identified as being ill or suffering from any specific disease per se; then it is safe to assume that diseases and illnesses appeared later as there was plenty of evidence of

---

*   Article written by Dr. John Morris relates to his visit and experience at the Chicago Field Museum captioned: "If its in the Museum Doesn't that it Right? Carried in the foundation for family and nation (back to Genesis, number 93 of the January issue of ICR [Institute for Creation Research] Acts and Facts, vol. 24 No. 1).

these later on. This was to be expected as a result of the fall of man that, as a consequence, ushered sin into the world.*

THE CONCEPT HEALTH (GOOD HEALTH)

When pain and suffering, as results of disease and illness, became givens in the human experience, they ultimately culminated in death.[10]

The following statement is attributed to Montaigne who said have once said:

> "Health is a precious thing and the only one, in truth, meriting that a man should lay out, not his time, sweat, labor and goods, but also his life, itself to obtain it."[11]

And Thomas Jefferson is also said to have once stated:

> "Without health, there is no happiness", that
> ". . . attention to health then should take the place of every other object" . . .,

and finally, that the

> ". . . most uninformed mind, with a healthier body is happier than the wisest valetudinarian."[12]

These quote, by the way, are great statements and plausible, given the level of importance that health and matters occupy in our lives. The scope of activities at the individual, community, national, and even global levels for and in the pursuit health is high regardless of the community or society one happens to live in. In addition, and agreement, with all the above observations made by Levey and Loomba, Hanlon and others have also observed the following:

Hanlon says this:

> Health is a state of total effective physiological and psychological functions, it has both a relative and an absolute meaning, varying

---

* This fascinating story and all that followed this course of events is depicted in Genesis chapter 3.

through the time and space both in individual and as a group, it is the result of the combination of many forces, intrinsic and extrinsic inherited and contrived individually and collectively, privately and publicly, medically, environmentally, and socially, and it is conditioned by culture, law and government. Public health is dedicated to the common attain-melt of the highest level of physical, mental and social well being and longevity consistent with available knowledge and sources at a given time and place. It holds this goal as its contribution to the most effective total development and life of the individual and his society (sic).[1]

Levey and Loomba make the following point:

The domain of the term "health" is as large and complex as the entire scope of human activities. Each and every human being is concerned with the concept of health—directly or indirectly, individually or collectively, consciously or unconsciously. The concept of health is intimately related to the idea of the quality of life, and is used to refer to the functioning abilities not only of individuals but also of organizations, societies and nations.[14]

The concept of "good health" is generally embraced by most normal people, even though not all normal people live healthy lives. As a matter of fact, most people live unhealthy lives and do so deliberately many, many a times. For instance, smokers, alcoholics, drug addicts, and automobile racers are considered normal folks who know the dangers inherent in the types of activities that they are involved in, yet they continue to be involved in those activities anyway. There are many more unhealthy behaviors, which most people know to be injurious to health but carry them out on a daily basis anyway, in every households of every day in every society—this is vis-à-vis a detailed level of knowledge at this present day of the twenty-first century.

The foregoing discussion, however, is just a scratch of the wealth of information that is available on this subject matter that deals with health.[15, 16] It is also noteworthy to point here that most people are functionally healthy when they are not sick in bed but up and carrying out their work or chores—i.e., doing those things they enjoy doing best. The issue of health comes up only when pain of any sort or when it is bad enough that they have stay in bed, then and only then, that health is called into question. Eugene C. Nelson et al. (1986) simply describes this functional health as

> ... the capacity to perform the normal activities of daily living in a natural home environment and the ability to enjoy life.[17]

And that

> ... good health is more than simply not having an obvious disease. It is realizing your physical, emotional, and social potential as an individual. It is being able to participate in your community and being able to enjoy it. It is an active effort to cut down your chances of suffering from disease.[18]

There are some definitions similar to these which also include other such concepts, as biological, social, environmental as well as ecological influences. Lawrence Corey et al. (1977) makes the following assertions:

> ... A state of equilibrium between humans and the physical, biological and social environments compatible with full and the active functional role of ecology. However, a good, broad and all-inclusive definition of health can be measured by its anatomic integrity.[19]

> ... The ability to work and perform family and other roles in the community, the ability to deal with physical, biological and social roles, the feeling of well-being and freedom from disease.[20]

The list of statements above is by no means exhaustive of the variously different aspects of the concept of health. But for these concepts to find any utility in health care, the scope must extend beyond conventional meaning as has been defined by WHO. For example, interwoven within the web of health concepts are factors like culture, attitudes, knowledge, values, acceptance, and acting on the knowledge of such aspects health concepts.

BRIEF AND GENERAL HISTORY OF HEALTH AND THE EVOLVEMENT OF WHAT IS REFERRED AS A HEALTH SYSTEM

Aside from the archeological evidence,[21] very little else besides conjecture can be said about the prehistoric hygienic practices of the people of those eras. Some hints, however, do still exist as to the hygienic practices of those periods, namely, keeping areas of dwelling places and sources of food clean. These same practices can still be seen in some of the so-called present-day so—"primitive" people or, as Hanlon chooses to call, the "not-so-Westernized civilization in some societies" or people who live their lives quite dissimilar to the Western lifestyle, even if this refers to a very few exceptions.

Primitive tribes have certain group mores regarding community hygienic practices, which are usually derived from the pragmatic past experiences and disease encounters. Rules against the fouling of family or tribal environments, for instance and as a rule, are universal. Many societies have taboos against depositing of human waste and other waste products near streams or campsites. Similarly, the burial of excreta and other dangerous products is at all not uncommon in some of these communities.[22] Furthermore, for most humans, including ancients who might be considered so faraway from the modern civilization, all instinctively have the feeling of hunger, thus the constant search for food to ameliorate it. The need for privacy, for such private acts such as defection or sexual intimacy and many other similar activities, is clearly another area that all human beings share in common.

Finally, all illness or disease encounters are usually attributed to some cause or causes with such beliefs varying from one society to another. Rachel F. Spector, 1985, for instance, makes the following assertion:

> A state of health is regarded by many people as the reward one
> receives from "good" behavior and illness as punishment for
> "bad" behavior. [23]

It is precisely because of such a belief or intuition, according to Levey, S. and N. Paul Loomba, that

> each and every human being is concerned with health concept.[24]

This relates to the quality of life that people live. Equally true, also, is the fact that organized health activities have, historically, been directed at stemming out diseases. The level of such activities may differ from one person to another and from community to community—i.e., the isolation of children with measles and people with smallpox are clearly good examples. The drainage of swamps, wastes, and other filthy and undesirable conditions or areas close to dwelling places that cause diseases and the digging of wells for fresh drinking water are all clearly other examples.

There is abundant archeological evidence that is indicative of these sentiments. For instance, the Minoans and the Cretan civilizations had drainage systems and water closets. The Egyptian civilization was advanced in the areas of personal cleanliness and the preparation of pharmaceuticals.[25] The Jews were the first to write the world's hygienic laws while the Greeks advanced the hygienic activities to include dietary changes and exercise.[26] The Romans included all the above, paved roads for quick military movements, and provided health benefits to soldiers and subjects alike in the Roman Empire. They constructed aqueducts for water supplies, passed laws to regulate building construction and inspected bad buildings, cleaned and repaired streets, and provided for garbage collection. They also constructed sewage drainage systems and regulated the construction of bars, public baths and were skilful engineers and administrators.[27]

The Christian era appeared in the scene couched in the philosophy of self-denial and service to others. This new philosophy was accepted and generally welcomed by many people following the decadent, palpable indulgence of the pagan practices and moral laxity of the Romans that led to the decay and fall of the Roman Empire that people were eager to forget. This, therefore, led to the eager embrace of the new philosophy that promoted self-denial, moderation, and hard work. The dawning of this new era was essentially the beginning of the Middle Ages,[28, 29] which lasted until Renaissance in the nineteenth century.[30] This period is marked by the ravages of sporadic diseases, epidemics, and pandemics, which were capped by the bubonic plague or "black death," the principal and most notorious disease of the period.[31] The human race came very close to the point of extinction and civilization, hitherto achieved in human history, that was nearly obliterated. It was also at that point that gains hitherto made in health and sanitary practices declined sharply and progress already made in the different areas of human endeavors ceased almost altogether. The setback and reaction to it were such that they included the following observation by Llyod F. Burton et al. (1980):

> A significant change in attitude towards sanitation and personal hygiene.[32]

And C. E. A. Winslow (1943), in agreement, explained it further in the following manner:

> "Refuse and body wastes were allowed to accumulate in and around dwellings. Slopes were customarily emptied out of windows, giving rise to the familiar outcry 'gardez I' care'. These and other insalubrious customs lasted until relatively recent times . . ." *in London and other places in Europe, writes Winslow.*[33]

However, the history of public health did not come to a total standstill during this period of the Dark Ages, as people were forced to face reality and to modify or change their lifestyles, habits, and customs or face the unpalatable consequences. Leprosy, for one, and other skin diseases had already offered some level of understanding of the transmissibility of certain diseases. Syphilis finally brought this point home, as it became abundantly clear that diseases were not only caused but were also transmitted.[34]

Islam arrived in the seventh century. Like Judaism, Islam placed much emphasis on cleanliness at personal level. However, the Islamic crusades resulted in the conquests of vast areas leading to vast numbers of pilgrims coming to Saudi Arabia, leading to cholera epidemics. Laws were promulgated to control and regulate immigration and the movement of people to Saudi Arabia. Lepers were banished into isolated camps and forced to wear uniform in order mark their presence in public places.

The quarantining* of ships for forty days at harbors, a form of isolation, that prevented the crews from any contact with the protected

---

*   *Quarantine* is the Islamic word for "forty." It was first introduced as a practice n the city of Venice in 1348 to isolate ships and passengers at the harbor for forty days. In 1377 in Reguda, areas were designated for travelers from plagued areas until they were freed of the disease or two months before they could disembark.

public to ensure they were free of diseases before they were allowed to disembark. This practice started in Venice, Italy, and became the fashion in Europe. This realization led to a vague understanding of incubation and incubation period for certain infectious diseases, thus the forty days' period of isolation to rule out the presence of the suspected infectious disease. In 1385 in Marseilles, France, the first laws of quarantining infectious diseases, like the plague, was first passed.[35]

THE RENAISSANCE

The Renaissance marked the period of knowledge expansion, free trade, and movement of people to areas with proclivity to concentration, which further increased not only the risk of infectious diseases but also peoples' consciousness of the infectious diseases. This consciousness gradually led to the belief in other source or origins of diseases and also helped in dispelling the long-held belief that diseases were results of punishment for sin.[36] By the end of the Middle Ages, certain infectious diseases had been identified and differentiated into classes. As a result, efforts in researching and treating some of these skin diseases—like leprosy, impetigo, smallpox, among other disease entities—were intensified.

Fracastorius, a physician in 1546, proposed the theory of contagion* (spread by air), direct contact or by some formites (inanimate articles), thus opening the way for such theories as each disease is caused by a specific agent. In 1723, Anthony Von Leeuwenhoek[37] discovered the cell in human body (i.e., blood cells and spermatozoa), bacterial protozoa, and spirilla. Toward the end of eighteenth century, William Petty[38] advocated the keeping of records of population (or vital statistics) of diseases and other related topics. By the end of that century, remarkable progress had been made in public health with such giant strides as the discovery of vaccination for smallpox made by Edward Jenner in 1798,[39] etcetera. These discoveries eventuated by culminating into what is today known as modern science, which has played a crucial role in modern medicine and public health.

---

*   Contagion is the spread of disease from one person to another from *Dorland's Pocket Medical Dictionary* (Philadelphia: W. B. Saunders Company, 1982) 142.

EMERGENCE OF HOSPITALS

Other public health endeavors and health care, but especially the hospital patient care progress, continued to mount and fast too. It is a well-known fact that the hospital has not always been the place where the sick were always cared for. While organized education can be traced back to ancient Egyptian civilization in 3000 BC, the care of the sick was, for a long time, relegated either to the family or for the sick to fend for themselves or were left to die.[40],[41] A dramatic change occurred with the arrival of the Christian era after the teachings of Jesus Christ, when caring for the sick shifted into monasteries and, eventually, into other church institutions as the monks assumed the role of caring for the sick.[42] Burton et al. (1980) make the following observation about the early beginnings of hospitals:

> ... Arising from the experience of military hospital of the Romans and from their valetudinarian for the sick poor, the Christian Church fostered the creation of Hote Dieu, a place for God's hospitality in many cities.[43] (sic)

On other fronts, the cause of disease prevention and treatment were advanced with the discovery of scurvy and its cure by James Lind, a Scottish physician who, in 1799, performed the experiment on the British seamen by giving them citrus fruits for their bleeding gums. Furthermore, some advances were achieved in technology with the use of anesthesia when Crawford W. Long first used nitrous oxide for tooth extraction in 1815. In 1868, the thermometer was first introduced for measuring body temperature by Carl R. A. Wunderlich. By the 1860s, the hypodermic syringe and needle were first used in the American Civil War.[44] This briefly summarizes the history and progress of public health in general. We now turn our attention to public health from the American public health's perspective.

A BRIEF REVIEW OF THE AMERICAN PUBLIC HEALTH SYSTEM

The Renaissance, as Garrison (1929) would have us belief, ushered in a new era as far as changes that relate to the public health and health care in general are concerned. The pace both accelerated as it was also more profound due to the bitter memory of the "black death" in the Dark

Ages. This prodded the people in the more civilized world, especially in Europe, to action.

The reaction to the plague ushered in the need to find both cure and prevention for future epidemics of diseases.

The lessons of hygiene were forced on Europeans as to how to live the everyday life in such a way as to prevent one from getting an infectious diseases or transmitting any. Hitherto, this had not been the practice, either due to ignorance or by sheer experience. However, while ignorance was not the main impediment that slowed human understanding and its ability to learn, as in some instances religious beliefs; nevertheless, it was the main cause which altogether hindered progress in the direction of public health. However, connections between diseases and their causes began to be made and on how to control these diseases and their spread. For instance, laws as to how to control the disposal of refuse and to improve other hygienic practices were enacted concurrently, as such movements as nationalism, imperialism, and industrialism began to hold sway in the Western world.[45]

In America, the British had a lot more influence than they did in health matters. The American public health scene, sanitation, medicine, and other health reforms were directly influenced by legislation and improvements taken through legislation in England. H. I. Bowditch (1986), the first president of the Massachusetts State Board of Health made in 1876, makes the following interesting observation:

> . . . By far the greatest influences have been exerted upon us in America by England, who by her unbounded pecuniary sacrifices and steady improvement in her legislation . . . The consummate skills in discovery, removal and prevention of whatever maybe prejudicial to the public health. [46]

The colonies had to be protected from the ravages of smallpox, yellow fever, and other infectious diseases as the toll in mortality had reached unprecedented proportion in colonial America. Some population of the native Indian tribes had been decimated by diseases introduced by the new settlers, and many of these early settlements had been totally wiped out.

Vital statistics is a major component of any efficient public health system and was used in the new colonies in 1659 in Massachusetts by enacting an act requiring the registration of death record. Subsequently, this led to other administrative public health procedures,[47] with subsequent laws enacted in 1647 by Massachusetts Bay Colony followed by laws in Boston, Salem, and Charleston in 1697 and 1708, respectively, which dealt with trades that were considered offensive to public health.

The quarantining of contacts, as earlier pointed out, and isolation of smallpox patients became law in Massachusetts. Effects of revolution and subsequent threat of yellow fever led to the abandonment of Philadelphia as the U.S. Federal Capital, an outcome of regulation by the established Permanent Board of Health.

Similar laws were subsequently enacted in all the other states of the Union, from Massachusetts by the end of eighteenth century[48] to Virginia by the close of the century (1800). All manners of laws dealing with public health, in one form or another, had been enacted in order to improve public health.

Comparatively speaking, progress in the public health field was rather stationary vis-à-vis progress that had been achieved in many other areas. The life expectancy in the colonies, for instance, was less than what was obtained in similar groups in Britain as a result of infectious disease epidemics such as smallpox, scarlet fever, and increasing infant mortality rate. By 1850, life expectancy in London was less than thirty-six (36) years. On this score, it is sad to say that this figure was not anymore glamorous in colonial America than it was in Europe, and as Hanlon points this out,

> ... The American social scene was the subject of scathing comments by visitors from abroad who were not impressed with crudity and barbarism of life in the United States and the generally unkempt appearance of its communities.[49]

In all the areas of public health reform in the United States, the Shattuck Report of the Sanitary Commission of Massachusetts in 1830 was the most revolutionary. It was because of it that the health boards were later established with other recommendations, including creation of sanitary inspection system, data collection, analysis of vital statistics, etcetera, which were instituted. It also included recommendation for studies on tuberculosis, control of alcoholism, supervision of mental diseases and migrant workers. These recommendations, at the time, were revolutionary and very well ahead of their time, as they remain salient even today. He also made recommendations on smoke control and called for training schools for nurses teaching of sanitary sciences in medical schools, to include preventive medicine in clinical practice, and for physical examination and family history records to be made mandatory in medical practice.[50]

The very first National Board of Health was formed in 1879, but four years later, it collapsed due to lack of funds and over "jurisdictional issue" or power struggle to control it between the Congress and local authorities. The Congress had established it and limited its existence to only four years but could not extend its continuation prior to its term expiration. This particular body, the National Board of Health, marked the beginning of official government-organized public health in the United States.[51, 52]

NOTES

1. Levey, S. and N. Paul Loomba, *Health Care Administration: A Managerial Perspective* (New York: J. B. Lippincott Co, 1984).
2. Edward W. Lehman, *Coordinating Health Care Explorations in International Relations,* vol.17 (Beverly Hills: Sage Publications Inc., 1975) 15.
3. S. Levey and N. Paul Loomba, *Health Care Administration: A Managerial Perspective* (New York: J. B. Lippincott Co., 1984) 3.
4. Holy Bible (KJV) (New York: Collin Clear-typed Press, 1984).
5. John J. Hanlon, *Public Health Administration and Practice*, 6th ed. (St. Louis: The C. V. Mosby Co., 1974) 13-14.
6. Ibid.,13.
7. Llyod E. Burton, Hugh H. Smith, and Andrew W. Nicols, *Public Health and Community Medicine*, 3rd ed. (Baltimore: Williams and Wilkins, 1980).
8. Ibid.
9. Holy Bible (NIV) (Grand Rapids, Michigan: Zondervan Bible Publishers, 1984) 1-3.
10. Ibid., 2-3.
11. Rhoda Thomas Tripp, *The International Thesaurus of Quotations* (New York: Harper and Row Pub., 1970) 412.
12. Steven Jonas, *Health Care Delivery in the United State* (New York: Springer Pub. Co., 1981), 21.
13. John J. Hanlon, *Public Health Administration and Practice*, 6th ed. (St. Louis: The C. V. Mosby Co., 1974), 4.
14. S. Levey and N. Paul Loomba, *Health Care Administration: A Managerial Perspective*, (New York: J. B. Lippincott Co., 1984) 3.
15. Rachel E. Spector, *Cultural Delivery in Health and Illness*, 2nd ed. (Norwalk, Connecticut: Appleton-Century-Crofts, 1985) 4.
16. John J. Last, *Public Health and Human Ecology* (Ottawa: Prentice-Hall, Appleton, Lange, 1987) 5.
17. Eugene G. Nelson et al., *Medical and Health Guides for People Over Forty* (Glenview, IL: Scott, Foreman and Co., 1986) 4.
18. Ibid.
19. John M. Last, *Public Health and Human Ecology* (Ottawa: Prentice-Hall, Appleton, and Lange, 1987) 6.
20. Ibid.

21. Llyod F. Burton, Hugh H. Smith and Andrew W. Nichols: *Public Health and Community Medicine*, 3rd ed. (Baltimore: Williams and Wilkins, 1980) 5.

22. John J. Hanlon, *Public Health Administration and Practice*, 6th ed. (St. Louis: The C. V. Mosby Co., l974) 13.

23. Rachel F. Specter, *Cultural Diversity in Health and Illness*, 2nd ed. (Norwich, Connecticut: Appleton-Century-Crofts, 1985) 4.

24. S. Levey and N. Paul Loomba, *Health Care Administration: A Managerial Perspective* (New York: J. B. Lippincott Co., 1984) 3.

25. John J. Hanlon, *Public Health Administration and Practice*, 6th ed. (St. Louis: The C. V. Mosby Co., 1974) 14.

26. Ibid.

27. Llyod F. Burton, Hugh H. Smith, and Andrew W. Nichols, *Public Health and Community Medicine*, 3rd ed. (Baltimore: Williams and Wilkins, 1980) 9-12.

28. John J. Hanlon: *Public Health Administration and Practice*, 6th ed., (St. Louis: The C. V. Mosby Co., 1974) 15.

29. Llyod E. Burton, Hugh H. Smith, and Andrew W. Nichols, *Public Health and Community Medicine*, 3rd ed. (Baltimore: Williams and Wilkins, 1980) 9-12.

30. Ibid.

31. Ibid.

32. C. E. A. Winslow: *The Conquest of Epidemic Diseases* (Princeton, NJ: Princeton Univ. Press, 1943).

33. G. A. Rosen: *A History of Public Health* (New York: M. D. Publications Inc., 1958).

34. John J. Hanlon: *Public Health Administration and Practice*, 6th ed. (St. Louis: The C. V. Mosby Co., 1974).

35. Llyod F. Burton, Hugh H. Smith, and Andrew W. Nichols: *Public Health and Community Medicine*, 3rd ed. (Baltimore: Williams and Wilkins, 1980) 16.

36. Ibid.

37. G. W. Burnett and H. W. Scherp: *Oral Microbiology and Infections Disease*, 3rd ed. (Baltimore: Williams and Wilkins, 1968) 4.

38. L. E. Burton, H. H. Smith, and A. W. Nichols, *Public Health and Community Medicine*, 3rd ed. (Baltimore: Williams and Wilkins, 1980) 33.

39. G. W. Burnett and H. W. Scherp: *Oral Microbiology and Infections Diseases*, 3rd ed. (Baltimore: Williams and Wilkins, 1968) 33.

40. J. B. de C. Sounder, *Transition from Ancient Egyptian to Greek Medicine* (Lawrence, Kansas: Univ. of Kansas Press, 1963).
41. Ruth M. A. French, *Dynamics of Health Care*, 3rd ed. (New York: McGraw-Hill Book Co., 1979) 21.
42. L. E. Burton, H. H. Smith, and A. W. Nichols: *Public Health and Community Medicine*, 3rd ed. (Baltimore: Williams and Wilkins, 1980), 11.
43. Ibid.
44. F. H. Garrison: *An Introduction to the History of Medicine*, 4th ed. (Philadelphia: W. B. Sounders Co., 1929) 431.
45. M. D. George, *London Life in the 18th Century* (New York: Alfred A. Khopf, 1925).
46. H. I. Bowditch, *Address on Hygienic and Preventive Medicine, Transaction of International Medical Congress* (Philadelphia, 1986).
47. H. D. Chadwick, "The Disease of Inhabitants of the Commonwealth," *New England of Medicine* 216 (June 10, 1937): 8.
48. John J. Hanlon: *Public Health Administration and Practice*, 6th ed., (St. Louis: The C. V. Mosby Co., 1974) 21.
49. Ibid.
50. L. Shattuck et al., *Report of the Sundry Commission of Massachusetts* (Boston: Bulton and State Printers, 1850).
51. W. G. Smillie, "The National Board of Health 1979-1983," *American Journal of Public Health* 33 (August 1943): 925.
52. F. M. Rogers and Lyon Svenring: *The Modernization among Peasants Impact of Communication* (New York: Holt Rinechart and Winston Inc., 1969).

CHAPTER TWO

GENERAL BACKGROUND

The definition of *change*, or a state of dynamism or flux, according Rogers and Svenring, (Ruth Sloan et al., 1967), is the absence of the status quo, but also alteration in status in the new state as well.[1] Education, on the other hand and from the perspective of civilization, is and has been used as a change agent, especially in this era of modernity. It has been so effectively used for these reasons and perhaps many more others, one may say.

Education was imported into Nigeria mainly through three major avenues. The first being through the explorers and the last two avenues were the following: the Christian missionaries who penetrated from the south and the jihadizing Islamists who penetrated through the north.[2] While education was the vehicle of change that the missionaries used, as earlier been alluded to, the main goal for such an education was only for the sole purpose of enabling the Africans to be able to read and then translate the Bible into their native languages or vernaculars. The invading Islamic jihadists, on the other hand, influenced and forced its way by coercion or sheer force (war—convert to Islam, or die) through jihads, which were carried out in the eighteenth and nineteenth centuries. The sole and only purpose of the jihad then, as it is even now, were purely for religious reasons and that alone. There was no scientific benefit to or behind it, none, zero, zilch!

Nigerian is a society with many segments and facets and has, since colonization by Britain in 1861[3] and from the perspective of civilization and modernization, experiences which change all the time. At any rate, whatever the motive for the change that was sought for Nigeria by using education, it did work and perhaps too well too!

The intended change was introduced piecemeal, a little at a time, with the sole intent of keeping the "wild Africans" at bay—under firm control. The introduction of education first began as teaching the African how to read and write, as the deeper recesses of knowledge, after all, belonged and resided with white colonizers as sole custodians of it. However, it was only a matter of time that the small changes that these Westerners had brought would fester and later on blossom as their commercial products and ideas would later on change these brute into a people who want more knowledge, but who want to live their lives like these white men. This change in lifestyle included the use of Western ideas of treating diseases by using Western or modern scientific medications.

In Nigeria, the pragmatic effectiveness of Western drugs led to the relief and/or eradication of many simple diseases that were wrecking havoc by killing thousands of people, with epidemics running rampant in community after community. If the steady increase in population were used as a measure of the state of health of the Nigerian society, from the inception of British rule to its merger (the North and South by the Royal Niger Company in 1900),[4, 5] then based on the Federal Office of Statistics figures, it should rightly be concluded that the Nigerian society has enjoyed better health with the consequent increase in life expectancy for its citizens because of it.[6]

The other question, however, that should also be raised is whether or not this conclusion is fair and correct. There were, indeed, more hospitals after the occurrences of these events—i.e., contact with the British, the introduction of education and adoption of Western ideas, etcetera—and certainly more so after the contact and certainly during the British rule than ever before. Just the mere change in population, on the upswing (positive side), justifies such a conclusion.

Nigeria today comprises of vast rural areas with numerous towns and villages therein scattered. The population of the country has, in a similar manner, increased, perhaps from a few millions at the beginning of colonization to over a hundred and twenty-five million today, by some estimations. These changes are definitely attributable to the pragmatic and miraculous effects of modern scientific medicine.

Some of these changes—and particularly having more drugstores, drug availability in drugstores, sophisticated medical equipments in hospitals, and a variety of medical gadgets—are all positive changes. Yet more is not always better as the aphorism "More is better" would have us believe. The health system in Nigeria today and its product (the health care services) in terms of dissemination of facilities and availability of these services—this quality, both in professional as well as layman's viewpoints, is a lot worse off today in spite of all so-called advances and improvements. And the irony is that with new and improved technology the quality of health care is supposed to also improve for the better, this is not the case, at least, not always.

Ordinary Nigerians still suffer unnecessarily despite these improvements," which, as far as these poor folks are concerned, do not exist, as most would feel more comfort if they knew these never existed in the first place!

SOCIO-CULTURAL, ECONOMIC, ECOLOGICAL AND POLITICAL BACKGROUNDS

The Nigerian society is a conglomeration of between 250[7] to 300.[8] Some estimates even place this figure at about 400 different ethnic groups[9] with a variety of languages, culture, traditions, values, and many a times, different backgrounds.

DeGoshe and the Federal Research Division of the Library of Congress estimate and place the population at a figure between 100 million or more people in 1990.[10, 11] There is the belief that Nigeria is the most populated country in Africa and the largest black nation in the world.[12] The current estimated figure is between 115 and 150 million by the decade of twenty-first century, leading to the speculation that one out of every eight (8) Africans lives in Nigeria and one out of every ten (10) black persons in the entire world is a Nigerian.

ETHNIC GROUPS AND DOMINATION

There are tree main or major ethnic groups that predominantly dominate the Nigerian social scene, namely, the Hausa/Fulani (the largest dominant group in the country with profound domination in the north), the Yoruba (the largest dominant group in the west), and the Igbo (the largest dominant group in the east).[13]

The north has the largest number of different ethnic groups with a land area of approximately two-thirds of the total land area of the entire country. The east and the west, about the same in size, are equally divided—the east into the former Eastern Region and the west into the former Western Region. The Western Region was later subdivided into the Midwestern Region in 1963.[14] Nevertheless, the social arrangement in each area remains such that the groups mentioned previously dominate all others subgroups in each regional area. This is the case, especially with the Hausa/Fulani groups in the northern regional area. The influence of these dominant groups is such that their languages serve as a sort of "lingua franca" in the areas of the regions of their dominance.

In the north, for instance, the Hausa language serves as the medium of communication and, was used in the past, as medium of instruction in elementary schools in the far north and parts of the Middle Belt in the north, both during and after colonial era (the first republic, the first and second military regimes). In the southernmost parts of the Middle Belt of the north where groups like the Tivs, Idomas, and similar others live, the Hausa/Fulani influence is less pronounced and so is the use of the Hausa language.

In both the east and west where the Igbo and Yoruba languages are used, they are not only used "lingua franca" for communication but also were used as media of instruction in the elementary school system both during and after the colonial era, as well as during the civilian rule of the first republic and the administrations of subsequent military juntas that followed.

CULTURAL BACKGROUND

John Friedl, (1976) defines culture as the

> . . . shared ways of life, common to a group of people and acquired as a member of society. This way of life is learned through interaction with other people and includes both material aspects and intangible knowledge (beliefs, attitudes, values, rules of behavior.[15]

21

While Anderson and Carter (1974) subscribe to this same notion, they, at the same time, also suggest that culture is:

> . . . those qualities and attributes that seem to be characteristic of all mankind. Those things unique to the species homo-sapiens as differentiated from all other forms of life[*][16] and that which binds a society together.[17]

Within the context of social norms and of the society ultimately, and from the anthropological perspective, the best definition of *culture* is perhaps the definition of B. Edward B. Taylor[*] who defines culture as

> . . . that complex whole which includes knowledge, beliefs, art, morals, laws customs and any other capabilities and habits acquired by man as a member of society.[18] (sic)

The Nigerian society certainly measure up to this definition and that of any group, either referred or in referred to, specifically, within the parameters of these definitions. Taylor's definition, for instance, is indubitably true that societies do have beliefs, art, moral code, laws, and customs peculiar to them, which John Friedl further elaborates in his definition of *culture*. This particular aspect, he maintains, makes people

> " . . . similar to some other people, yet different from majority of people in the world".[19]

> We are all basically the same physically in that we are members of the same species. And we are all different in that each of us has an individual personality that cannot be duplicated. It is culture that binds us together into a group sharing a certain degree of similarity overcoming the individual differences among us, yet setting us apart from other groups.[20]

On that score, therefore, Nigeria and the overabundance of tribal marks (for most tribal groups) and the traditional dances in all groups, for example,

---

[*]   Edward Burnett Taylor is referred to as the father of anthropology since he was the first to publish researches of early history of mankind in 1865, thus establishing himself as a force in the field.

are both customary and mark each tribe as separate from the rest in the society. It is, however, unfortunate that Nigerians have added into this mix of cultural gems, corruption which they unabashedly and, many a time, proudly announce to the world as the "Nigerian factor" during business transactions, implying that graft or bribe as integral part of the business process. Duty and responsibility to most, if you are a Nigerian, must translate into a palpable paper called "naira," or they are not interested or are they duty bound, or responsibility or accountability.

OTHER MORE OBVIOUS CULTURAL ASPECTS

Other cultural practices that have salience at this point include farming, food and food preparation, cattle rearing, language, courtship and marriage ceremonies, etc.

1. Food and Food Preparation
Tuwo da miya, for instance, is the main dish especially in the north and parts of the Middle Belt. *Eba* and pounded yam are similar in the style of preparation done mostly in the southern Middle Belt, the southern regions and people who originated from that part of the country, but have migrated to parts of the north.

2. Arts
Artwork has its place in the Nigerian society as it also varies from one ethnic group to another. Some of the areas that artwork is both expressed and displayed include pottery, household utensils, farming and garden instruments or implements. A good and quick way to see as well as learn about the artistic ingenuity of Nigerian is to visit or tour a marketplace where these articles are on constant display. The methods used in crop cultivation and a host of other daily aids of living are cultural aspects not peculiar to the Nigerian society only, but pervasive in other human societies.

Nigeria has, through its moderately long history, produced a rich oral tradition and poetry by such world-renown as Wole Soyinka, the 1986 Nobel Prize winner in Literature, J. P. Clark, G. Okpara, Cyprian Ekwensi, Chinua Achebe, to mention just a few among many others, which is almost purely uncontaminated by the so-called imported influences. Time and space will not permit the tabulation or in-depth analysis of the many other aspects available of the Nigerian culture. However, materials still abound on this particular subject as specifically displayed in great details in the works of Dr. Yusufu Turaki, *History of SIM/ECWA in Nigeria* (1993), and the British legacy in Northern Nigeria (1993), which are "must-read" in the phraseology of the Honorable Chief Solomon Lar, former governor of Plateau State, as they are expansive and exceptionally explanatory.

GEOGRAPHY AND ECOLOGY

Nigeria is located on the West Coast of Africa with an approximate land area of over 923,700 square kilometers.[21, 22] Its country sits within the tropical zone and borders with the Gulf of Guinea, which comprises the Bights of Benin and Biafra, of the Atlantic Ocean, in the south. On the west, it share borders with the Republic of Benin, on the north and Niger; Chad on the Northeast, Cameroon on the east and Togo on south-east. It is about 800 miles in length from the northernmost tip to southernmost borders and approximately the same in width.[23] The current estimates of the population of this tropical nation by some place it in the neighborhood of 125 million people or more; this makes it the most populous nation in Africa and the biggest black nation in the world. Out of every five Africans, one is believed to live in Nigeria.

TOPOGRAPHY

The country is basically a flat land with minor exception of hills, even mountains, mainly in the northern parts of the country.

Two main rivers—namely, River Niger, which divides the northwestern half of the country, and River Benue just about the other half of the northeastern portion—both make their way to the middle of the country where they converge to unite just off the center to the south to form the River Niger. The River Niger then flows toward the Atlantic Ocean where it empties on the south, but before joining the Atlantic Ocean, it breaks and forms the riverine delta area in the southern part of the country.

The climate is tropical and equatorial on the southernmost while it is subtropical further inland from the coastline areas where vegetation is coarse and dense. In the hinterland, it is savanna, especially in the Middle

Belt areas with milder vegetation and is ideal for agriculture; semiarid in the far north, but arid at the northernmost border areas that border the Sahara[24, 25] Desert or where it begins and/or ends.

Because it is tropically located, the Nigerian climate has two main seasons, namely, the dry and rainy seasons. The rainy season begins in the spring around April and ends in October while the dry season begins around November and ends March or April, in some instances.

ECONOMIC BACKGROUND

Before money was introduced into the Nigerian way of life and the commercial aspect of the economy, agriculture was the mainstay of the economy while the hatter system, a system of exchange—i.e., the exchange of one set of goods given in exchange for another—was the method of the transactions of commerce.

An estimated 99.5 percent of the population were, and perhaps are still, farmers who either lived on or near the farm. This was the situation until colonization and subsequent to the mining of coal, tin, columbite, and other minerals, which eventually emerged as avenues or ventures for making money, and replaced the agricultural venture for a very small percentage of the population. Following the barter system and with the introduction of money, excess food and cash crops were, and still are, being sold to procure domestic goods such as furniture, other necessities, and entertainment during festive occasions. Cash crops or agricultural products cultivated purposely for trade, exported for money and foreign exchange are soya beans, rubber, cocoa, kola nuts, palm oil, and nuts.[26]

Oil drilling and mining have recently emerged as very important aspects of the economy in the last three or so decades, and while agriculture remains a major part in the lives of many Nigerians, the combination of mining and oil drilling represents about a fourth of the gross domestic product (GDP) and petroleum products, which represent about three-fourths of the gross national product or total Federal revenue.[27] Accordingly, building and construction are just about one-fourth of a growing economy while the government sector, which employs about 50 percent of the total labor workforce in the country, represents about a sixth.

This is hard to believe, and I, for one, do not believe it! How can an entity that is responsible for most of the employment in the country, including the military services, police, coast guards, parastasals, and all but adds up only to about one-sixth of its total revenues? Not a chance, except of course and only if the explanation for this anomaly is tacit admission as to having factored in the corruption quotient, which Nigerians have become notorious of, but continue to publicly deny and/or defend!

VALUES

The values of the many Nigerians, as it pertains to health and related health issues, can be summarized by this quintessential Hausa adage, "Lafiya uwar kome." The literal interpretation of this is "Health is everything." A spiced paraphrase version would sound something like this: health is the "mother"—everything to everyone, regardless of where we happen to live in. Put another way, health tops the list of every human aspiration and the central concern of each and every normal human activity. How true! This maxim is not only trans-cultural in application, but indeed, an axiom universally accepted! However, words and actions are two separate areas distinctively separate, and without action, words alone certainly have little or no consequences. Accordingly, and consonant with this idea, Ruth French makes the following point:

> . . . Throughout the world, the health of every nation is predicated upon the health of its people. Obviously material resources, productivity and consumption of goods and services are without meaning if the health of the people is such that prevents their maximal utilization and activity. Economic prosperity is intimately associated with health.[28]

She maintains that there is no aspect of life that the value system of each individual—but ultimately that of society as well eventually—is not affected, and profoundly so by the state of the individual's health. Similarly, G. Viekers (1984) also points out how the goals of public health are set by each individual based on their state health and social values also. Along a similar vein, Yusufu Turaki (1993) defines values as the "conception of that which is desirable" and that values are then

26

> . . . the conceptual social variables which influence the selection from available modes, means and ends of action by persons in society.[29]

Turaki specifically specifies as he emphasizes how the world's view of a people, of necessity, reflects their values[30] and, I might add, also their concept of health, which would directly impact their behavior.[31]

Plainly stated another way, the argument that Dr. Turaki is advancing here is simply this: the concept and to cherish any of the values we for long have had—i.e., those aspects that positively influence our image as individual and a society—these are the drives that propel any group of people in the direction of self-preservation and, ultimately, self-perpetuation. These also lead toward comfortable living[32] conditions, and I dare interject that these assumptions are only true in so far as the health of the individual is and remains the basis and focus of a society's leadership. Otherwise, all else is useless should that not be the case.

However, sad to say, this is indeed not so in Nigeria as it is most certainly exemplified by the living standards of citizens of most developed societies. Societies with individual high values and with individuals enjoying good health regardless of the level of their economic status elevate the entire living condition or standard of its citizenship. The provision of such necessities as running water, electricity, good roads, as exemplified by what obtains in the developed societies, is where all this begins. The exact opposite obtains in Nigeria.

A clear example is how only the privileged few have access to what are considered the most basics of living conditions for survival in most of the developed societies that Nigerian leaders aspire for the Nigerian society to look like. However, even the ancient Roman Empire had more sense of duty, responsibility toward its citizenry and knew the importance as well as the value of good drinking water for the health needs of its citizens than does this new group or crop of modern leaders of Nigeria who continue to brag of Nigeria as being the "giant of Africa." The Roman, as ancient as they were, did not only knew what was good and, health-wise, beneficial to their citizens but also provided it by all odds and cost. Were that not the case, the Roman Empire's decline and demise would have occurred a lot sooner than when it did in 476 A.D.[33] I wonder if they truly believe in this so-called giant. Or perhaps they meant the "pygmy of Africa!" I could be wrong, but it seems they do really mean "giant," as they seem to like the title so bad that it is used very often with the slightest hint of any remorse. At any rate and as I have indicated before, words and actions do exist in two, totally separated into two different hemispheres. Of course, in this instance anyway, these are empty words are completely worthless and devoid of any meaning! Nigeria is yet to earn a place among a modern world community of nations; it is then, and only then, can it "begin" to aspire for the titular "giant of Africa" title.

Nigerians certainly has values as this is painfully obvious in its culture, customs, and traditions. However, whether or not these foregoing definitions and discussions—but also in addition, whether or not these values—do influence the people's conduct and thus the conduct of politicians, the style of governing by its leaders remains to be seen. However, based on the very obvious and that by observing the lack of basic necessities for living a healthy decent life as well as the state of the health system, in its operation, administration, and delivery of health care to its citizens, one must have to gainsay that there is any positive influence that the values has on the citizens of this very society.

There is no question that Ruth French's statement—which indicates that "the health of every nation is predicated" on the health of its people—is right on target! The health of the citizens in every society serves as the crux and basis for judging it! This is so because it is always a conscious decision by leadership (government) of the society to make it paramount and so.

POLITICAL BACKGROUND

There is no doubt that politics in Nigeria continues to change, even if those that govern and play politics still cherish ideologies and values of yesteryears' societies come and go. The promotion of division among tribes so as to gain or remain in control necessitates treating some, in most instances, dominant groups better than others in order to achieve this end. Some may consider this strategy as "moving with the times" or a component of good and effective governing style. I, however, beg to differ, and this is based on my observation of an intractably intransigent ethnocentricity attitude coupled with a psuedo-pious religion and its religious ideology. The provision of such basics as pipe water, good roads,

28

electricity to some areas, but none for others, furthers the ball along the line of this argument. The aim is to keep people outside the ethnic group so that they could remain subjugated; this action enables the dominating group dominant and in complete control.[34]

There have been failed attempts at uniting the Nigeria's dominant tribes: Hausa/Fulani, Yoruba, Igbo. This has been the case since the colonial period, but this subject is worthy of some level of discussion, yet not at this time. At any rate, serious attempts started during the very first republic of a civilian government and right after the colonial era and before the civil war of the mid-1960s.

However, these efforts did not only failed but have, categorically, been abandoned and continued to fester to the present day is criminality of no equality as there is this level of adamant recalcitrance being displayed by the dominant groups with the so-called power, not only in numbers but also of numbers. You see, unity among them would relegate some of them to the minority status, and therefore, according to them, the struggle must continue. These struggles culminated into civil and religious unrest situation that have come to characterize the 1980s all the way to the middle of first decade of the twenty-first century. These unrests were clearly avoidable, but the regimes in power at the time showed no desire in quelling these civil unrests. Neither did they intend to handle them justly with injustice, clearly because of the dominant religious tones these had assumed. Moreover, because the military leaders were themselves Muslims and the dominant perception then was that Muslim were not only in power controlling the reigns of government (including the police and the military), but Muslims were in majority and ready to teach the "infidels" a thing or two for daring to challenge Allah's representation and gift of the Nigerian nation. This level of irresponsibility of complicity, as displayed in some of these attitude and actions, clearly testifies to the banal nature of the Nigerian situation.

Greed and corruption are other phenomena that might have been quiescent in the colonial era, but started surfacing shortly after the inception of the first republic civilian administration. The Northernization Policy was instituted by the then former Northern Region premier Sir Ahmadu Bello, the Sardauna of Sokoto, who primarily used it to "advance" the cause of educationally lagging behind northerners who then and now still

29

are behind their southern counterparts in education in almost every field of study. Regardless of the good intentions of the policy, it did not, for sure, further the cause of unity between the tribal groups; if anything, it further deepened the rifts of divisions among tribes and set the cause for unity several decades back.

The army meddling in politics carried with it the audacious aura of emancipation and the panacea from all the evil and corrupt politicians. The irony, however, proved that the treatment and medicine was worse than the disease, as it was deadly because testing power by the men in uniform was similar to handing over the guarding of the sheep's pen to a pack of hyenas or, worst, lions. A few years down the line, Nigerians woke up to an empty treasure with the nation's defense system in utter shamble, and the culmination of this state of affairs saw its zenith during General Ibrahim Badmosi Babangida's regime of junta from 1983 to 1993 after toppling Alhaji Shehu Shagari, a whim of a president, who handed running the affairs of the federal government of Nigeria to the Nigerian version of a mafia group of the ilk of Umaru Dikko, who carted what was left in Nigeria's treasure: Europe, and Britain in particular.

Corruption became full-fledged during the Babangida's regime as it had been firmly institutionalized[35] in every aspect of Nigeria's social life and institutions to the point of glamorization, even veneration. Nevertheless, corruption scaled to new heights just few short years after the Babangida administration had exited its grip on the reigns of governance.

People can and do make mistakes, as they would sometimes, many times; after a mistake has been made, they should be forgiven and be excused if forgiveness is sought. A new direction is then called for as it is necessary, but no one has the right to be wrong, especially if it is deliberate all the time and is expected to be excused for doing so.

THE HISTORY AND BACKGROUND OF MEDICINE AND HEALTH CARE IN NIGERIA

Traditional medicine men have always played a role in the medical history of Nigeria for as long as the society has existed. The *wombais* the *bokas or bokaye* of the Hausa/Fulani tribes; the *gozans* of Nupes; the *adahunses*

30

of Yorubas; the *edebias* of Igbos; and so on were all players in traditional medicine and, thus the health status of these respective natives. All have provided care, given dietary advice and sanitary suggestions to all who patronize their services for the purpose of seeking cure from diseases or for promoting healthy living to avoid becoming sick. Such service provision has been going on even before the arrival of the Western explorers into the society.

The history of "native" health care services in the country, on the other hand, cannot disavow the very fact that contacts with the west and outside civilizations served as impetus or were even responsible for organized existence of modern medical care services, at least in Nigeria, if not the entirety of West Africa. It is in that vein that the health system of Nigeria was fashioned after its archetype model in Britain.[36] The influence and legacy of the British, after almost a century occupation, affected the lifestyle of Nigerians in almost all areas of their existence and was far more pervasive than was initially realized. For decades, the educational system was a carbon copy of the British system, even after the colonial rule, until General Olusegun Obasanjo's decree of universal education in the mid—1970s.[37]

Scientific and modern medical health care services in Nigeria owe their origins to contacts with the West and Western civilization, which dates back some five hundred years or so ago. Earlier contacts with Mediterranean and Near East civilizations such as the Phoenicians and Carthaginians had little, if any, effect in this specific area. Even the arrival of the Islamic culture around the thirteenth century AD, some seven hundred or so years, brought nothing of substance in this area. These early contacts with Western traders and subsequent arrivals of the Christian missionaries, perhaps in the nineteenth century, date as far back as the early 1470s through Benin and Warri areas at the time.

Other contacts with the Portuguese, Spaniards, Danish, French, British, etcetera, by venue of slave trade via trading ships to the Americas via Europe of the transatlantic routes (the great triangle) further intensified these contacts. These ships carried medical personnel and supplies for the medical care and health needs for crews, staffs, and the slaves, the main ware of the expeditions. The efforts of people like William Wilberforce and other parliamentary figures in the British Parliament—concerned on the welfare of the slaves and trading slaves in the 1800s—resulted in the simple treatment, vaccination programs for slaves and coastal towns that were then reachable.

Through these efforts, eventually they were supported by the British government in the Niger Delta areas in 1807. Subsequent to which, some temporary medical care service contacts were made with the natives in the seventeenth century. Such efforts ended at the Delta areas with no ventures any further inland due to lack of roads, hostile climatic conditions, yellow fever, malaria, and several other disease epidemics. Some Scottish explorers and missionaries in the ilk of David Livingstone, Mungo Park, John Kirk, and others inched their way inland. With the use of prophylactic drugs against malaria and other diseases, they succeeded in making contacts with the people further inlands. Subsequently, however, after the colonial occupation, colonial governors of Nigeria began to improve the sanitary services in the Lagos area.[38, 39]

It has been pointed out before that the efforts of Christian missionaries played a key role for the efforts of education in Nigeria. Most certainly, the pace of the educational efforts would definitely not have been the same, minus the role of all Christian missionary groups that came to the country in those of education dearth. Equally true is the fact that the missionaries contributed to building hospitals and health centers—planting such health care facilities was not only tremendously enormous but pioneering, to say the least.

They were first in erecting hospitals along the coastal areas with the very first hospital in Sao mine in 1504, at Abeokuta in 1860s, in Lagos and Calabar in 1888.[40] As for the northern parts of the country, it took much longer to penetrate due to Islamic and Arab influence and bad or no motor and non-pliable roads, as a result of tropical vegetation. The north, however, was later penetrated by the persistent intransigence of some of the missionary groups, namely, the SIM (Sudan Interior Mission), Anglicans, the SUM (Sudan United Missions), the Roman Catholic missions, and others.[41]

The colonial government arrived at the health scene very late and, rather, as a matter of adjustment than an initiative to improve the health lot of its subjects. At any rate, it is "better late than never," so goes the aphorism. The first medical services were established for the military and their families, but evolved eventually from what was then known as the "garrison" or "barrack" medical care, to what later became the Colonial Medical Services in the country. This was the forerunner to what later became the Nigerian Medical Service.

REVIEW OF LITERATURE

There is generally very little in history books on the history of medicine, health and health services in Africa and even fewer on Nigeria. The few that do exist on Africa include such works as the *History of Medicine in South Africa* by Edmund H. Burrow (1958), *The Sudan Medical Services* by Squire (1958), *History of Medical Service in Tangayika* by Gelfand (1964), and *A History of the Nigerian Health Services* by Schram (1971).

Specific to Nigeria, Ralph Schram (1971) gives a general historical background beginning with early contacts with the European and their various missions, some for trade, others on exploration, yet for others it was mission work and lastly and by no means the least, this last came for territorial conquest in a period that spans over five hundred years. He alludes to the fact that health care and medical service started as services for ship crews, military men in the form of garrison or barrack medical service, which became the Colonial Medical Services. This was then later adopted by the colonial administration and eventually become the Nigerian Medical Service.

DeGoshe's (1984) dissertation in analyzing a Nigerian television drama series first gives a historical perspective of the country, its geography, cultural perspective, population, and a brief mention of its various ethnic tribal groups. Many of Schram's descriptions are in agreement with DeGoshe and others, although Schram's account predominantly is slanted toward the historicity of medical care as opposed to the descriptive analytical nature of the cultural heritage of Nigeria by DeGoshe. French and Lome (1985) trace the origins and progress of medicine from ancient times to the tenth century with, of course, some with emphasis on the modern medical care in the West. They give a human perspective on medicine, surgical practices, the current curriculum of medical training and practice in the West.

Turaki (1983), in his introductory section of the *History of SIM/IECWA in Nigeria*, deals in-depth and specifically with that topic with only a token mentioned of the Nigeria society. However, in the British legacy in Northern Nigeria (1993), he treats that subject and the history of the Nigerian society with such uncanny thoroughness and superb analytical display. Others, who have dealt with the country's history, have done so with respect to socio-economic, cultural, values, geographical, and some other aspects, even if on a cursory level, they include Omolewa (1991), Falola et al. (1970), Nanguang (Dissertation, South Western University, 1990), Rogers and Svenring (1962), Mobobinje (1968), Abernethy (1969), and Hatch (1970).

On medical care and/or health care in general, Willgoose (1974) presents a methodological approach to teaching and the implementation of health care in any elementary setting. Shorter (1987) briefly describes the progress of a century of medical care in general between 1887 and 1987, dubbing the period as the "health century" but especially in the United States where most of the milestones were achieved or reached. Doreen Nagy (1988), in her book *Popular Medicine in 17th Century England*, focuses her investigation on the system of health care sustained by the nonprofessional health care workers in the seventeenth-century England. She contrasts her views with some of the paraprofessional and professional health care services.

NOTES

1. Ruth Sloan et al., *The Educated African* (New York: Fredrick A. Praeger Pub, 1967).
2. John Fried: *Cultural Anthropology* (New York: Harper's College Press, 1976) 42.
3. Alvin R. Bobabinje, *Urbanization in Nigeria* (New York: African Pub. Corporation, 1968).
4. John Hatch, *Nigeria: The Seeds of Disaster* (Chicago: Henry Regnery Co., 1970).
5. Federal Office of Statistics—The Health of Nigerians (Lagos, September, 1984).
6. Joe DeGoshe: *A Content Analysis of a Nigerian TV Drama Series "Cock Crow at Dawn"* (Chicago: University of Chicago Press, 1984).
7. Yusufu Turaki, *The British Colonial Legacy in Northern Nigeria: A Social Ethical Analysis of the Colonial and Post Colonial Society and Politics in Nigeria,* (Jos, Plateau State: Challenge Press, 1993).
8. Federal Research Division Library of Congress, *Nigeria: A Country Study* (Washington D.C: U.S. Government. Printing Office, 1992) 205.
9. Joe DeGoshe: *A Content Analysis of a Nigerian TV Drama Series "Cock Crow at Dawn"* (University of Chicago Press, 1984).
10. Federal Research Division Library of Congress, *Nigeria: A Country Study* (Washington D.C: U.S. Government. Printing Office, 1992) 205.
11. Joe DeGoshe: *A Content Analysis of a Nigerian TV Drama Series "Cock Crow at Dawn,"* (University of Chicago Press, 1984).
12. *The Europa World Year Book* (London: Europa Publication Ltd., 1994).
13. *Research Division Library of Congress Nigeria, a Country Study* (Washington, D.C.: U.S. Government. Printing Office, 1992) 51.
14. Yusufu Turaki: *The British Colonial Legacy in Northern Nigeria: A Social Ethical Analysis of the Colonial and Post Colonial Society and Politics in Nigeria* (Nigeria, Jos: Challenge Press, 1993).
15. John Fried: *Cultural Anthropology* (New York: Harper's College Press, 1976) 41.
16. Ibid., 42.
17. Ibid., 46.
18. Ibid.

19. *Colliers Encyclopedia*, vol.12 (New York: MacMillian Educational, 1981) 546.
20. Ibid.
21. Federal Research Division Library of Congress, *Nigeria: A Country Study* (Washington, D.C.: U.S. Government. Printing Office, 1992) xvi.
22. Ruth Sloan et al., *The Educated African* (New York: Fredrick A. Praeger Pub., 1967).
23. David Abernethy, *The Political Dilemma of Popular Education: An African Case* (Standard Univ. Press, 1969).
24. Federal Office of Statistics, *Annual Abstract of Statistics* (Nigeria, 1982).
25. Michael Omolewa, *Certificate History of Nigeria* (Lagos, Nigeria: Longman, 1990) 33.
26. Alvin R. Mobobinje: *Urbanization in Nigeria II and Nigeria in the 19th Century* (Lagos: Longman, 1991) 61.
27. Toyin, Falola et al., *History of Nigeria* (New York: African Publication Corp., 1968).
28. Federal Research Division Library of Congress, *Nigeria: A Country Study* (Washington, D.C.: U.S. Government. Printing Office, 1992) xvi.
29. Ruth M. French, *Dynamics of Health Care* (New York: McGraw-Hill Book Co., 1979) 4.
30. Yusufu Turaki: *The British Colonial Legacy in Northern Nigeria: A Social Ethical Analysis of the Colonial and Post Colonial Society and Politics in Nigeria* (Jos: Challenge Press, 1993).
31. Ibid.
32. Ibid.
33. Halley's Bible Handbook (Grand Rapids, MI: Zondervan Publication House, 1965) 758.
34. John Hatch, *Nigeria: The Seeds of Disaster* (Chicago: Henry Regnery Co., 1970).
35. Yusufu Turaki: *The British Colonial Legacy in Northern Nigeria: A Social Ethical Analysis of the Colonial and Post Colonial Society and Politics in Nigeria* (Jos: Challenge Press, 1993).
36. R. A. Schram, *A History of Nigerian Health Services* (Ibadan: Ibadan Univ. Press, 1971).
37. Federal Research Division Library of Congress, *Nigeria: A Country Study* (Washington, D. C.: U.S. Government. Printing Office, 1992) 142 & 107.

38. R. A. Schram, *A History of the Nigerian Health Services* (Ibadan: Ibadan Univ. Press, 1971).
39. Federal Research Division Library of Congress, *Nigeria: A Country Study* (Washington, D. C.: U.S. Government. Printing Office, 1992) 144.
40. R. A. Schram, *A History of the Nigerian Health Services* (Ibadan: Ibadan Univ. Press, 1971).
41. Ibid.

CHAPTER THREE

DEFINITION OF TERMS AND GENERAL PRINCIPLE OF HEALTH AND HEALTH CARE

INTRODUCTION

The Hausa proverbial saying "Lafiya uwar kome" comes from common sense and literally means that health is the "mother" of everything. This has already been referred to elsewhere in the previous chapters and, without any equivocation, refers to the fact that health is the center of all normal human activity. Normal individuals everywhere—regardless of location, beliefs, or ideology—enjoy living healthy lives with all, or almost all anyway, activities directed and revolving around the aim to achieve this particular end.

Paradoxically, however, some activities of normal individuals are antithetical to physical well-being. Smoking, car racing, and other risky behaviors are clearly good examples. In Nigeria, before the shift in beliefs toward the "magical" powers of the Western medical cure, which happens to be very recent and just in the last century, medical care, healing, and other health activities were the trusted domains of traditional medical practitioners. By the way, this group is still around, albeit in much smaller numbers than was the case at the turn of last century. There is a resurgence, however, as they are beginning to make a comeback, as a result to the ever-increasing disaffection, to the point of even giving up, on the modern methods of medical care, as its quality has been declining and cost for such care skyrocketing.

As has already been stated, the care and healing activities of traditional medicine men and women centered in the area and the idea of appeasing ancestral spirits, i.e., to drive away evil spirits. These were credited with either causing diseases, illnesses, and/or upsetting the ecological balance in the ambiance of the sick and, of course, the ecological environment in general. Traditional care included practices of abstention from certain food products and/or their alteration, i.e., taking of concoctions prepared by the traditional practitioners, privation of certain food products (dieting), sprinkling of animal blood over certain foods or articles, burning of incenses (to appease or drive away evil spirits), use of roots and leaves, etcetera, to appease these departed ancestral spirits. Furthermore, the invocation and/or incantation of psychic powers, behavioral modification, etcetera, were all also other aspects of the traditional medical care craft.

Quite similar to modern medicine in some of its practice presentation, traditional medicine is equally fragmented with all kinds of specialists in many different areas of practice. Some specialized in internal diseases, similar to the internists in modern medical care; others treat backaches, while yet others set broken bones, reduced fractures, a specialty that is similar or resembles that of the orthopedic doctors. Other native medical craft practitioners (*bokaye*) attempt to modify "crazy" behavior similar to practice of psychiatrists in the areas of mental illness, malnutrition, and so on.

The benefits of medical care to the average Nigerian were, at the very onset, magical when compared to the effects of traditional medical care. The results wrought by the new system were simple, direct, and dramatic, with very few, if any, rules that camouflaged the obvious results or outcome as far as they were concerned. The use of antibiotic drugs to treat bacterial infections, for instance, or the use of anti—malarial to treat malaria, with the accompanying results not only speedy but dropped the level of fatality significantly. The results were the same regardless the facility in which the treatment was given—albeit a hospital, clinic, dispensary, or health center. Such results solidified the belief and trust in modern medical care, thus a consequent drop in the patronage for the traditional medical craft.

Modern medical care cost, however, started graduating from the initial free care, especially in the mission facilities, to small charges; then the cost started getting excessively expensive, to the point of surpassing that of the traditional services which, hitherto, were considered very expensive. This fact, coupled with the steady decline of both the accessibility and the quality of care delivered in these modern medical facilities, made it necessary for the return to the detested traditional medicine and women/men again. Now the surge in that direction is real and dramatic. The skepticism and cynicism toward health system as a whole is both obvious and very sad, and modern medical care in Nigeria has failed the most vulnerable in Nigeria. This is all true because of greed, dishonesty, corruption, tribalism, and the like, which are responsible for the failure and all because of the moral decay and values in the Nigerian society.

Fundamentally, according to Steven Jonas (1986),[1] there is a general belief that health care, in effect, deals with health promotion.*1 * This is may not be very correct, since most health care activities center around getting rid of an illness or a disease state. The premise of his argument does not square off quite well with the education and general orientation of health care professionals and especially physicians. I subscribe to the latter notion even as I differ with the first one. Health activities ranging from prevention to the treatment for cure of diseases are all health promoting activities. Getting rid of a disease, cure if you will, returns the individual to health, no matter how you look at it. This, to my mind, is so since the cured person will return to some level of health even if that will not mean attaining total health for whatever reason, probably many hidden unknown reasons.

In chapter 1, the general background of Nigeria has been presented, including the cultural diversity of its cultural and the historical perspective as to how its health system developed. A synopsis of some aspects of chapter 1 has received added emphasis in chapter 2, based on the perceived level of their importance. In chapter 3, attention needs to focus on the definition of some health concepts, both conventional as well as some invention peculiar to the Nigerian society. The general conclusion from these various definitions is that health represents the functional state of life, while the dysfunctional state represents an illness or a disease state.[2,3] We also now know, as it must be evident, that not every disease is curable or even preventable.[4] As Nicholas Galli (1979) would admonish when he says that what we call health care is a misnomer, this is because the health system, he maintains, is in reality concerned with illness and designed to combat deviations from health [5] This, indeed, is the case, empirically!

At any rate, the fundamental principle that governs most health care delivery systems is, generally, altruistic as it pertains to pain and suffering relief, since by curing disease and by restoring or prolonging life.[6] This observation applies to all health care activities regardless of the level at which activity takes place, whether at the personal, communal, or societal level. Furthermore, there is a profound difference between the availability of health care, which implies availability, accessibility, and affordability of the service health care provided. Russell Coile Jr. (1990) captures the thrust of this idea as he succinctly portrays it when he says that health services should be available at a reasonable cost and that their procurement ought to be

> quick and convenient appointments, accommodating attitudes, responsive service, a pleasant seating and a short wait, the best equipment, and someone to listen who cares. Better yet, the medical encounter results in a therapy that works or at least makes the patient feel better.[7]

Health care providers, he cautions, should endeavor to work primarily for the services of sick customers whose satisfaction should be raison d'être for care providers.[8] Basically, therefore, this outlines and underlines the basics, thus the measuring criterion of success for any health care system. It must also provide health care services in a quick, convenient, accommodating, empathetic, responsive, and pleasant a manner as possible. In addition to all that has been said on account, careful consideration to the unique cultural differences that might exist in the population being served must also be a primary area of focus.

A brief review of the history of health services in United States shows that the modern health service system that is placed developed directly from effective means of treating diseases. Medical technology, for example, created the system, as it became a necessary part of health care services with the required standards for all health care personnel. From the middle of nineteenth century, a period of sanitary awakening resulting in such demands as the environmental sanitation, safe drinking water, and many more others, which ultimately led to the creation of public health departments in state after state in not only the United States, but Europe as well.

Health endeavors—i.e., hospital organization, etcetera—also became realities before the end of nineteenth century. Private, not-for-profit institutions and even local government sponsorships of some of these hospital organizations started to surface. Other sponsorships, such as run by local governments, departments of public health with mental health systems by states or federal agencies, which were also rare and without effective organization, also came into existence.[9]

DEFINITION OF TERMS, SOME GENERAL HEALTH AND HEALTH CARE CONCEPTS

Cleveland R. Hickman (1968) defines health concept as a

> " . . . hygienic knowledge "corresponding to some health experience that influences ones health practice."[10]

Already, we are aware that certain activities prevent or slow disease progress, while others promote health. To understand the different health concepts, therefore, it is important to understand how some of the diseases are acquired as well as ways to prevent them. The factors that influence the health of people at individual and ultimately at the community, or even societal, levels include heredity, environment, education, psychology, and other factors. All of these, to some extent, influence the development and maintenance of physical, emotional health, well-being, and stability.[11]

In an environment with hostile conditions, heath concepts are usually acquired with some creativity and imagination. We see this trait of behavior in every group of people since God placed man on earth right from ancient times up to our modern era. Man has been blessed with complex and yet useful biological tools, namely, intuition, natural defiance mechanisms (immunity), and a nervous system—all of which work in concert to help man deal with many disease entities. These mechanisms have enabled man, regardless of the period of history in which he lived, to remember and interpret feelings, events, unfriendly conditions—pleasant one as well as the unpleasant—from all sorts of sources and to harness them into ways that would provide protection or some form of it. Man has, in that process, been able to acquire knowledge that is vitally necessary to adjust when he is required to do so, to distinguish harmful things in the environment, and to solve current problems based on the knowledge so gained from his past. Thus this helps in the preparation for future encounters or combats.

Our current health and disease concepts as well as our reaction to these derive from our peevish past experiences and early brushes with disease or even death encounters. Because of these encounters, we were forced to learn more about diseases, but also our own bodies. Our health concept, therefore, have been built on disease and medical knowledge about the body which then enable us to project and prepare for the future. Knowledge does not, however, necessarily always translate into correct action. Otherwise, behaviors like smoking, driving without a seat belt, or driving under the influence of drugs or alcohol would not be the problems that they have become nowadays. These and many other examples have become not only solid empirical evidences but also solid scientifically (as some of these can be duplicated and reproduced) by showing how certain human behavior can be iconoclastic,[12] in causing deadly diseases, but also how to prevent them.

HEALTH: This word derives from the English word *hal*, which means "sound," "healthy," "healed," or "whole." Other definitions of *health*, including the one by World Health Organization (WHO), are presented in the first chapter. It is a state of equilibrium, taking into account the ecology of man and his bio-physio-social environments that need to be functionally compatible. The interrelationships set the rules, define all the various aspects of the other relationships, including all conditions that govern the variables that are in interplay here. Man as the beneficiary must, of necessity, adhere to the set rules that govern his relationship with his environment[13] if he is to maximally benefit from it.

HYGIENE: This deals in general with cleanliness and the sciences of health, which also means the preservation of health. Cleveland P. Hickman (1968) states that hygiene is

> . . . a discipline formulated from a knowledge of biology, physiology, bacteriology, chemistry, psychology, physics and many other branches of learning, concerned as it is with all information pertinent to healthful living.[14]

Put another way then, hygiene, as a health concept, is a product of the efforts of human beings who interact with their environment by manipulating and extracting from it the maximum benefit by staying disease free. To that effect, therefore, Ruth M. French (1979) interjects that disease

> . . . is a manifestation of life through the reaction of a total living organism to abnormal stimuli . . . a consequence of interactions between organisms and environmental stimuli (which maybe chemical, physical, biological, and sociological, etc) stimuli which exceed the adaptability of the subject.[15] (sic)

SANITATION: There are many concepts that apply to sanitation, yet it simply means the disposal of injurious to health wastes in a human environment. In public health, it means the development and application of measures that contribute in making the environment healthier for people living in it.[16] Hanlon (1974) says that sanitary

> . . . activities aimed at the preservation and improvement of the environment will always represent a major part of community health programs

or initiatives. This is particularly true, since without sanitation, it is virtually impossible to keep people and communities safe from rodents and so healthy, as disease epidemics are almost always sure to follow. Sanitary efforts and measures began to be organized in earnest, in public health as a result of effort that started in nineteenth century.[18]

The vivid portrayals of the sanitary conditions or their lack in Britain and London to be specific as Edwin Chadwick, the first public health director in Britain reveals,[19] or in America and elsewhere is a cogent testimony to the necessity of hygiene and sanitary measures in all human societies. Imagine a world with no sanitation or sanitary measures and the effects of such a situation even in our today's world!

HEALTH RISK: A health risk or hazard is any condition that, a contact with or exposure to, heightens the likelihood of getting injured by contracting a disease that destabilizes the state of one's health. The control of such factors and conditions results in discomfort for people, thus causing pain or discomfort.

Paradoxically, though, the basic essential for life are air, water, and food, which provide the organism the means of survival, i.e., breathing, eating, drinking, transportation, shelter, etcetera. While these same elements are very basic to human survival, it is through their media that teaming numbers of bacteria, capable of causing injury to humans, are transmitted into the human body. The air we breathe serves as a good example. It is the source by which all kinds of microorganisms are cargoed into the human lungs with every gulp of air taken during the act of normal breathing. Human efforts to control disease, pain, and suffering, however, have not always centered on preventive measures in controlling the environmental sources. In mid-nineteenth century, eminent figures like Edwin Chadwick of Britain and Lammuel Shattuck of Massachusetts,[20] in colonial America, linked the causes of disease directly to disease epidemics and that to the unsanitary living conditions that was pervasive in human environments of those days. Their efforts and recommendations resulted in improved living conditions and therefore the health of the people of their periods that have reverberated to our day.

HEALTH PRACTICE: Health practices are those activities that enhance health. Major areas of health activities and practices are in the hygienic practices of individuals or communities and the environmental control methods used by individuals, in preventive medicine, public health, and other curative incasures.[21]

ENVIRONMENTAL HEALTH: This is considered by Morgan (1993) as the first line of defense mechanism of human against disease invasion. This endeavor involves the treatment to produce quality water, proper lighting, disposal of wastes, adequate management of hazardous waste materials from industrial plants and waste products.

Pest and insect controls are also part of this particular endeavor as it is a major avenue of human torment by hordes of little rascal, rodents, mosquitoes, flies, to name just a few from this army of nature's tormentors.

Milk sanitation and food management also rank very high in the equation of disease control. Others include interstate and international travel regulations, good occupational health regulations, air/water pollution control, environmental safety measures, prevention programs, housing, land use, recreation, and many more areas, which all constitute the first line of action against diseases and their causing agents.

The second line of defense against disease is the public health and preventive medicine, which involves the adaptation of the body by equipping it with antibodies (Ab) via "immunity" (active and passive) that antagonize disease agents that gain entrance into the body. This particular method prevents the establishment or reestablishment of the foreign agent that might subsequently subject the body to disease onslaught. One major way of doing this involves the fortification of the body with good and proper nutrition, followed by good personal hygiene, routine checkups (for diabetes, dental diseases, hypertension, etc.) and the employment of health education in every available situation that requires a health decision.

The third line of action involves public health and medical prevention, which entail early diagnosis and treatment of disease conditions, easy access of care and affordability of such care. Finally, curative efforts such as treatment—medical care which might involve chemotherapy, radiation, surgery, laboratory and other diagnostic processes, corrective rehabilitation such as speech or respiratory therapy, and so on.

HEALTH PROMOTION: This refers to individual and community efforts with actions that are aimed at advancing the state of well-being at individual's level by preventing certain health
Hazardous conditions, in order to obtain the optimal level of health for all involved.[23]

Anderson and Langton (1961) believe that personal health promotion centers on individual safeguards with dynamic health status encompassing activities leading to the improvement of health. The efforts in such a pursuit involve utilizing community health resources as important health practice. They list the following as important steps in health promotion: periodic health assessment of needs; understanding of action adopted and based on hereditary traits; concern and care of those organs of the body most susceptible to diseases such as teeth, skin, ears, and eyes; avoiding products harmful to health like cigarettes smoking and excessive alcohol. Beverages and adherence to proper nutrition, moderation in exercise are good examples, the avoidance of fatigue, getting adequate sleep and rest, the avoidance of health hazards, the prevention of infection, and so on.[24]

Finally, Rubinson and Wesley (1984) assert that health promotion is an activity that encourages behavior which leads to good health, like exercise; immunization; screening (for diabetes, hypertension, etc.); and similar other activities directed at living healthy.[25]

DISEASE: *Disease*, according to Marshall and Pearson (1972),

> may be defined as any condition which actually or potentially impedes individual function.

Health, on the other hand, is that mental state that provides the individual with the maximum potential to function.[26]

Ruth French (1972), on the other hand, postulates that

> . . . disease or trauma is a threat to homeostasis, a threat which calls into action that is protective and restorative mechanisms of the body.[27]

Disease, however, according to *Dorland's Pocket Medical Dictionary* (1982), is,

> . . . any deviation from or interruption of the normal structure or function of any part, organ or system that is manifested by a characteristic set of symptoms and signs and whose etiology, pathology and prognosis as it may be known or unknown.[28]

This latest definition is a lot better, as it is more broad and inclusive. A disease state always exists when the normal function of the body or any of its subsystems is abnormally interrupted by injury or the invasion by parasites. For example, a disease state exists when the pancreas fails to secrete insulin (diabetes) resulting in the excretion of high content of sugar in blood and into the urine, or anemia as a result of prolonged blood loss from hookworm infestation and so on.

PARASITE: A parasite is any organism that is harbored at the expense of the host regardless of the nature of their symbiotic (a close association of unrelated subjects) relationship.[29] In other words, the host loses benefits while the invader gains or benefit(s). Microorganisms that cause infection such as plasmodium in malaria and worm infestation of the ilk of infestation like lumbricoids in ascariasis (roundworm) are clear examples of parasitism or parasitic relationship. However, Jawetz, Melnick, and Adelberg (1972) claim that the relation of parasite and the host does not always imply harm to the host,

. . . on the contrary, the most successful parasite achieves a balance with the host which ensures the survival, growth, and propagation of both parasite and the host.[30]

PREVENTION: This means the use of a prophylactic measure in the effort to guard against or in anticipation of something unpleasant about to happen. The main objective in prevention is to prevent disease occurrence by taking steps and avoid activities that are known to cause disease.

Major steps in prevention include environmental and personal hygienic measures, sanitation, as well as other approaches that could be effective in the attenuation of disease establishment. Environmental manipulation is designed to prevent contact between people and the agents of diseases, while the reverse works when disease agents are in contact with people, even when such irritants are harmless. The manipulation of the environment is one of the primary concerns of prevention.[31]

Vaccination is also another considered to be a primary preventive measure, as it protects a person from contracting a disease when contact has been made with a disease agent. The treatment of a disease situation is considered secondary prevention, a curative measure, and rehabilitation programs are tertiary preventive measures geared toward limiting any disability that would occur by increasing the functional potential of the individual during and after the disease.

Preventive medicine or medical prevention has to do with the medical approach that is concerned with the general preventive measures aimed at improving the health of the environment and the relationship of the people that live with it. This means early detection, diagnosis, and treatment of diseases so as to prevent serious consequences that could follow.[32]

INFECTION: The simple definition of *infection* is the ability of germs or bacteria or their products to invade the body and multiply. Accordingly, Jawetz, Melnich, and Adelberg (1987) maintain that

> ... infection is the process whereby the parasite enters into relationship with the host . . .,

with two necessary components, namely, entry and an established multiplication in the victim.[33]

IMMUNITY: This is one of the several ways of protection acquired either due to resistance or security obtained against certain disease agents after a bout with the disease. Having had a certain disease, like measles or smallpox, the individual is conferred permanent immunity, an inoculation of antigens (Ag) and will enable the body to form antibodies (Ab), which confer protection against future disease episodes.[34]

DIAGNOSIS: Diagnosis of a disease refers to the determination of the nature and cause of a disease. This is based on observed symptoms, signs, and the laboratory findings to confirm the diagnosis.

EPIDEMIOLOGY: This involves the study of disease occurrence in human population, which focuses primary on groups of people.[35] There is, therefore, more to epidemiology, than the mere or simple preceding description. Friedman, (1994) and Wilner, et al (1973) refer to *epidemiology* as the description of the distribution of "human health problems" that endeavors to establish causation of the problems and the means of establishing effective control measures. An aspect of epidemiology would focus on the aspect of investigating a disease, while another might lay emphasis on measurements or circumstances under which a disease occurs in one population and not in another. In general, according to Wilner et al. (1973), epidemiology focuses on the "total health disease spectrum," indicating the multi-factorial nature of this subject.[36]

ENDEMIC: This means the presence of any disease entity in a human population on a continuous basis.[37] A good example of an endemic disease is the perennial presence of malaria in some tropical countries, among which Nigeria ranks as one.

EPIDEMIC: This term refers to the excessive, prevalence of a disease in a community due to spread from somewhere else or a temporary increase in the number of epidemic cases. Wilner, et al, (1993) speculate that epidemics have, over the human history, killed more soldiers than have weapons of war.[38]

PANDEMIC: This is an epidemic on a grand scale affecting other regions of the world.

SPORADIC: This refers to the occurrence of a single-disease entity, which is scattered over a wide area range. A sporadic disease is neither epidemic nor pandemic with cases spread appearing over long intervals of time.

INCIDENCE: This refers to the number of new cases of a specific disease within a specific population per year.

MORBIDITY: This means that the incidence, severity of sickness and its accident(s), that is a "chance of occurrence" in a defined group or a class of people.

PREVALENCE: This word refers to all the numbers of a specific disease episode within a population at a given time.

RISK MANAGEMENT: This refers to the control of circumstances or events that pose threats related to health and other occupations which are not safe or comfortable to anyone that is in close contact or in their vicinity. Risk management eliminates the threat to injury and financial loss or liability that may be associated with such risks.

HEALTH CARE: Any advice, educational instruction, and treatment by a qualified professional that is for the expressed purpose of improving or maintaining the health of people, i.e., both well and the sick people.

PRIMARY CARE: The primary care aspect of personal care places emphasis on first contact between a health professional and a patient with a professional who assumes responsibility on an ongoing basis for the patient's health needs. These needs may range from checkups to treatment; coordination of cases, needs, and referrals with other source groups; and referral to secondary and tertiary care providers under the definition of prevention for secondary and tertiary cases.

ANTIBODY (Ab): This is a modified protein in the serum of animal's or people's blood, so formed in response to antigens (Ag—foreign inoculates) that accords the recipient immunity from a particular disease or group of diseases.

ANTIGEN (Ag): This is one of a number of different protein substances that stimulate animal immune response in the tissues. It primes the body in readiness to identify an invading organism and marshals its resources to fight the invasion.

PATHOLOGY: This deals with the medical science of all the essentials, i.e., nature and function of change that is due to disease and its processes, while a *pathogen* refers to bacteria or other disease-causing substances. *Pathogenesis* refers to the origin or mode of development which a disease takes, from development to cure; therefore, *pathogenic* simply means the ability for an organism or substance capable of causing disease and is able to do so.

DISABILITY: This word refers to partial or total physical or mental handicap that results from an injury or illness. Partial disability limits one or more functions for a particular job or role.

AMBULATORY CARE: This refers to that branch of health services that provides diagnosis, treatment, and/or rehabilitation, which patients come for on their own and return home after the care or service.

MANAGED CARE: This is a health care concept that refers to a health care system which integrates health care delivery, and its incurred cost to beneficiaries by prearrangement with certain providers who, on a set standard, provide comprehensive health care to a particular clientele.

HEALTH SERVICE SYSTEM: This is the organizational structure or arrangement through which different health care services are provided to patients. Hospitals, clinics, or health care centers within a community are examples of health service system.

HEALTH EDUCATION: This refers to the process of assisting people to make informed decisions about matters affecting individual or group health.

CARE: The management of a sick person to improve or cure them of a disease or state of illness. The caregiver can be a professional, nonprofessional, or both[39] or any of these combinations.

COMPLICATION: This refers to conditions that arise after an initial disease condition. For example, conjunctivitis in a frequent complication of measles in children and pneumonia after bad cold or influenza, a fracture with limited mobility in any age group, can cause pneumonia in any group.[40]

TREATMENT: This means the care and management of patients with diseases or disorders.

There are different modalities of treatment programs, like the conservative approach (using limited measures), radical approach (using every permissible means), palliative treatment (designed to alleviate pain), preventive approach (prophylactic or preventive), empirical approach (from proven or pragmatic evidence or experience) that have proven effective, supportive, symptomatic, and rehabilitative (restorative) treatment modalities.

Besides these, medication, diet, and exercise are also commonly used in combination with most of the preceding treatment approaches or modalities, but especially in treating chronic disease conditions like diabetes mellitus and a few others.

REHABILITATION: The main goal of rehabilitation is restoring lost function due to whatever cause. Main efforts, according to Wilner et al, (1973), do involve assessment of abilities and skills that are appropriate to the needs of the disabled.

> . . . Rehabilitation may consist of restoring the patient to the activities of daily living, teaching him or her to live within his or her limitations or retraining for other types of occupations (vocational rehabilitation). Special living and work

arrangements may be an appropriate part of rehabilitation of some patients and may be found in cooperative living centers, shelters, workshops and selected placement in industries.[41]

Rehabilitation programs are usually formed in hospitals with orthopedic units, long-term care facilities, and orthopedic hospitals.

TRANSMISSION: Transmission is a very appropriate topic in health discussions and refers to the transfer of disease among people, from one individual to another. Transmission of pathogens is done either in direct or indirect manner.

In a direct transmission, the pathogens are communicated directly from the carrier to the recipient without any intermediaries. A clear example is a droplet particle from a tuberculosis patient's cough or sneeze directly on the face of another person, as the recipient inhales particles of the infected discharge. In an indirect transmission, there is an intermediary, such as a fly in a dysentery outbreak or mosquito in malaria fever.

HOMEOSTASIS: This literally means a state of balance or equilibrium, that ideal and functional state, for most organisms. The body is made up of billions of cells which form its very basic units that maintain the right internal environment and equilibrium for a normal person. Edward D. Frohlick (1981) describes by defining homeostasis this way:

> . . . Cells are continually bathed in extra-cellular fluid, which is sometimes called internal environment of the body. The constituents of this fluid are very exactly controlled, and, as long as they remain within the normal range, each cell is capable of living as an individual unit and performing its respective tasks for the body. A very large portion of our discussion of human physiology will deal with this exact regulation of the constituents in the extra-cellular fluid; this is called "homeostasis" which simply means "*maintenance of constant conditions in the internal environment.*"[42] (emphasis added)

All the various systems in the body do need the steadiness guaranteed only by a state of homeostasis, a state of balance. On the other hand, there is also an immunological homeostasis which confers immunity to one's antigens within the body. Without this, the body's own antibodies could wreck havoc on the same body by destroying the very cells that they are meant to protect because from birth, these "self-antigens" have been imbued with this capability of doing this.[43]

SUSCEPTIBILITY: *Susceptibility* refers to lack of resistance that makes a person an easy prey to infection. Put another way, it is a direct opposite that runs counter to immunity (state of the body that prevents one from getting infection). Like immunity, it is also specific, as a person can be immune to one disease and be susceptible to yet another. Wilner, Walkley, and Goerke (1973) explain it in this way:

> . . . Even though a pathogen gains entry to the body it does not necessarily result in infection or disease. In order to fall victim to the disease, the new host must be susceptible to it. However, the body has certain defense mechanisms, which help protect against invading pathogens and may aid in the destruction of the latter. Such mechanisms are called resistance, and if sufficiently great, they constitute immunity.[44]

QUARANTINE: This refers to that period of contact with a disease agent and up to the very first signs of the disease beginning to manifest. It also means the period when the movement of those in contact with an infectious disease is restricted—until the period of that disease is known to have developed is over with no signs or symptoms of the disease—before contact with the general population is allowed. Wilner et al, (1973) describe quarantine as a process of detecting infectious agents, infected person, or other implicated hosts and vectors and preventing their introduction into a susceptible locality or population.[45]

CARRIER: A carrier is someone who has been in contact with a source of infection and is capable of passing the infectious agents to virtually every susceptible individual that comes into contact with him or her. However, carriers do not necessarily come down with the disease, the germs of which they carry.

ISOLATION: This is the physical separation of a patient with an infectious and/or communicable disease from every person who does not have disease. This was commonly in practice in the days of smallpox infections, or currently with measles, and other virulent infectious diseases. Quarantine deals, apparently, with the well or healthy, whereas isolation affects only the sick, ill, or people who have the potential to be "carriers" of a disease.

REVIEW OF LITERATURE

In most countries, especially in the West, there is a plethora of literature in both the health and non-health fields alike, replete with health ideas, which constantly undergo discussion and debate in all circles, academic and nonacademic, and information media settings. On the surface, such terms as *culture, environment, environmental health, ecology, trauma, epidemics, nutrition, habits, lifestyle, prevention, disease* control, [46, 47] and many others all deal with some aspect of health. Many of these terms have health implications on such grand scales as to involve major chunks of national and even international budgets.

According to Levey and Loomba (1990), the U.S. national health cost in the 1990s was over 400 percent over the cost of the decade of the 1980s, which was then estimated at well over 400 billion dollars,[48, 49] approximately 10 percent of the national budget[50] at the time. This was not the case or the same for Nigeria at the time of these estimates and most certainly not even close today, as Nigeria's health budget is sure not what it should or ought to be, in view of the health issues facing the citizens of Nigeria. Greater interest is focused elsewhere to other less-important matters with greater expenditures.

In the third edition of her book *Cultural Diversity in Health and Illness*, Rachel Spector (1979), to some degree, describes the various factors reflected in modifying the health beliefs of people. Among these are experiences that result from action-benefit cycle, disease condition and its level of seriousness, and threats from other socio-cultural variables specific to each society.

Charles Austin (1988) spells out some ways that make it possible for both the health system to function in service organizations which he likens to the human body and mechanical system organization in the *Information System for Health Services Administration*, 3rd edition. This analysis elicits some striking similarities between the principles of health services and that of the general system theory, which further sheds light on the dynamics of the concepts of equilibrium, feedback, open and close systems, environmental control, etcetera, and integral parts of a system.

The interdependence of parts and their relationships with each other leads to a good product (health care, good or bad) for the health service organization. In *Health Care Management: A Text in Organization Theory and Behavior*, Stephen Shortell and Arnold Kaluzny (1983) discuss the enormity and size of expenditure of the health care system, as well as its share in the U.S. gross national product, complexity, and the diverse nature of its professionals. They further delineate a succinctly descriptive profile of its various services. The criteria for organizing, administering such organizations, their goals, mission for both open and closed systems are all very well laid out and discussed.

In the book report, *Dimensions in Health*, Abraham Horwitz (1964) discusses the ideals and humanitarian efforts in dealing with health issues that lead to the implementation of such programs as prevention programs, treatment programs, and health promotion programs. Guild, Fruisz, and Bojar (1969), on the other hand, deal with the concepts of environmental health, holistic health, health examination, interviews, history taking, and physical examination. They use case histories to illustrate the concepts of the science of health.

In *Health Principles and Practice*, Anderson and Langton (1961) list some fifteen ways of promoting personal health, which can range from individual regular inventory of health status, to restoration, and referral to appropriate and available community resources, in a timely manner. They suggest ways of both extending life and enjoying it to its fullness. They include indices of personal profile which could lead to freedom from disease, disabilities, good sleep, rest, relaxation, good appetite, maintenance of right weight, emotional stability, and so on. Finally, they emphasize the need to pay avid attention to personal hygienic factors like dental, hearing, visual care, and frequent examination.

Bailar, III et al. (editors, 1987), in *Assessing Risks to Health Methodological Approaches*, lists the various agencies involved in risk assessment and the analysis of key components involved there. In the eleventh chapter of the

17th edition of the *Review of Medical Microbiology*, Jawetz, Melnick, and Adelberg (1987) describe and discuss infections, their various agents and attributes that enable them to cause disease. They also discuss the mechanism that determine resistance, natural, acquired immunities and genetic influences. Hickman (1968), in the second chapter of the third edition of *Health for College Students*, explains the formation of health concepts. He provides a list of health and disease concepts in a detailed discussion of some of the disease entities that go back to ancient times.

Marshall and Pearson (1972) give general definitions of health and health concepts. They discuss by detailing the cost of maintaining health in America in their book *Dynamics of Health and Disease*. They list three major activities that could ensure good health for people and ways of prevention, restoration, and organization.

Last (1987) states the scope, goals, methods of public health, giving its historical perspectives and details the meaning of primary, secondary, and tertiary prevention with explanation on the national and international health policies, some aspects of the ecology in a global context and their implications for politics.

Frohlick (editor, 1981) describes the organization, physiology of the body, concepts of homeostasis, cell function, body fluids, kidneys, blood immunity, respiration, circulation, and other functions.

Wilner, Walkley, and Goerke (1973) outline in chapter 9 those components that constitute vital statistics, their demographics and then analyze the experimental aspects of the subject. Blum (1983), in chapter 1 of *Expanding Health Care Horizon: From a General System Concepts of Health to a National Health Policy*, 2nd edition, describes the relationship of the health system, subsystems aspects of the ecology, from its health function to the balancing or the homeostatic effect that moderates the circle of the dynamics in its eco-ambiance.

Dever, (1991) discusses his philosophical concept and analyses of holistic health, the methodology, involved in multidimensional process in *Public Health and Policy in Community Health Analysis: Global Awareness at the Local Level*, 2nd edition. He explains the value system and its profound effect on health attitudes, habits, and hygiene. He further explains and inks the global nature of these concepts to some of the planning methods in health management. In the *Management Information Systems for Public Health*, the spelled-out details are designed to encourage and involve individuals in health activities. He suggests ways for computer innovations and programming. This "farming out" of the health programs to other agencies, outside of the health field, is an issue worthy of consideration.

John Gentry (1978) highlights the definition of some health concepts and health care plan for care practices. In *Primary Health Care More than Medicine*, Rosaline S. Miller (1983) takes a look at organization, policy, problems, and care issues that confront ambulatory care services, and she spells out a variety of health care models that providers can use to improve the quality of care to their consumers. She emphasizes, however, that these are by no means panaceas to problems that bewitch the ambulatory care system.

The principles and guidelines for risk management through improvement in communication are discussed by Cavello, McCallum, and Pavlova (editors, 1989). They spell out the route and ways for educating the public on risk management by health officials and list the various risk factors, government communication programs through paradigms of case analysis. In the third edition of *Dimensions of Community Health*, Dean Miller (1984) provides an overview on numerous community health issues over the last two decades of the twentieth century by focusing on community health structure from the local, state, national, to the international level and emphasizes the importance of providing health care relative to the health problems confronting the average citizen. This important point that is particularly salient to the Nigerian situation must be stressed here.

Lee and Estes (editors, 1990) discuss factors that influence the health of a U.S. citizen in *The Nation's Health*. Central to the financing of health services depicted by failure to develop comprehensive programs that could control cost is the advocacy issue to ensure accessibility. Other contributing factors include government abdication of responsibility, rising cost due to overtreatment brought about by increases in malpractice suits. The unexpected as well as unwelcome arrival of AIDS, the most dreaded disease since the black death of the Middle Ages, further compounds health problems and matters in general.

Roger Birnbaum (1976) describes in some detail the health maintenance organizations concepts, delivery systems, benefits and limitation to both patients and physicians. Steven R. Eastaugh (1992), in *Health Economics: Efficiency, Quality, and Equity*, discusses with emphasis placed on health economics and focuses attention on health care efficiency and quality in public health policy. In chapter 1, he deals with the analysis, production, and functional aspect of health cost.

The rest of the book deals with economic mode of hospitals, physician behavior, cost containment, gate-keeping and managing health care in long-term facilities, and so forth. Wilson and Neuhauser (1985) summarize the major components of health care in the United States in *Health Services in the United States*.

Murray Grant (1981), in the third edition of *Handbook of Community Health*, discusses the fundamentals of epidemiology and genetics, health statistics, principles of preventing communicable diseases, geriatrics, medical sociology, environmental factors in disease prevention, maternal and child health, nutrition, dental, mental occupational health, accidents, retardation, and several other health topics. Finally, Abram S. Benenson (editor, 1990), in *Control of Communicable Diseases in Man: A Handy Ready Source of Information for Health Workers*, describes communicable diseases found in humans, their sources, incubation periods, treatment and describes the pertinent terminology and concepts that are related to the particular area of health.

NOTES

1. Steven Jonas, *Health Care Delivery in United States*, 2nd ed. (New York: Springer Pub., Co., 1986) 12.
2. Ibid., 18.
3. Carter L. Marshall and David Pearson: *Dynamics of Health and Disease* (New York: Appleton-Century-Crofts. Educational Division, Meredith Co., 1974), 2.
4. Steven Jonas, *Health Care Delivery in United States*, 2nd ed. (New York: Springer Pub. Co., 1981) 18.
5. Nicholas, Galli,: *Foundations and Principles of Health Education* (Santa Barbara: John Willey and Sons, 1978) 39.
6. Daniel M. Wilner, Rosabelle Rand Walkley, and Lenor S. Goerke, *Introduction to Public Health*, 6th ed. (New York: MacMillan Publication Co. Inc., 1973), 71.
7. Russell C. Coile Jr, *The New Medicine: Reshaping Medical Practice and Health Care Management* (Rockvile, MD.: Aspen Pub., Inc., 1990), 355.
8. Ibid., 357.
9. Jonathan S. Rakich, Beaufort B. Longest Jr., and Kurt Darr, *Managing Health Service Organizations*, 2nd ed. (Philadelphia: W. E. Saunders Co., 1985) 29-31.
10. Cleveland P. Hickman: *Health for College Students*, 3rd ed. (Englewood Cliffs, NJ: Prentice-Hall, Inc., 1968), 14.
11. W. R. Guild, R. E. Fuisz, and S. Bojar: *The Science of Health* (Englewood Cliffs, NJ: Prentice-Hall, Inc., 1965), 2.
12. C. P. Hickman: *Health for College Students*, 3rd ed. (Englewood Cliffs, NJ:. Prentice-Hall Inc., 1965), 15.
13. J. J. Hanlon: *Public Health: Administration and Practice*, 6th ed. (St. Louis: The C. V. Mosby Co., 1974), 517.
14. Cleveland P. Hickman: *Health for College Students*, 3rd ed. (Englewood Cliffs, NJ: Prentice-Hall Inc., 1968), 14.
15. Ruth M. French: *Dynamics of Health Care*, 3rd ed. (New York: McGraw-Hill Book Co., 1979), 3.
16. __The Random House Dictionary* (New York: Random House, 1980) 779.
17. J. J. Hanlon: *Public Health: Administration and Practice*, 6th ed. (St. Louis: The C. V. Mosby Co., 1974),545.
18. Ibid.

19. B. W. Richardson: *The Health of Nations: A Review of the Works of Edwin Chadwick*, vol. 11 (London: Longmans, Green and Co., 1887).

20. Monroe T. Morgan: *Environmental Health* (Madison, WI: WCB Brown and Benchmark Pub., 1993) 24.

21. Ibid., 25.

22. Ibid.

23. Snehendu B. Karr, editor: *Health Promotion Indicators and Action* (New York: Springer Pub. Co., 1989), 1.

24. C. L. Anderson and C. V. Langton: *Health Principles and Practice*, 3rd ed. (St. Louis: The C. V. Mosby, 1961),30-31.

25. L. Rubison and A. R. Wesley: *Health Education: Foundations for the Future,* (St. Louis: Times Mirror/Mosby College Pub., 1984) 258.

26. C. L. Marshall and D. Pearson: *Dynamics of Health and Disease* (New York: Appleton-Century-Crofts, 1972), 2.

27. R. M. French: *Dynamics of Health Care*, 3rd ed. (New York: McGraw-Hill Book Co., 1979), 3.

28. __Dorland's Pocket Medical Dictionary*, 24th ed. (Philadelphia: W. B. Saunders Co., 1982), 79.

29. Ibid., 452.

30. Ernest Jawetz, Joseph L. Melnick, and Edward A. Adelberg: *Review of Medical Microbiology* (Los Altos, CA: Lange Med. Pub., 1912), 128.

31. C. L. Marshall and D. Pearson: *Dynamics of Health and Disease* (New York: Appleton-Century-Crofts, 1912), 4.

32. L. Rubinson and A. F. Wesley: *Health Education: Foundations for the Future* (St. Louis: Times Mirror/Mosby College Pub., 1984), 258.

33. W. E. Jawetz, J. L. Melnick, and E. A. Adelberg: *Review of Medical Microbiology*, 7th ed. (Norwalk, CT: Appleton and Lange, 1987), 160.

34. W. E Waters and K. S. Clift: *Community Medicine: A Textbook for Nurses and Visitors* (London: Groom Helm, 1983), 110-111.

35. Gray D. Friedman: *Primer of Epidemiology*, 4th ed. (New York: McGraw-Hill Inc., 1994), 1.

36. D. M. Wilner, Rosabelle P. Walkley, and Lenor S. Goerke: *Introduction to Public Health*, 6th ed. (New York: MacMillan Pub. Co. Inc., 1973), 286-287.

37. L. E. Burton et al.: *Public Health and Community Medicine*, 3rd ed. (Baltimore: Williams and Wilkins, 1980), 577.

38. D. M. Wilner, Rosabelle P. Walkley, and Lenor S. Goerke: *Introduction to Public Health*, 6th ed. (New York: MacMillan Pub. Co., Inc., 1973), 303.

39. C. C. Meisenheimer: *Improving Quality: A Guide to Effective Programs* (Gaithersburg, MD: Aspen Pub. Inc., 1992), 505.

40. Marcus A. Krupp et al: *Physician's Handbook*, 21st ed. (Los Altos, California: Lange Medical Pub., 1985), 425.

41. D. M. Wilner, Rosabelle P. Walkley, and Lenor S. Goerke: *Introduction to Public Health*, 6th ed. (New York: MacMillan Pub. Co., Inc., 1973), 345.

42. E. D. Frolich, editor: *Rypins' Medical Licensure Examinations: Topical Summaries and Questions* (Philadelphia: I. E. Lippincott Co., 1981), 139.

43. J. S. Thompson and M. W. Thompson: *Genetics in Medicine*, 4th ed. (Philadelphia: W. B. Sounders Co., 1986), 59.

44. D. M. Wilner, Rosabelle P. Walkley, and Lenor S. Goerke: *Introduction to Public Health*, 6th ed. (New York: MacMillan Pub. Co. Inc., 1913), 310.

45. Ibid., 311.

46. M. T. Morgan: *Environmental Health* (Madison, WI: WCB Brown and Benchmark Pub., 1993), 16-28.

47. J. M. Last: *Public Health and Human Ecology* (Ottawa: Prentice-Hall, Appleton and Lange, 1987) 1-24.

48. S. Levey and N. P. Loomba: *Health Care Administration: A Managerial Perspective*, 2nd ed. (Philadelphia: J. B. Lippincott Co., 1990), v.

49. S. M. Shortell and A. D. Kaluzny: *Health Care Management: A Text in Organization Theory and Behavior* (New York: John Wiley and Sons, 1983), 1-24.

CHAPTER FOUR

THE HEALTH SYSTEM IN NIGERIA

INTRODUCTION

The development of health care system in Nigeria was, after all, accident, considering the fact that white people did not come with the purpose of helping Africans get rid of the diseases that were killing us left, right, up, and center. The main purpose of their sojourn has been briefly alluded to in the previous discussions. Although some of the discussion is rather perfunctory, shallow if you will, nevertheless, it reveals certain profound facts and a level of a mind-set about these early Western explorers and colonially minded wealth hunters. Helping the African out of his ignorance, misery, and development were the furthest things from his mind at that point, it was only later that some of them decided to the precious little as an afterthought!

The trade, commerce, and missionary efforts, especially their pioneering role and efforts in starting hospitals, eventually culminated in what was then known as the "garrison" medicine or "barrack" medical care.

Diet constitutes an important part of any people just as the culture and traditions. It is in that vein that a quote from a nutritionist is in order here. This prominent nutritionist is quoted as once having said that "man digs his grave with his teeth."[1] This statement is based on what we eat or not eat. This statement is an aphorism that Americans know a thing or two about, this is because American are overweight and consequently suffer from a variety of diseases like high blood pressure, diabetes, and few others because of it. Therefore, the statement or saying that "you are what you eat" is so very true. Of course, there is more to health than the idea expressed in this simple statement, since personal hygiene, exercise, and environmental factors are all necessary components, which play critical roles in the scheme of overall health status.

THE HEALTH SYSTEM IN NIGERIA

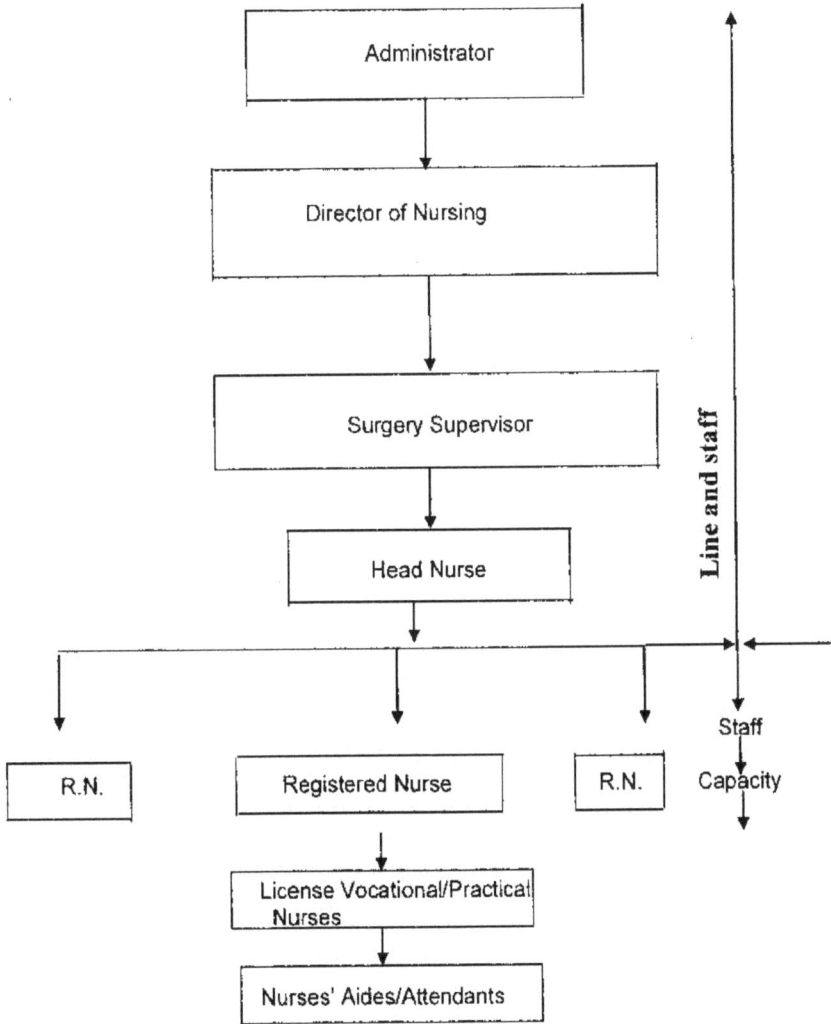

Diagram: A standard model for Line and Staff Authority-
Nursing service in a hospital organization

The various definitions of *culture* have been described in chapter 1. Anderson and Carter define culture as qualities and attributes that are characteristic and uniquely human behaviors that differentiate us from other forms of life.[2] The way of life for a people and some of the transmissible behavioral elements that bind citizens of a society include manners, habits, morals, modes of the transmission, tools, and how they are used.[3]

From these cultural and anthropological perspectives, and because Nigeria is a heterogeneous society with many customs and traditions, there is hardly a pure culture with traditions that are 100 percent and unique only to the Nigerian society alone. The culture is an amalgam of customs and traditions that have been adopted from other cultures, namely, the Western culture, and the incorporated over time and now claimed as Nigerian culture. The way Nigerians dress with shirt tie, suit or coat "cover," shoes and socks; white wedding dress, wedding cakes, etc., even our native languages are now spattered with English words (a good example is the pidgin English); and there are a host of others that dare not attempt to try detail here, or that would be all that the rest of this book will have to be devoted to. This particular aspect has been touched on earlier as well.

However, with regards to food and food preparation, there seems to be some general similarities in the type of food stuffs and their preparation in many regions of the country. No food substance or stuff is peculiar to any particular ethnic group since most foodstuffs—e.g., rice, beans, yams, maize, cassava, etcetera—are consumed by almost all the ethnic groups. *Tuwo da miya*, for example, and *hura da nono* are the main dishes of the Hausa/Fulani groups on the northern segment of the country. *Tuwo*, the main course, is prepared from guinea corn, maize, millet, or accha—all cereals and predominantly carbohydrates in constitution. Accha is similar to rice and wheat and grown in a similar manner, albeit its grain is a lot smaller than either rice or wheat. Furthermore, rice and wheat may be grounded, but their grains are usually cooked whole-size. Accha, after the removal of its husk, is always prepared a whole grain without pulverization except making gruel or *kunu*. The *miya* segment of the *tuwo da miya* is prepared from a concoction of vegetables mixed with beef, fowl meat, or fish. The *tuwo* segment looks like a pudding or stuffing-like, which a portion is taken then dipped into the *miya* as the dish is being consumed. In the southern region and sections of Nigeria, *eba* or *teba,* is e., the equivalent of *tuwo*, a common and favorable dish in the north. It is prepared in somewhat a similar manner and eaten in like manner as *tuwo da miya* by both the Yorubas and Igbos and their subgroups of ethnic tribes respectively. It is eaten with soup or *miya* called *dege-dege. Eba* or *teba* may be prepared from *gari* (made from cassava) and pounded yam from yams.

Hura da nono, on the other hand, is prepared from guinea corn (*dawa*) or millet (*dauro* or *gero*) with sour milk (*nono* or yoghurt) added. It is cherished mostly in the north predominantly by the Hausa/Fulani mostly, but also other subgroups of ethnic tribes. The equivalent of this food stuff is the soaked ground cassava (*garin kwake*) granule or farina with water, milk, or sour milk and sugar added. It is consumed mostly by the Yoruba and Igbo groups. Other dishes like *kunu* (gruel), *akamu* (pap), *fate, brabisco* (bean cake), *kosai,* or *moimoi* are made from beans with eggs, pepper, some meat, and some other vegetable added. These are all common food preparations by most ethnic groups in every region of the country. Pounded yam is one of the major dishes of the Igbo groups and several other tribes in the Middle Belt area of the north, especially the Tiv, Idoma and Igala, Ninzom, Mada, and other tribal groups.

Because the majority of Nigerians are farmers, their diet comprises mainly of carbohydrates, a steady source of energy for the hard manual labor that is involved, i.e., the manual filling of the soil that farming requires in most third world countries in Africa. It is, however, a balanced diet with adequate nutrition, which, according to Harvey et al. (1976), plays a very crucial role in human life[6] and Nigerians are by no means exempted. The ordinary Nigerian usually eats a balanced diet even if it has a high content of carbohydrate.[7] Frequently, however, this leads to malnutrition, especially in the very young and elderly, with its attendant complications and also low resistance to disease[8] in these same susceptible groups.

A. THE HEALTH CARE SYSTEM

Health Concepts Unique to Nigeria

The health concepts that are used idiomatically in Nigeria and discussed here are the ones mostly used by Nigerians as only a few have been selected for the purpose of hand.

67

1. General Terms and Concepts Used in Nigerian Health Care Facilities

a. General Hospital

A general hospital is a health facility and a multi-treatment setting that generally includes an outpatient department, an emergency room, medical and surgical inpatient units, which may include pediatric, maternity sections, and a pharmacy. It may also have a laboratory, perhaps x-ray or radiology sections and sometimes a few other ancillary services. A lot of general hospitals in Nigeria are in such deplorable conditions that the meaning "general hospital" does not do justice to the concept, except for the fact and for the implication that there does not seem to be any evidence to link the two. These are at variance with the original meaning of the concept of a hospital altogether. This noble concept, a general hospital as used in Nigeria, it seems, has changed considerably, that it has come to mean things like "demand center," "privation unit," "butcher's house," or "robbers' den." These implied meanings have absolutely nothing to do with the care of the sick and for good reasons shouldn't because they do not connote any sense or idea of care whatsoever.

The above polemics are ardent description of what Nigerian hospitals have turned into and the kind of hardship visited on the sick people, who are supposed to be cared for by health care professions. These hospitals are "demand centers" because sick people face all kinds of demands, rational and otherwise, that all center on money.

They are "butchers' centers," "robbers' dens" because of the high rate of casualties that result in death because of surgical complications. Equally true, they are robbing units because of similar reasons, as it is in these hospitals that the sick are deprived of their possessions and livelihood to pay for very bad level of health care. And of course, the term *privation center* is self-explanatory.[10]

b. Management

This word *management* is a concept that is at variance with everything that it stands for, especially when you are in a health facility in Nigeria. Those who use the conventional definition will be disappointed because of its application in Nigeria, which is so strangely different. Here, the word *management* means "manage it," "improvise," "make do" as it stands for all kinds of distorted meanings.

The word *management* can mean to manage with less than what is ideal or, altogether, the absence of what is reasonably needed for treatment, but not available because of professional misuse or abuse. For instance, nurses are known to give intramuscular injections (IM) and start intravenous (IV) treatment without the benefit of cleaning the sites, first with an alcohol swab (bacteriocidal or bacteriostatic) preparations, sometimes not even water is used to prepare an injection site! These items are not available either because they have been stolen, i.e., taken to private clinics for use at the patients' expense.

However, in other circumstances, *management* may also mean someone—a nurse or a hospital attendant in place of a doctor—coming to the aid of a suffering patient by giving them an illicit injection or prescription, provided they have been or expect to paid by the patient's relative.

c. Doctor

The title *doctor* is so loosely used, as it may refer to any of the following definitions: a well-trained medical doctor or a physician (the conventional definition); a nurse, midwife, or any other paramedical professional in possession of a stethoscope (not only nonconventional, but also unacceptable definitions); in some rural areas, anyone who works in a hospital, a clinic, a dispensary, or a drugstore, or even anyone with a syringe qualifies as a doctor. As Uchenna Nwokolo, (1960) indicates,

. . . Unqualified laymen with stethoscopes, lancets, and syringes were far worse than witch-doctors. Even nurses, technical assistants, chemists and radiographers would join in the preference of being medically qualified. Infection, drug resistance, toxic effects, anaphylaxis and death were all too frequently the result . . . 11

Of course, there is another group of doctors that is different from the preceding group that is referred to as the "acada," "book," or "paper" doctor. This is the group whose knowledge has nothing to do with medicine or pharmacology, but in philosophy of all other fields of study, i.e., history, geology, mathematics, etc., and "lecture" in Nigeria's institutions of higher learning.

c. Business

The word *business* could and does refer to a legitimate business enterprise arrangement, such as having a government license to sell drugs at a drugstore, for example, is a business enterprise.

The word *business* also refers to any shady business activity, like the selling or charging patients for medications, in government hospitals, where this is meant to be free is referred to as "business." It could also means diverting medications from the hospital's pharmacy to private drugstores, which technically is thievery or bluntly put is stealing, as it is the conversion of government property or equipments to private use. In other societies, these fraudulent and criminal activities are dealt with severely; but in Nigeria, thieves of this caliber have been given chieftaincy titles and sometimes the highest national award! They wield a lot of power and are the biggest guests at social gatherings and other public receptions.

e. Health

What this concept conjures up to the ordinary Nigerian is more than the mere ability to be free from pain and discomfort, both physically and mentally. Rather, it is the ability to carry on with the ordinary activities of daily living, a definition that is in consonance with the various definitions discussed in others chapters.

However, health is a myth in present-day Nigeria. The Obasanjo government or factor was supposed to change this situation for the better, but it has come and danced and is now gone with no palpable change whatsoever! "Soja muscles" and all! In case, just in case you are nursing a grudge about my obtuse approach here, I ask you to just take a look at the NEPA and Electricity or Water Board and the water services situations in your area, areas that bobcat promised "changes" and soon too! Even today, they still demand payments for services that they have not rendered or intend to render, and this has been going on for over the past decade, since General Olusegun Obasanjo came to the presidency in 1999. You be the judge yourself!

f. Nurse

A nurse may be any individual that cares for the sick and the ill in the hospital, dispensary, or other health settings. Nursing mothers are also nurses, but on a different plane and level. The role of the nurse is, more frequently than not, confused with that of the physician, but especially by the illiterate populace in rural areas. This does not preclude the fact that this same mentality obtains even in cities where literacy is a lot better. More often than not, nurses have been and, still, are called "doctors" as ordinary people do not know, neither do some of them care to know, the difference between nurses and trained physicians.

g. Drugstore or Chemist

These are terms that are frequently used interchangeably in places where drugs and other approved medicaments are sanctioned to be sold, even in an open area in a marketplace.

In societies where the rule of law exists, drugstores are manned and run by pharmacists and trained pharmacy technicians or attendants, even in rural areas. In Nigeria, however, this is not so as most drugstores and pharmacies are run by untrained personnel, the majority of which has never attended any formal training in the pharmaceutical discipline or, for that matter, any of the health professional training. Occasionally, you will find some who have never attended school of any kind and yet sell powerful medications that are complex and capable of altering human constitution, or even kill, under the supervision of people trained in that discipline. This is the area that most of the untrained hawkers peddle drugs and medications to the unwary public for consumption and constantly suffer the horrible consequences.***

h. Midwife

This is a profession, in the strict interpretation of the word, for older women who help other women during delivery. Because they are older and more experienced, yet without the benefit of any formal training, these midwives (or *unguwar zoma* in Hausa) help women in labor to deliver their babies safely.

Most female nurses in Nigeria are also trained nurse-midwives with the so-called dual qualification or preparation in nursing and midwifery. It is interesting to note that before the advent of modern medical care and the avalanche of medical technology, the good old-fashioned midwife was not trained but gave good care to both the mother and the baby. Of course, the lack of training was also attended by a high infant mortality rate.

i. Pharmacy

This is where all drugs and medication for the hospital use are stored and dispensed to all the treatment units of the hospital. The pharmacy is supposed to be run by a trained pharmacist. In some instances, however, some hospitals in Nigeria have a pharmacy or dispensary attendant who mans this department. Pharmacists are also found outside the hospital in commercial settings where they are supposed to supervise or control all transactions that deal with the purchase of drugs for commercial purposes.

j. Hawker

This is an individual who peddles drugs and medications that he or she has absolutely no knowledge as to their pharmaco-dynamics, as far as the human body is concerned. The little knowledge that he might have about these dangerous drugs he probably heard secondhand from someone with no clue, like himself. While these drugs are meant for the cure of certain medical conditions, these too he has no knowledge of their pathogenesis, yet he sells these to the public and openly with no consequences whatsoever!

In marketplaces and other public settings, hawkers or peddlers are, more often than not, outlets of fake or expired drugs, which is yet another wrung on the level and degree of menace that this group is to the Nigerian public. Their wares are advertised frequently and freely. The proverbial saying "Little knowledge is dangerous" is so true and serious, in this instance, that it is not even funny—not even in a country like Nigeria! And this is an understatement to say the very least!

k. Native Doctor

A native doctor is someone who thinks he is well versed in his particular area of expertise, as far as traditional medicine and care are concerned. The majority of people from these groups, who mostly are illiterate, as most of them cannot even read or write, but have, in many instances, saved lives. The areas that they prominently prove most useful include bone-setting (reduction of fractures) and emotional issues.

The craft of native doctoring is usually passed on from one generation to the next, i.e., from father to son, but the art can also be learned by some other member(s) in the clan, depending on arrangements in some special circumstances.

The main advantage of this art is that it sometimes cures those cases that conventional medicine has tried unsuccessfully and to no effect. On the other hand, this group's so-called practitioners fail to recognize instances and conditions that are outside the purview of their scope of practice. Their inability to help in healing the ailing only spurs them diabolical moves and insinuations, as they refuse to come to terms with their inabilities and/or failures. They rationalize their failures instead by blaming not others but members of the same family by turning members against one another, solely for gluttonous and wanton greed. This demonic behavior creates tension, strife, intense animosity, and downright violence at a time that the family needs help and support.

All this, after having bled that family dry of their precious little resources, as result of exotic demands, with very little result to show for it, family members themselves are going through a trying period in their devotion and care of the sick person, but have suddenly found themselves torn apart by such baseless accusations. In other words, they hold themselves on a high and unimpeachable pedestal, a level much higher than the society is willing to allot to them. To ensure that they are held blameless, these evil merchants, harbingers, and missionaries of pandemonium only profess to wish their clients, when the opposite is the case, not by any means professional but counterfeits, as it has shown that it has no moral or ethical campus whatsoever! This is the case because when such conditions which are inimical to their patient's recovery and well-being, they definitely earned the name "profession" for this shameful behavior, and this is so unfortunate.

2. THE NIGERIAN HEALTH SRVICES

A brief history of health care in Nigeria as already discussed has not discussed all there is to discuss about the subject, so further description and discussion is warranted here. Hospitals and other health care facilities were started through the tireless efforts of missionary groups in the eighteenth to nineteenth centuries, which climaxed during the colonial era of rule. The Roman Catholic missions dominated the missionary efforts in Nigeria with approximately 40 percent of the total number of 118 of mission hospitals by independence in 1960.

The number of mission hospitals of 118 surpassed the number of government-owned hospitals of only 101 by twenty-four percentage points for the same period. Catholic mission hospitals held sway or dominated in the south, while the Sudan Interior Mission and Sudan United Mission hospitals concentrated in the Middle Belt and sparsely in the northernmost areas of the country. The combined total number of hospitals and health facilities operated by both the SUM and the SIM in the north were twenty-five. These played an important role in shaping the health system network and the training of health care workers for the entire country. They played an immense role in the training and education of nurses and other paramedical personnel, some of whom were sponsored to study overseas in advanced training programs for certain areas of specialties. These efforts are responsible for both the acceptance and distribution of modem medical care in the country. This thrust played a key role for the dwindling with the ultimate ebbing, significantly, of the so-called native medicine in the country.

Comparison and Contrast of the Colonial and Missionary Medical Care Efforts

The colonial administration behavior, in a sharp contrast to that of the missionaries, started the construction of government hospitals much later and only after missionary efforts had been well in progress. It followed the example of such efforts by also giving free medical care, first, only to expatriates in government service, in government-owned hospitals in Lagos, Calabar, Abeokuta, and coastal areas in the mid-1870s. These government health care facilities later on expanded to other areas of the country, as they filtered down further to the native government service officials and their families.

During the first and second world wars, these efforts were curtailed as medical personnel were deployed to other African or European countries. Government schools for the training of medical personnel in Nigeria, however, were expanded after these wars, but Nigerian medical graduates could not practice in any of the government hospitals even if they were trained in Europe, except of course only when they treated native Nigerians. This type of discrimination and other social injustices led to agitations and protests by the pioneering nationalist movements of these early days.

Out of such movements emerged the version of modern health care facilities and institutions to train health care workers in the country. The

Richards's administration in 1946 established the Ministry of Health to coordinate health services throughout the country. That particular colonial administration instituted a ten-year health development program plan for the nation, the outcome of which produced the University of Ibadan, which found University College Hospital that included a faculty of medicine by 1934.

Seven schools of nursing and/or midwifery and two schools of pharmacy, one in Lagos and the other in Zaria, were also established. By independence in 1960, there were over sixty government nursing and midwifery schools in the country. The health development program budgeted funds for hospitals, clinics, and health centers, most of which concentrated in metropolitan areas of the country, while little funding was provided for rural areas where the majority of the population lived. Similarly, there was a sharp imbalance between the north and the south in terms of the distribution of the health facilities, as there were fewer of these in the for northern population and more, a lot more, for the southern populace. The imbalance affected the rural areas where over 80 percent of the population resided and still does even today.

However, by 1980, there were even more government-owned hospitals and health facilities in the country, this was brought about as a result of a steady economic growth of the 1970s that came with the oil boom, which were not only seen in the health industry and care facilities but also in education. Secondary and tertiary levels of education witnessed immense growths also. All these changes led to sharp increases in the numbers of privately owned or for profit health establishments with parochial interests, trend that has continued ever since. The steady exodus of physicians from government services in droves and in favor of personal practice is a clear testament to this trend.

The health system in Nigeria was fashioned after the socialized health system of Britain. Now, however, the two systems do not look anywhere close to resembling each other, as they so radically look different, that it is difficult to believe that this was modeled after the former.[10] The British health system, while a socialized one, does provide health care and other health services to all citizens, with virtually no payment. On the other hand, it is dogged by a very high price tag to the British government, which is paid for by exacting heavy taxes to the working class. In all fairness, it means that it ranks very high in the government's budget; the opposite of this, of course, is true in Nigeria. Say what you will, the British health system works very well in meeting the basic health needs of the British citizens, at least that much can be said about it.

The Nigerian health systems, on the other hand, bear merely a faint semblance, even if at that, of a socialized health system. And the zinger is, it does not even work! Areas of any similarity are the voluntary and private endeavors present in both systems. Why is it that the British health system works, while that of Nigeria doesn't, when one is the replica of the other?

British health system is the archetype controlled by health professionals, especially physicians. The other health professionals—namely, nurses, pharmacists, and others (paraprofessional:
technical nurses, pharmacy attendants, and so on)—are, to some degree, participants in the policy-decisions making. They are entrusted with daily operations of the health facilities as "supporters" of the professionals because of their integrity and adherence, not only to the moral code but also to professional ethics and standards.

This group of professionals is represented at the very highest echelon of decision-making body of every government that comes to power. The minister of health is a cabinet member of the ruling party, the military regime in power with the president or the head of state as the chairman of that body.

There seems to be some similarity of this kind of a setup in Nigeria, as the Federal Minister of Health is also a cabinet member of any government or administration in Nigeria. This same Federal Minister of Health is chair of the Ministry of Health of the entire federation which supervises the activities of all the states, Ministry of Health and all their commissioners, including the Federal Capital Territory of Abuja with all states' ministries of health permanent secretaries. However, this is where the resemblance with Great Britain ends. Why? Why, because the British system works while that of Nigeria does not!

All the states' medical directors in Nigeria (all physicians and/or any other appointees deemed necessary by the various states) participate in policy matters of the federal Ministry of Health as do permanent secretaries, heads of the national medical, nursing and pharmacist associations or their deputies, who are also members of this body.

While the minister of health is usually a medical doctor, yet the position is a political-appointed position, as it is at times filled by a selection from a list of experts within the health field, yet this is not always the case. This body, the federal Ministry of Health is responsible for advising the party in power over technical on health matters and is also charged with developing, as well as recommending health policies and programs for the nation. It also oversees the planning, coordination, execution, and funding operations of all government health facilities in the nation as it does this by the following: [11]

1. Planning and finding ways that would serve as an effective system of delivery of health care services for the entire population,
2. Integrating preventive and curative health measures,
3. Implementing and promoting effective health services, and
4. Rehabilitating and preparing individuals for services to the general public.[12]

The states' ministries of health, their commissioner at the state levels are replicas of the Ministry of Health at the federal level. The chief officer, the commissioner, supervises this section of the state government by ensuring that all health programs' operations in the state are within the framework that has been prescribed by the national health policy.
Health management boards are subordinate arms of the state ministries of health, charged with overseeing all the health care facilities in the state. A health management board is an agency that is specifically meant to circumvent most of the bureaucratic processes that states' ministries of health are known for. This process aims and assists in the decentralization in order to reduce the bureaucracy that tends to become bureau-crazy, but this, however, has turned out to be an exact opposite and antithetical to the original intended purpose. Even under the HMBs, with the tendency to operate under bogus machinery of red tape, the amount of red tape in the system is just over the top.

The health management board's other functions include employment and the staffing of health facilities, promotion and staff discipline, ascertaining and maintaining stipulated health care standards. It is also responsible for staffing all the health facilities; professionals and their conduct, accountability, education, and training; staff in service; procurement and distribution of operating materials like drugs, chemicals, medical equipment, etc. It also carries out periodic reviews of revenues and assesses venues of services that hospitals provide.[14]

The Zonal Management Committees arm the health management boards that operate at the district level and serve as avenues of decentralization to promote efficiency. These zonal committees monitor health activities closer to the loci of such activities in communities. The zonal office oversees the running of health facilities under the auspices of the health management board in the zonal area.

Zonal Committee membership consists of a chairman, a depute chairman, a secretary, and a member from each of the "wards" of the zone, appointed by the governor, the commissioner of health. Rural Health Committees operate under the jurisdiction of the zonal office. This is a quasi-ministry with different departments similar the arrangement of ministries at the state government level.

Finally, the Local or Rural Health Committee is a part of the local government that runs health centers, clinics, maternal/child clinic centers, dispensaries, and special clinics of tuberculosis, leprosy, etc., of local government.

Voluntary Organizations

Voluntary organizations such as the United Nations and especially the mission societies' organizations organize and run health program in hospitals, health centers, dispensaries, and other clinic systems. These voluntary organizations usually charge fees for services, but most of these organizations are subsidized through government grants, both state and federal, who maintain some control to ensure quality of care. Parochial endeavors, in which individuals own and run hospitals, clinics, both or some combination of both, to make a profit also exist. Health services in these settings are rendered for free by a practitioner or a group of proprietors.

Finally, we have reviewed the organization of the health system in rather broad generalities. For the sake of brevity, only the hospitals, health centers, and dispensary organizations will be further discussed in this section.

Of all the health care facilities in Nigeria, the hospital is one of the most recognized. This is as a result of its multidimensional and multifaceted nature. The hospital has the highest concentration of health professionals than in any of all the other health institutions in the country as this is also true in most societies in the world.

Above all, major surgeries are performed in the general hospital on top of the other health services available in it. Besides variety, the availability of expert services in the general hospital makes it ideal for the care of the critically ill during any given period of the day. There are more other reasons, which are not all that very convenient in these other facilities, but rather, it is the hub health care activities in the health system.

General Operations and Administration

The general hospital, whether governmental, voluntary, or proprietary, is usually administered by a medical director or superintendent, a physician. Under the medical director are all the medical doctors and other health professionals. Under the administrator are all the departmental heads, i.e., the departments of surgery, medicine, pediatrics, outpatient and clinical services, obstetrics and gynecology, radiology, laboratory, etc. There are rarely more departments or services than those listed above in a general hospital. Under the department heads are residents—one or two depending on the particular circumstances of the hospital—who have completed their internship or house-manship and finally those clinical students in their third, fourth, and fifth years of studies, if the hospital is a teaching hospital.

The Role of the Nurse in This Arrangement

Medical care depends heavily on nursing staff and the nursing care that they perform. The matron or director of nurses runs the show as the nursing department is biggest with the largest number of employees than any other department in the whole of health system. This person is charged with staffing all nursing units, provision of proper nursing care to all inpatients, outpatients, and clinics that the hospital operates.

Basically, the director of nurses has an assistant, who is also a nurse under whom the supervision of all nursing and ancillary staff, such as the kitchen and others, falls. Decisions pertaining to hiring, staffing, promotion, training, and discipline of nurses are made by nursing. Under these, two or more individuals are staff nurses of different designations—technical nurses, ward attendants, or orderlies, all in that order. They help with the simple and menial unit work of nursing care.

Health centers usually are administered, usually by nurses, with the most seniority (except in exceptional situations) as officers in charge and who are responsible for staffing, discipline, decision-making, and seeing to the daily smooth running of the various clinics at the centers. The health center usually has midwives and other health workers who are not nurses. For example, dispensary attendants, community health workers, laboratory attendants are not nurses or midwives and are referred to as such for the lack of a better term.

The dispensary setting, on the other hand, is usually headed by a dispensary attendant who, by nature of his/her training, has a good alchemical, some level of diagnostic knowledge and some administrative abilities. The dispensary attendant usually has an assistant and one or two orderlies trained to do specific tasks such as the cleaning of wounds, dressing, etc. The dispensary is equipped with a laboratory with an attendant for some limited diagnostic abilities.

In summary then, the health system consists of all the health institutions and facilities, the programs and regulators, the health professionals and the entirety of the health professional groups. Para as well as nonprofessionals, the educators and those training the health professionals are all part of the health system.

B. THE BRITISH HEALTH SYSTEM

The British health system or the British National Health Service was established in 1948 and reorganized in 1974[15, 16] under the jurisdiction of the Department of Health and Social Security. It provides free and comprehensive health services to all British citizens and is funded by the British government, which controls certain aspects of health services. The Secretary of State for Social Services, a cabinet member in the British government, heads the department and reports to the prime minister.

Directly under the Secretary of State for the Department of Health and Social Services is the Central Health Services Council. This body is comprised of health professionals (medicine, nursing, pharmacy, dental, health administration, and community health, about thirty-one members in all) that advise and report annually to the secretary of state on all significant issues that concern national health services. There are other special advisory committees which report and advice him or her on matters like child mental health and special areas' matters. The secretary of state, from time to time, appoints a special ad hoc committee on special subjects. Department of Health exercises control over the funding of health facilities on a continuous basis, but the construction of facilities and the purchase of equipment are usually done only once. This means that the initial building of a facility and its equipment are paid for by the department of health; however, maintenance, repair, and modification issues after construction become the purview and responsibility of facility and its administration thereafter.

In comparing the two systems, it is very clear that there is a great deal of resemblance between the Nigerian and the British systems—the Nigerian health system is, indubitably, a copy of the British system. The overall setup is similar, so is the hierarchical order of organization, the bureaucratic arrangement and processes for both systems—these leave no room for denying the fact that one of the two systems is the archetype (the British's system) and the other, a copy (the Nigeria's system).

Nigerian Health System: Efficient as Designed Or A Debacle in Shambles and Tatters?

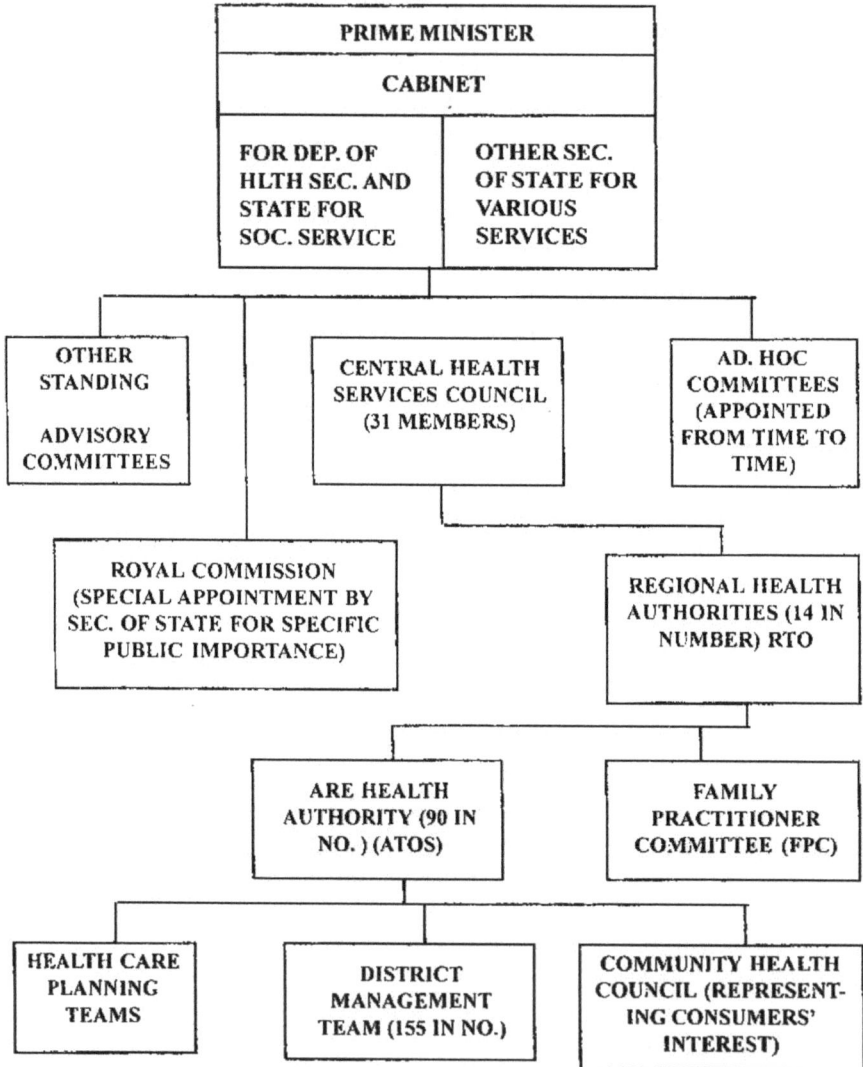

| PRIME MINISTER |
| CABINET |

| FOR DEP. OF HLTH SEC. AND STATE FOR SOC. SERVICE | OTHER SEC. OF STATE FOR VARIOUS SERVICES |

| OTHER STANDING ADVISORY COMMITTEES | CENTRAL HEALTH SERVICES COUNCIL (31 MEMBERS) | AD. HOC COMMITTEES (APPOINTED FROM TIME TO TIME) |

| ROYAL COMMISSION (SPECIAL APPOINTMENT BY SEC. OF STATE FOR SPECIFIC PUBLIC IMPORTANCE) | REGIONAL HEALTH AUTHORITIES (14 IN NUMBER) RTO |

| ARE HEALTH AUTHORITY (90 IN NO.) (ATOS) | FAMILY PRACTITIONER COMMITTEE (FPC) |

| HEALTH CARE PLANNING TEAMS | DISTRICT MANAGEMENT TEAM (155 IN NO.) | COMMUNITY HEALTH COUNCIL (REPRESENT-ING CONSUMERS' INTEREST) |

Figure: A simple diagram of the hierarchical representation of the British health system

C. THE U.S. HEALTH SYSTEM

The United States health system is a four-tier system of operation that comprises of federal, state, local, and municipal levels. In each tier, the hospital is the biggest organization and/or arrangement, a fact that seems to be an international practice.

There is some level of international connection or cooperation, if you will, with participation by the world community of nations in controlling pandemics and the commercial aspect of the health industry.

The U.S. Department of Health Education and Welfare (D1-IEW), created in 1953, five years after the institution of the British health system, is responsible for the health of the population and health services in the United States. Wilner, Walkley, and Goerke (1973) list six different functions of the U.S. Department of Health to the general population and another six for special groups of the population. The six functions for all citizens are the following:

1. Protection against hazards that affect the entire population that cannot be imaged by the state.
2. Collection of vital statistics and related data.
3. Promotion and the advancement of biological, medical, and environmental sciences.
4. Promotion improvement and increasing the number of health facilities and personnel to certain groups.
5. Support of state and local governments in maintaining public health services.
6. Disaster relief and civil defence.[23]

Other functions, but for a special population groups include the following:

1. Protection of certain categories of workers against certain hazardous occupations and adverse conditions of work.
2. Provision of special services for children, the aged, mentally ill, mentally retarded, economically deprived, the blind, and the handicapped.
3. Funding medical care of local and state governments for certain categories.

4. Funding special services for farm families.
5. Provision of medical care and hospitalization for veterans, merchant seamen, the native American Indians, native Alaskans, federal prisons, narcotic addicts, leprosy patients, uniform services and their dependents, injured civil service employees on duty.
6. Provision of medical and hospital insurance for civil service employees of the federal government.[24]

. . . The U. S. government participates in the international health endeavors by collecting, experimenting and shares the gained scientific knowledge and making it available to developing nations with poor health and sanitation systems, poor health programs and malnutrition.[25]

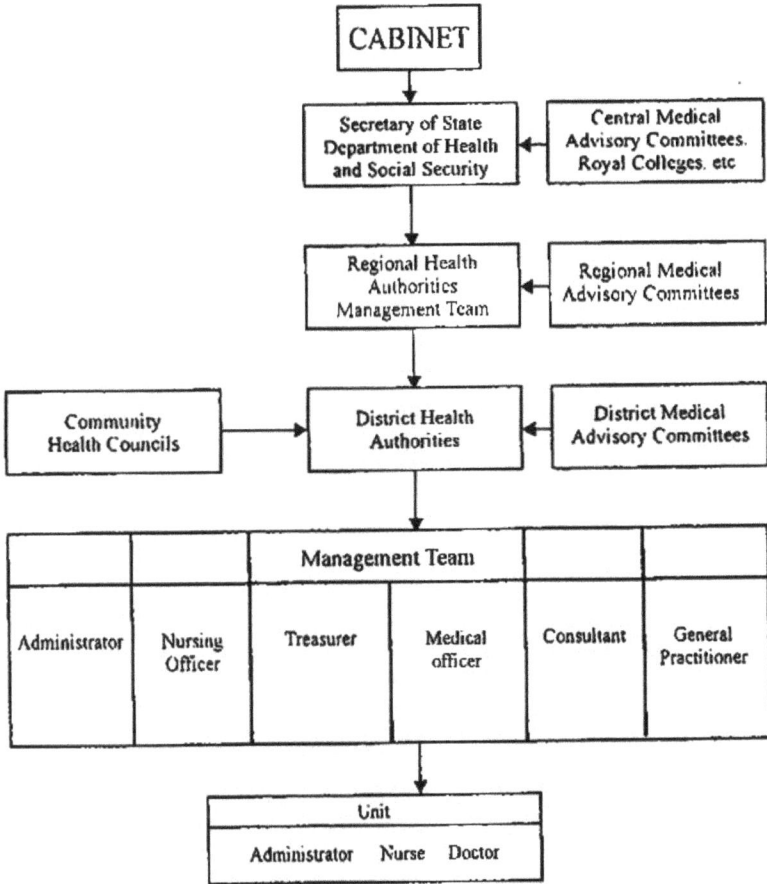

From Marshal W. Raphael: *The U.S. Health System: Origins and Functions*, 1984 edition., 207.

Adopted by some alteration and other modification, i.e., the addition of other levels. Last layer presented in model-supervision level (C/nurse, coordinator, etc.), RN/staff nurse level, practical nurse level, assistant/orderly level.

The Health System in Nigeria

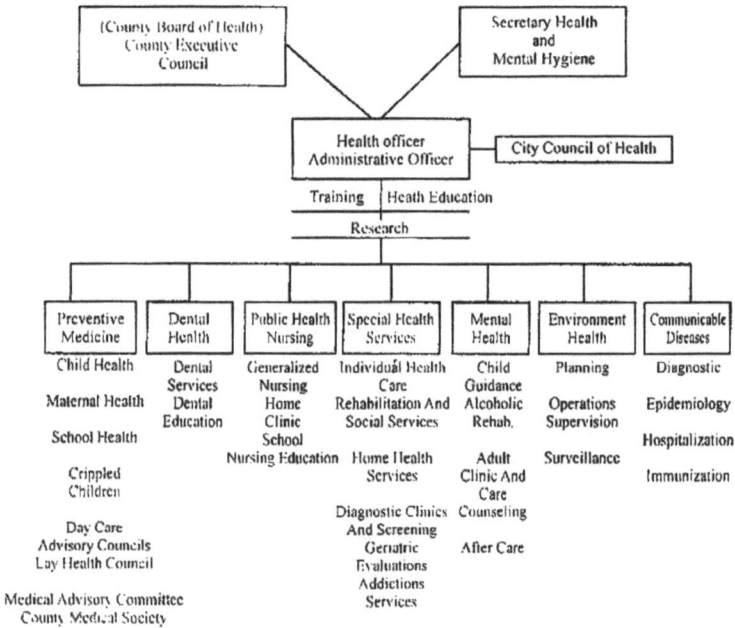

From M. W. Raffel (1980) p. 480 - for modification prior to adaption

Nigerian Health System: Efficient as Designed Or A Debacle in Shambles and Tatters?

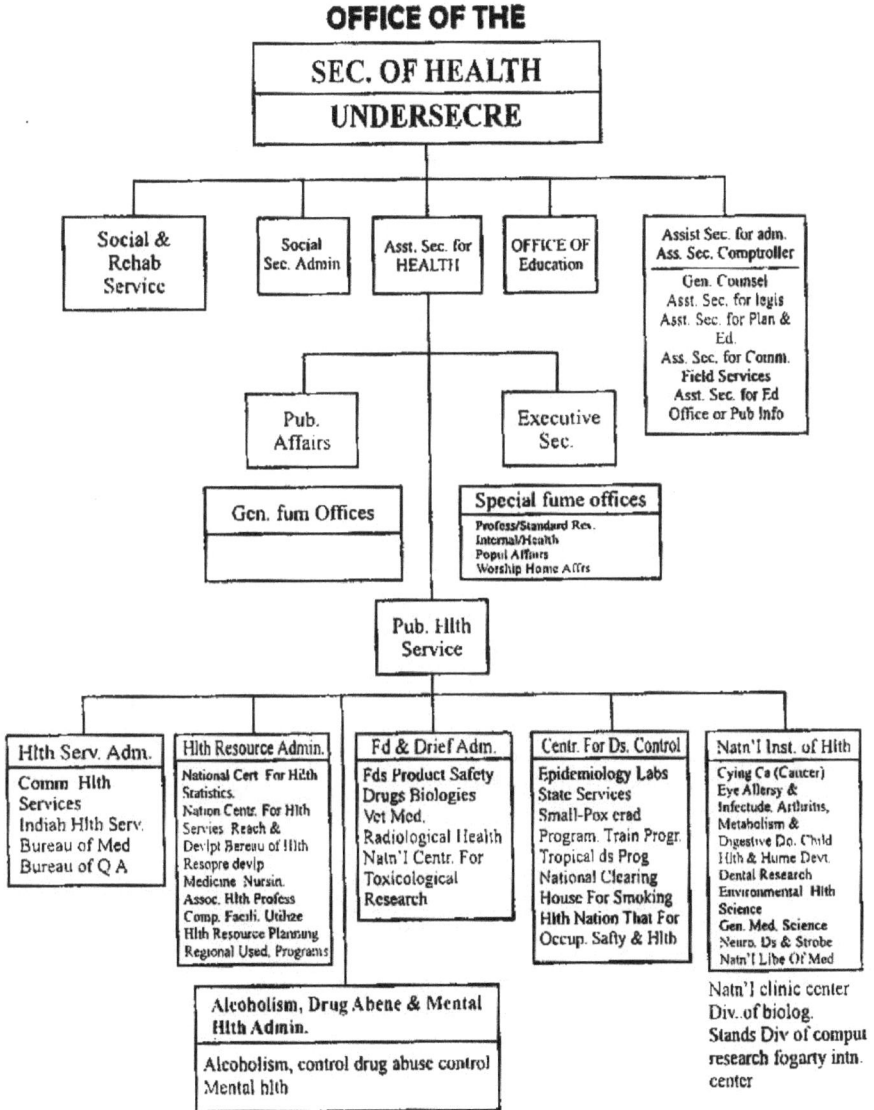

OFFICE OF THE

SEC. OF HEALTH
UNDERSECRE

Social & Rehab Service	Social Sec. Admin	Asst. Sec. for HEALTH	OFFICE OF Education	Assist Sec. for adm. Ass. Sec. Comptroller

Assist Sec. for adm. Ass. Sec. Comptroller
Gen. Counsel
Asst. Sec. for legis
Asst. Sec. for Plan & Ed.
Ass. Sec. for Comm.
Field Services
Asst. Sec. for Ed
Office or Pub Info

Pub. Affairs

Executive Sec.

Gen. fum Offices

Special fume offices
Profess/Standard Res.
Internal/Health
Popul Affairs
Worship Home Affrs

Pub. Hlth Service

Hlth Serv. Adm.	Hlth Resource Admin.	Fd & Drief Adm.	Centr. For Ds. Control	Natn'l Inst. of Hlth
Comm Hlth Services Indiah Hlth Serv. Bureau of Med Bureau of Q A	National Cert For Hlth Statistics. Nation Centr. For Hlth Servies Reach & Devlpt Bereau of Hlth Resopre devlp Medicine Nursin. Assoc. Hlth Profess Comp. Faeili. Utilize Hlth Resource Planning Regional Used. Programs	Fds Product Safety Drugs Biologies Vet Med. Radiological Health Natn'l Centr. For Toxicological Research	Epidemiology Labs State Services Small-Pox erad Program. Train Progr. Tropical ds Prog National Clearing House For Smoking Hlth Nation That For Occup. Safty & Hlth	Cying Ca (Cancer) Eye Allersy & Infectude. Arthritis, Metabolism & Digestive Do. Child Hlth & Hume Devt. Dental Research Environmental Hlth Science Gen. Med. Science Neuro. Ds & Strobe Natn'l Libe Of Med

Alcoholism, Drug Abene & Mental Hlth Admin.

Alcoholism, control drug abuse control
Mental hlth

Natn'l clinic center
Div. of biolog.
Stands Div of comput
research fogarty intn.
center

Figure: Diagram of the schematic representation of the U.S. Federal Department of Health Welfare (adopted from J. J. Hanlon, 1974)

THE HEALTH SYSTEM IN NIGERIA

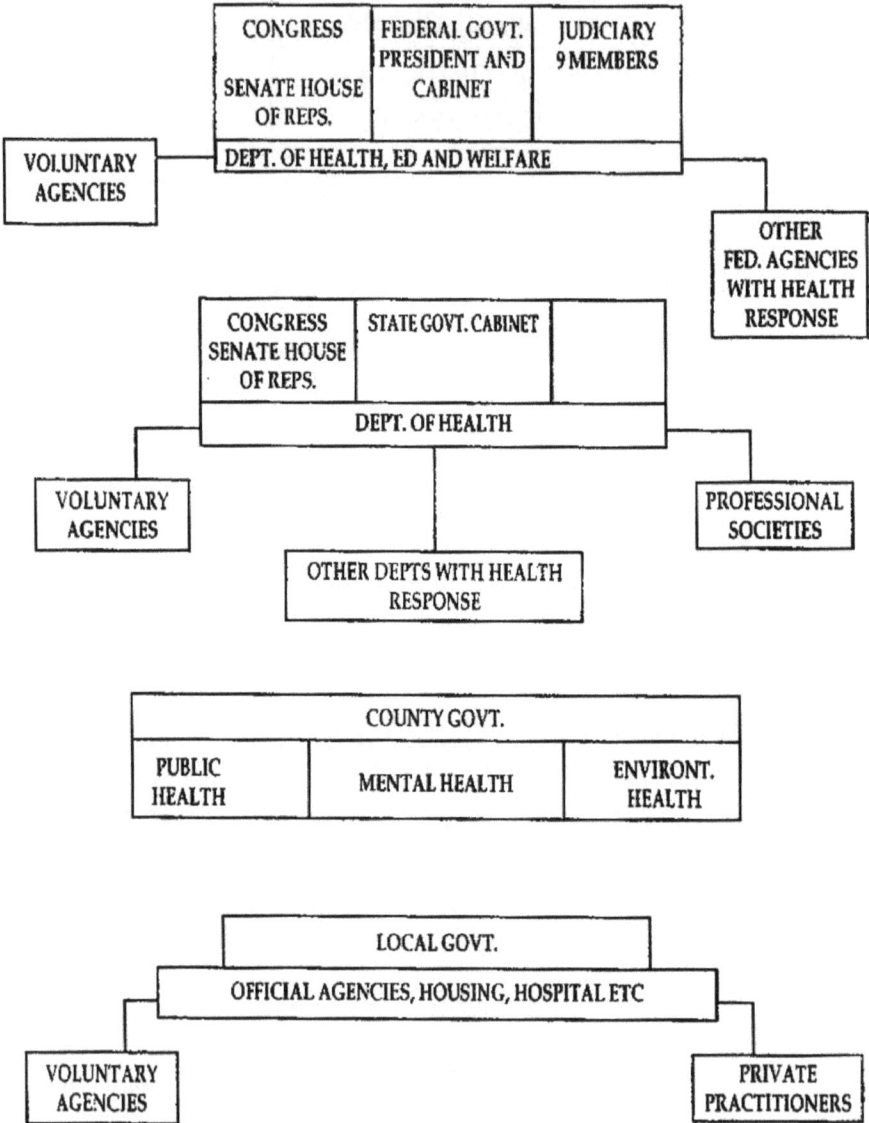

CONGRESS	FEDERAL GOVT.	JUDICIARY
	PRESIDENT AND	9 MEMBERS
SENATE HOUSE OF REPS.	CABINET	

VOLUNTARY AGENCIES	DEPT. OF HEALTH, ED AND WELFARE

OTHER FED. AGENCIES WITH HEALTH RESPONSE

CONGRESS SENATE HOUSE OF REPS.	STATE GOVT. CABINET	
DEPT. OF HEALTH		

VOLUNTARY AGENCIES		PROFESSIONAL SOCIETIES

OTHER DEPTS WITH HEALTH RESPONSE

COUNTY GOVT.		
PUBLIC HEALTH	MENTAL HEALTH	ENVIRONT. HEALTH

LOCAL GOVT.
OFFICIAL AGENCIES, HOUSING, HOSPITAL ETC

VOLUNTARY AGENCIES		PRIVATE PRACTITIONERS

A simple graphic representation of the U.S. health system

Nigerian Health System: Efficient as Designed Or A Debacle in Shambles and Tatters?

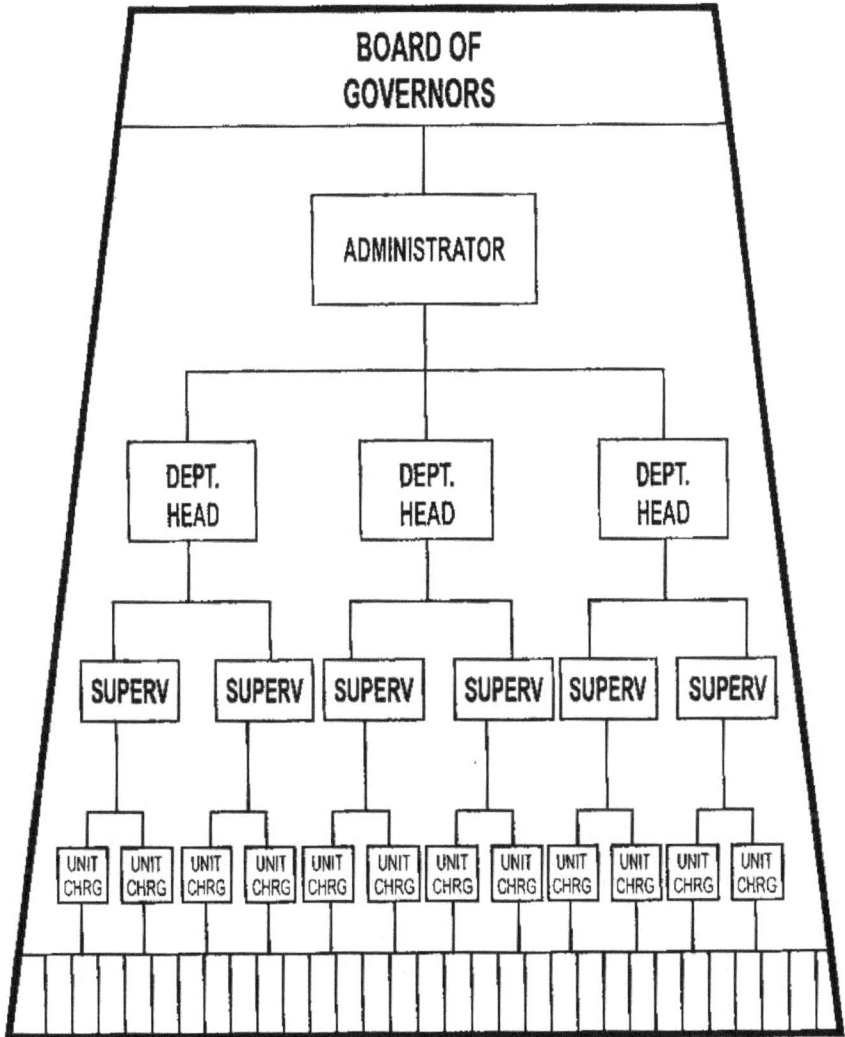

Figure: Organizational chart: Levels of management in scalar
form as representing the classical theory

Major functions of public department of health and its activities are carried out by DHEW, although there are various health organizations and some government departments whose roles overlap and some of the functions unnecessarily duplicated. There are six agencies that execute the DHEW programs, three of which are components of the public health services, i.e., Food and Drug Administration (FDA), Health Services and Mental Health Administration (HSMHA), and the National Institute of Health (NIH). The other three are the Social Security Administration (SSA), Social Rehabilitation Service (SRS), and the Office of Education (OE), which are indirectly health-related programs. For example, the OE, together with Public Health Service, deals with the training and education for the health manpower while the SSA administers the medical care programs.

The United States is divided into ten regional areas with DHEW offices in each of the ten regions charged with coordination and programs consultation within that region. Refer to the organization charts on page.

The Public Health Service (PHS) is the main organization with the delegated responsibilities to protect, improve the general health of citizens, and cater for the health needs of everyone. Therefore, it supports through its agencies, health programs, state and local levels, scientific research efforts and the development of programs for all personnel.

The Food and Drug Administration is responsible for the safety and the effectiveness of all devices used in health care, food, drugs, and cosmetics. The Health Services and Mental Health Administration (HSMHA) is responsible for a wide range of activities, seventeen major components—ranging from prevention to the rehabilitation programs of alcoholics, drug users, etc. At the head of the Department of Health Education and Welfare (DHEW) is the secretary who is a member of cabinet of the executive branch of government of the day. Under this department is the office of the surgeon general, who is the assistant secretary of the DHEW. The next on a top-down level of ranking are the National Institutes of Health, Food and Drug Administration, Health Services and Mental Health Administration, and all the subdivisions or sections that are under their control. Next are the Regional Food and Drug directors and the Regional Health directors.[26]

Other federal agencies with significant health responsibilities include the Department of Justice; the Department of State; the Environmental Protection Agency (EPA); the Department of the Army, Navy, and Air Force; the Department of Labor; and the Veterans Administration.

3. THE NIGERIAN HEALTH CARE SERVICES

Health care is a part of the health system, and it is delivered in a number of ways and in different settings in Nigeria just as it is the case in other parts of the world. The hospital is by far the biggest of all the health facilities in Nigeria, a fact that also corresponds to findings in other nations.[28] The health center in Nigeria is next in terms of size, then the dispensary, the clinic, and all others. All these make up the health care facilities within the health care system.

Subsequent discussion will attempt to analyze each of these settings. Health care in proprietary settings, such as in mission or private hospitals or other care settings, is given on a fee-for-service basis. Voluntary organizations such as WHO, UNESCO, Red Cross International provide free services as it once was with all indigenous Nigerian governmental agencies, i.e., federal, state, and local government health care facilities. This is no longer the case except for immunizations for certain diseases, but even then, money changes hands between the provider of care and the recipient as bribery is a form of payment.

Before delving into the analysis of these facilities, there is also the need to mention efforts in Nigeria that are directed at health for all, a national goal by AD 2000, involving all health agencies at federal, state, local, and voluntary agency levels. This noble effort, albeit a universal one for that matter, has proven illusory and at least in Nigeria, anyway, that was adopted by the United Nations some two or more decades ago. As a result of such an effort, Nigeria adopted the basic health service scheme (BSS) or primary health care (PHC) in 1979 and set up some objectives to serve as the vehicle and to guide in the achievement of that goal. However, the year 2000 has come and gone, as we are now in 2009, and yet no state is anywhere close to achieving that goal. Guess what, the ideals of such a lofty goal have not only fallen by the wayside, but have actually been supplanted by greed and love money.

There is plenty of wisdom in the old saying, "Prevention is better than cure," but it is only true if the reader is (a Nigerian with the willingness to suspend credulity by believing that the current crops of Nigerian leaders will do what is right for all Nigerians) ready to heed this warning. It was the plea of this wisdom that goaded the health ministries and the administrators of health facilities of the country in 1981—about 10,020 of them—to engage, directly or indirectly, in the quest for this process and setting such lofty a goal that was never to b e realized.[29]

A maternity hospital is a facility strictly for the delivery of babies and obstetrical situations, a rehabilitation hospital for the rehabilitation and restoration of function lost as a result of illness or injury. An eye hospital is for eye diseases treatment and surgical procedures. Others types of hospitals include veterinary hospital for the treatment and/or care of animals; and a teaching hospital is essentially the same as a general hospital, except for the fact that it is also used as a place of formal instruction for health professionals but especially of physicians and nurses.

General hospitals have departments other than the ones already mentioned, as they have to include a pharmacy where drugs and medications are stored for general use of the hospital. A typical general hospital bed capacity, on the average, ranges from 30 to 100 beds or more. Moreover, a general hospital also has to have a laboratory, a department that is very necessary for diagnostic purposes, and radiology or x-ray department, also very necessary and crucial aspect of diagnosis, except in Nigeria.

Outpatient services like the emergency or casualty section and clinics in most general hospitals are used for emergency, medical and surgical conditions. A variety of clinics that operate during the day in a general hospital include pediatric; surgical; eye, ear, and nose (ENT) clinics, most of which operate during the day.

There also ancillary services that are part of the hospital system, and these may include security, telephone, physical therapy or rehabilitation, library services, patients' records, ambulance, morgue (or mortuary), and kitchen or dietary. It should be noted here also that some general hospitals in Nigeria do not necessarily have all of these departments. However, essential services may be available in outpatient and inpatient services or any combination of the two. A typical hospital bed capacity on the average ranges from 30 to 100 beds while larger ones may range from 130 to 200 beds or more.

Other health care facilities that are models of what obtains in the British health system include the health center and the dispensary, both of which share some similarity with the general hospital. The health center is a multiple of clinics with no impatient unit. Normally in this setting, patients are screened, tested, treated, and then sent home or referred to a hospital or some other treatment settings for complicated medical situations or procedures that may require specialized skill care.

However, some of these facilities have limited bed capacity and patients may be admitted, as some clinics have, between four (4) to fourteen (14) beds for observation, for a few days of care, but if the area is too remote to a hospital. Usually nurses and paramedical personnel run these settings except for the dispensary, which is run by specially trained medical auxiliary such as the dispensary attendant who has some training in diagnosis, mixing and dispensing of drugs administration. In many instances, pharmacy attendants know how to run these drug rooms or stores. Registered nurses have played, and continue to play, a big role in the running of these health centers. These settings place emphasis on the preventive (primary) care that are simply treatment adjunct facilities.

Dispensaries and its network of operations came into being in the 1930, but later on were merged with the maternity home, which never really was a success. They were, and still are, poorly administered aside from the fact that they were better built with lighting and a lot different surroundings. Medications in them were stored in refrigerators following drugs manufacturer's directives, but NEPA is a new distraction to content, and this is as a result of atrociously erratic electrical services to all localities in the nation. However, these facilities serve as the only medical aid to and for a host of towns and villages with teaming populations in such localities.[31] They usually constitute the only health care facilities in these local areas.

4. HEALTH DELIVERY OF HEALTH CARE

Nurses and midwives run the inpatient units, the clinics, and carry out the actual patient care. Over the past decades or so, registered nurses have played the roles that only physicians play in most developed societies. They have also done so admirably well considering the level of their education and training. They give bedside care for inpatient units and act as consultants in ambulatory and, in some instances, in outpatient care settings as well.

Therefore, the accusation leveled against nurses by Ralph Schram, (1971) that even the nurses who are being misused "join in the pretence of being medically qualified" as not only unfair but altogether self-serving and wrong. This is because nurses in the Nigeria work under stringent conditions and the threat of losing their livelihood. That they do tolerate such level of abuse, under such conditions in the Nigerian health care system, is totally understandable. They are deliberately abused and misused by the doctors and other employers, without whimper of protest, not even from the board of nursing or the medical board or by the government, in the guise that there is "a physician shortage." Nurses have, in effect, been thrust into these roles without any option, and to suggest that these dedicated nurses are in this "cabal" of conspiracy is a false premise for the start! If they are judged as ill qualified, the solution is not to add to their responsibilities, they should instead be educated and trained to help them cope with these new added roles. But blame? No!

Midwives give gynecological, maternal, and infant care but are also used as regular nurses in certain areas as a result of profound "nurse shortage." These so-called shortages of physicians and nurses are nothing but a contrivance, as a lot of nurses graduate from nursing schools operated, run by state governments and all expenses paid, who then refuse to employ them for some unknown reasons, or ones best known to them. This applies also to physicians as well.

Community and psychiatric auxiliary nurses are as well similarly used. They are equally limited in their education preparation and training, but they are misused, as nurses and just as abused, without caring about the possible harm they can cause to human life. I have heard of auxiliaries referring to themselves as "doctors," and this stems from the weight of the responsibility that they are given. However, I must say it stems directly from the institutions from where they received their training. In a similar manner, the dispensary attendants' training does not include bedside care or a lot of other care procedures, but in certain places and some very unique circumstances, they are used to staff inpatient units as nurses.

Furthermore, nurses or midwives with the so-called double qualification, meaning that a staff nurse is trained as a staff nurse but, in addition, returned to train as a midwife and vice versa. After this, she is then dually qualified in both areas. I am not sure or aware whether or not male nurses with an orthopedic, psychiatric, nursing administration, anesthetic, or any other nursing subspecialty training to qualify for the term *double qualification*. However, this kind of orientation can be traced back to the British system and its legacy that was bequeathed to the Nigerian heath system.

This is not the case in the Canadian or American systems. Further training following any of the three methods to become a nurse does not change the basic designation of the staff nurse. For example, all nurses, including those with PhDs, are all referred to as registered nurse (RN), first and foremost before any other designation that might follow. Moreover, education in a graduate school following a baccalaureate degree (BSN), depending on the area of specialty, enables the nurse to become a nurse practitioner and so on. All are basically nurses, registered nurses (RN) and are so recognized despite further training level of or education. Even here, no one is referred to as a "doubly qualified" nurse. It is necessary to point out the profound so-called nurse and physician shortage that has plagued the Nigerian health scene for so long, which thus makes it possible for non-physicians to both practice medicine, with no repercussions, as though the behavior is sanctioned by the society.

5. METHODS FOR BECOMING A NURSE IN NIGERIA

Until recently, there were three different methods of becoming a registered nurse in the United States[32] which follows:

1. The hospital training model where a high school graduate or someone with equivalent qualification spends two to three years in training in the hospital.
2. The two-year college program usually in a community college setting.
3. The baccalaureate program in a university[33] where a high school graduate spends four years.

All the three different levels of preparation take the same qualifying examination for registration as a staff nurse in all the fifty states of

United States. These different levels of preparation will be developed and discussed further in the following chapter under the nursing profession.

Further down the ladder and at the very bottom of the health care professions are the attendants and orderlies. These categories or terms of describing these groups of workers are synonymous as they are essentially one and the same, but except that one designation of "attendant," refers to a female category, while the other, "orderly," refers to male attendants. Their work essentially encompasses helping nurses and, at times, physicians with simple nursing care, as well as environmental cleaning of inpatient units, the clinics and other hospital areas including the theater, laboratory, x-ray, morgue, and so on. In the United States, orderlies rarely engage in environmental hygiene as this duty belongs to housekeeping personnel, they are mainly used for lifting patients in and out of bed.

The type of care given by all the health professions at the direction of physicians, referred to as medical care model, is given by doctors, nurses, pharmacists, laboratory and x-ray technicians, nurses, attendants, and orderlies. This model of care is usually carried out in a hospital setting while that which is carried out in other settings differs significantly, this is because of the location and where care is given. In the hospital, a patient stays twenty-four hours a day for care until discharge. In an ambulatory setting, the patient comes for treatment at a specified hour or time and returns home after the treatment every day or as scheduled.

Health care in ambulatory settings is essentially secondary prevention, which means that a disease and the treatment for a disease state that does not require an around-the-clock supervision. Patients come to these settings as a result of a disease process already advancing into an illness process. Most of the time, effective treatment can be given, but oftentimes, it is extended delay before sending help is too late.

At any rate, care is initiated after a complaint to either a doctor or a nurse, or a dispensary attendant. This is followed by diagnosis, after laboratory tests and/or radiological examination, where and when these facilities are available. The next stage is the prescription phase, which begins the management or treatment phase or process with the initiation of the first dose of medication. Injections are given at the ambulatory facilities with instructions or directions for follow-up where and when that is necessary. In the hospital, prescriptions are filled within the confines of the facility in the pharmacy, if and when drugs are available. However, if this is not the case, patients or relatives are advised to purchase medications at a local drugstore, and usually, a specific drugstore is recommended for that very purpose. After the purchase and the medicine is brought to the health facility, the nurse then administers the drug to the patient or the patient suffers. In an outpatient situation, prescription is given and the purchased medication is taken home with the directions on how to self-administer the drug including injections.

As for community nurses, their work entails acting as sanitation and environmental officials and advisors to communities in addition to giving vaccination to forestall disease epidemics in the rural areas. Most of the time, rural dwellers do not worry about disease epidemics until it is too late, but community nurses are charged with the responsibility and of giving basic instructions on personal and communal levels about hygiene in designated areas to heighten awareness of disease epidemics. They may help deliver babies; treat simple diseases (wounds, infestation, scabies, etc.); and mobile antenatal care.

The psychiatric nurse on the other hand, like the community nurse, is not a nurse in the traditional sense and so limited in providing only inpatient care to psychiatric patients under the direct supervision of a staff nurse or physician in clinics. Incidentally, though, obstetrics and gynecology, psychiatry, orthopedic, pediatrics, and community nursing are all part of the nursing curriculum of nurse preparation in the United States. This is different from the training program for nurses in Nigeria and Britain concerning areas mentioned above.

Finally, health care in private and voluntary sectors is quite similar to what it obtains in the government health care facilities. However, a major difference that is quite significant and worth mentioning is the question of quality, efficiency of care given, the equipment and quality of the instruments with which that employee uses in giving care. In most higher or tertiary institutions of learning, there are special clinics for students. Treatment for the institution's staff and their defendants in these clinic settings is hardly any different from what it obtains in the society generally.

REVIEW OF LITERATURE

The general but brief history and evolvement of Nigeria from dark ages began with its early contacts with the Europeans. This history is portrayed as well as discussed to some extent by Joe DeGoshe (1989), Obafemi Awolowo (1968), Helen Metz, Ralph Schram (1971), Alan Burns, Yusuf Turaki (1993), Michael Omolewa (1970), and Toyin Falola et al. (1991). The historical development of health services in the country began with the early contacts with Europeans that dates as far back as five hundred years or more. This is well chronicled by Ralph Schram, who paints fairly clear and perhaps accurate beginnings of the nation and its early efforts in establishing medical services in the country.

Folorunso, Abudu (1983) discusses the planning priorities for health care policies and methods of effective delivery of it in his "Health and Development in Africa" by an International Interdisciplinary Symposium on African Countries' Health Services. He argues that health planning policies and prerequisites, which he terms *objectives*, need a "prompt re-evaluation and reordering of priorities" if the health of citizens is considered that important and to be realized. The health needs of the majority, he maintains, have taken a secondary or even lesser priority to other projects.

Collins Airhihenbuwa and Ira Harrison (1993) defend the method of traditional practice in Africa, pointing to its pivotal role in the medical care and practice. The objective, besides the relief of suffering, they argue, should also strike a balance between the individual and his environment. Their argument concludes by attributing the negative attitude of the West and science toward traditional medicine as due to ignorance and misunderstanding on the part Europeans, which causes suspicion and misrepresentation. They cite examples of traditional medical practices in several African countries, including some major cities in Nigeria, where traditional practice has exerted positive effects on the health of citizens. I think this claim is a myth, or the proponents of the theory have very active imaginations, as there is no evidence or basis for this claim! To argue that the essential differences between the two methods of medical care are scientific and based on Western recognition, which was caused by slavery and colonial subjugation of Africans.

Good grief! So the West is now to blame for the harsh treatment of Africans by Africans themselves, which has resulted in their suppression and the inhibition of African intellectual development? [47] Yet slavery was outlawed and stopped nearly two hundred years ago!

Here I take exception to this pejorative attack on reasonable intelligence as a gross display of naiveté. I would submit that Africans have been treated far more harshly than any slave master ever even imagined to treat black slaves. We cannot ignore the fact that it was the Africans themselves that sold fellow Africans to the slave masters who bought these Africans, considered then as humans rejects by their own brothers. They were whisked and horded away from their natural domiciles and taken to Europe, other foreign destinations and hostile environments. Furthermore, only Africans can be blamed for not developing their own "medical practice" or the so-called native medicine by failing to make it creditable. It is not anyone's fault that this so-called native medicine is so shrouded in secrecy, neither is anyone to be blamed other than Africans themselves who have failed to properly organize. Besides, it is neither opened for public scrutiny like its Western counterpart, nor does it lend itself to be used for the benefit of all Africans as scientific medicine benefits all people and not just Europeans!

Maurice King (editor, 1966) points out in chapter 2 of his *Medical Care in Developing Countries* the discrepancies in educational and economic resources; the differences in organization, planning, and the delivery of health care to poor areas, which he claims are poorly organized and utilized in certain areas. He then gives some practical suggestions a sort of road map that should be used in the process of organization, planning, and the development of health care to a targeted population.[48] John Bryant (1969), in chapter 8 of *Health and the Developing World*, discusses the dilemma of quality, quantity, cost of medical education, and medicine in developing countries. He briefly describes the demographics, their medical applications and implications in Nigeria spanning the period of three decades, from 1950 to 1980.[49, 50, 52] Patience Barefoot and Jean Cunningham (1977) give a brief description of terminologies commonly used by health professionals in the British system.[53] Margot Jeffery gives a similar description, just as do Barefoot and Cunningham, on the British health system. He then critiques its achievements and failures by nature of its huge escalating cost.[54]

In *The U.S. Health System: Origins and Functions*, Marshal Raffael (1980) details the different training programs that nurses and the paramedical professions undergo in order to be able to fit in and take on the responsibility of caring for the sick. In chapter 4, she points out how the nursing profession started as a "helping profession" with training of nurses in the hospital for three years, which she refers to as the diploma program. The baccalaureate four year program in the university setting began about the time of the first World War, while the associate degree program staled in the early 1950s for two and a half years in community colleges. All these programs led to the licensure for the registered nurse post completion and passing of the licensing examination in any of the fifty states in the United States.[55, 56, 57] In chapter 10, Raffael analyzes the U.S. health system from the state to the local level, discussing the functions of these various agencies.[58]

Steven Jonas (1981) describes the three different programs for becoming a nurse in the United States in his book *Health Care Delivery in the United States*.[59] In chapter 11 of *Health Principles and Practices*, Anderson and Longton (1961) also gives an in-depth account and analysis of the U.S. health system at every level from the local up to the federal level. Chapter 12 lists voluntary agencies with international connections and their trends in health care responsibilities at giving details of organizations, policies, funding, roles, and the effect on the lives of the members of the human race.[60, 61]

Douglas Mackintosh (1978) takes a look at the general system theory approach and its application to the health care delivery system. He pays particular attention to its application in terms of the input-output framework.[62] Robert Kohn and Ken White give a similar and yet more in-depth exposition of the general system theory, as it is applied to health care system in *Health Care: An International Study*. In chapter 2, they describe the framework for the system theory, orientation and modality components for the system.*[63] Rakich, Longest, and Darr (1985) discuss in the second chapter of *Managing Health Services Organizations*, 2nd edition, the conceptual framework in understanding health care, goals of the system, types of ownership, organizations, providers, workers, education, licensure, and certification by local, state, and federal regulatory bodies.*

Finally, in Mercy-Rosenan's *Public Health and Preventive Medicine*, 11th edition, Last et al. [64] gives the basics and general components of hospital organizations, the care services rendered and health services on a personal level.

NOTES

1. M. King, *A Medical Laboratory for Developing Countries* (London: Oxford Press, 1973).
2. R. E. Anderson and I. E. Carter, *Human Behavior in the Social Environment* (Chicago: Aldine Pub. Co., 1974).
3. M. Jacobs and B. J. Stern, *General Anthropology* (New York: Barnes and Nobles Books, 1955) 2-3.
4. M. L. De Fleur, V. D. William, and L. B. De Fleur, *Sociology: Human Society* (Glenview, IL: Scott, Foresman and Co., 1973) 117.
5. McGehee A. Harvey et al., ed., *The Principles and Practice of Medicine* (New York: Appleton-Century-Crafts, 1976).
6. *The Nigerian Household*. Federal Office of Statistics 1983/84, 1985.
7. *The Democrat*, Thursday, September 29 1988.
8. M. A. Harvey et al., edition, *The Principles and Practice of Medicine* (New York: Appleton-Century-Crofts, 1976).
9. D. M. Nanguang, *Causes of Problems for Nursing Administration in Nigeria* (New Orleans, Louisiana: South Western University, 1990) 48 & 49.
10. Ibid., 49-51.
11. R. A. Schram, *A History of the Nigerian Health Services* (Ibadan, Nigeria: Ibadan Univ. Press, 1971) 347 & 349.
12. D. M. Nanguang, *Causes of Problems for Nursing Administration in Nigeria* (New Orleans, Louisiana: South Western University, 1990) 54.
13. Ibid.
14. J. B. Meredith Davies : *Community Health, Preventive Medicine and Social Services*, 4th ed. (London: Bailliere III, Tindall, 1979), 1.
15. M. M. Rosenthal and M. Frenkel, *Health Care Systems and Their Patients: An International Perspective* (Boulder, Colorado: Westview Press, 1992) 221.
16. P. Barefoot and P. J. Cunningham, *Community Services: The Health Worker's A to Z* (London: Faber & Faber, 1979) 186.
17. J. B. Meredith Davies; *Community Health, Preventive Medicine and Social Services* (London: Bailliere III, Tindall, 1979), 5.
18. P. Barefoot and P. J. Cunningham, *Community Services: The Health Worker's A to Z* (London: Faber & Faber, 1977).
19. J. B. Meredith Davies: *Community Health Preventive Medicine and Social Services* (London: Bailliere Tindall, 1979), 21.
20. Ibid., 25.

21. P. Barefoot and P. J. Cunningham: *Community Services: The Health Worker's A to Z* (London: Faber & Faber, 1977) 189-190.

22. D. M. Wilner, R. P. Walkley, and L. S. Goerke: *Introduction to Public Health*, 6th ed. (New York: MacMillan Pub. Co., Inc. 1973) 33.

23. Ibid., 34.

24. Ibid.

25. Ibid., 35-44.

26. Ibid., 45.

27. J. J. Hanlon: *Public Health Administration and Practice*, 6th ed. (St. Louis: The C. V. Mosby Co., 1974), 277 & 298.

28. Ibid.

29. __Annual Abstract of Statistics, Federal Office of Statistics, Lagos, Nigeria, 1982.

30. __*The Democrat*, vol. 1, December 24, 1988.

31. S. Jonas: *Health Care Delivery in the United States* (New York: Springer Pub. Co., 1981) 93-96.

32. M. W. Raffael: *The U.S. Health System: Origins and Functions* (New York: John Wiley & Sons, 1980) 163-167.

33. Ibid.

34. J. DeGoshe: *A Content Analysis of a Nigerian TV Drama Series "Cock Crow at Dawn"* (Chicago: University of Chicago Press, 1989).

35. Obafemi Awolowo: *The People's Republic* (Ibadan: Oxford Univ. Press, 1968).

36. Helen Metz: *Nigeria: A Country Study* (Washington, D.C.: Library Congress Cataloguing Pub. Data, 1997), 4-56.

37. R. A. Schram, *A History of the Nigerian Health Services* (Ibadan, NG: Ibadan Univ. Press 1971).

38. Sir Alan Burns: *History of Nigeria* (Old Working Survey: Urwin Brothers Ltd., 1972).

39. Y. Turaki: *An Introduction to the History of SIM/ECWA in Nigeria, 1893-1993* (Jos, Nigeria: Challenge Press, 1993).

40. Y. Turaki: *The British Colonial Legacy of the Colonial and Post Colonial Society and Politics in Nigeria* (Jos, Nigeria: Challenge Press, 1993).

41. M. Omolewa: *Certificate History of Nigeria* (Lagos: Nig. Longman, 1970).

42. T. Falola: *The History of Nigeria* (Lagos, NG: Longman 1991).

43. D. M. Nanguang: *Causes of Problems for Nursing Administration in Nigeria* (New Orleans, Louisiana: South Western University, 1989).

44. R. A. Schram: *A History of the Nigerian Health Services* (Ibadan, NG: Ibadan Univ. Press, 1971).

45. __ "Health and Development in Africa, June 2-4, 1982" (Internationales Interdisciplinares Symposium, Universitat Bayreuth, 1983).

46. Ibid., 324-334.

47. L. Conrad and E. B. Gallagher, eds.: *Health and Health Care in Developing Countries: Sociological Perspective* (Philadelphia: Temple Univ. Press, 1993) 122-132.

48. King Maurice, ed.: *Medical Care in Developing Countries: A Primer on the Medicine of Poverty and a Symposium from Makerere* (Lusaka, Zambia: Oxford Univ. Press, 1966).

49. I. Bryant: *Health and the Developing World* (Ithaca, NY: Cornell Univ. Press, 1969) 257-265.

50. Ibid., 262.

51. D. M. Nanguang: *Causes of Problems for Nursing Administration in Nigeria* (New Orleans, Louisiana: South Western Univ. Press, 1989).

52. J. B. M. Davies: *Community Health, Preventive Medicine and Social Services* (London: Bailliere Tindall, 1979) 1-40.

53. P. Barefoot and P. J. Cunningham: *Community Services: The Health Worker's A to Z* (London: Faber & Faber, 1977).

54. *Jeffery Margot* All information quoted from this particular source while it was available in initial manuscripts, has some been lost either during transit or a combination of other factors that were outside the control of the author.

55. M. W. Raffael: *The U.S. Health System: Origins and Functions* (New York: John Wiley and Sons 1980).

56. Ibid.

57. S. Jonas: *Health Care Delivery in the United States* (New York: Springer Pub. Co., 1981) 93-96.

58. C. L. Anderson and C. V. Langton: *Health Principles and Practice*, 3rd ed. (St. Louis: The C. V. Mosby Co., 1961) 344-376.

59. Ibid., 376-405.

60. D. R. Mackintosh, *Systems of Health Care* (Boulder, Colorado: Westview Press, 1978).

61. R. Kohn and K. L. White, *Health Care: An International Study* (London: Oxford Univ. Press, 1976).

62. J. M. Last et al., eds., *Macy-Rosonace Public Health and Preventive Medicine*, 11th ed. (New York: Appleton-Century-Crofts, 1980).

CHAPTER FIVE

THE HEALTH PROFESSIONS AND THEIR TRAINING PROGRAMS

INTRODUCTION

This chapter will delve into that not only crucial but necessary part of the health system, the professions and the professional (who make the system work), their education and preparation. Without these professionals and their dedication, the health system and the care facilities are of no value or of any importance to anyone, including the sick. The net result of such a tragic situation would see the return of most diseases, which would run rampant by nature of plagues, disease, epidemics, and pandemics that would devastate communities in every society and to the degree that even the periods of the dark ages could not rival.

Therefore, the main goal and objective of any health system is to maximize health benefits to and for every citizen by preventing diseases through the cheapest means possible. So that when sickness does strike, the quality of live, during and after it, is preserved and the quality of care becomes the yardstick by which the health system is measured.

A good understanding of the definition of *health*, therefore, is in order at this particular juncture. While some definitions have earlier been advanced in the previous chapters, some reference to this topic is again warranted at this point.

The concept of health implies an idea that is dialectic, that is, it has its pros and cons. *Health*, according to F. F. Heidgerken (1965—Kostrzewski, 1991) represents the absence of disease—a state of balance and normality in performing its activities, playing the roles with all the necessary biological processes of the body's organ systems in steady, working order. This state of normalcy is homeostasis, which *Anatomica's Body Atlas* refers to as

> the tendency to stability in the normal physiological state of
> the human body, while "metabolism" refers to all the physical
> and chemical processes that take place in the body.[1]

Of course, what is normal is, usually, what is average for populations in general, in most instances. For example, the average body temperature of man is 98.4°F,[2] a body temperature above this is considered abnormal and below it a sort of a hypothermia, but this depends on how high or low it is and so normal or abnormal.

Alternatively, the other dimension or the pros aspect of the health concept deals with the apparent normality. For instance, an individual who performs his or her normal functions as prescribed by society, when in fact, he/she is far from being well or healthy, is still considered "healthy" and "normal." Or an individual with high blood pressure who does not have the usual signs and symptoms that normally accompany a serious health condition is healthy, as far as the rest of his/her surrounding world is concerned, since he/she is up and about performing his/her regular roles in the community. It is little wonder then that the nicknamed Silent Killer was invented and attached to diseases like high blood pressure and its ilk. A disease in this "silent killer" category, like the high blood pressure, I prefer to call the "pseudo" health disease because it is a disease, which many who have it do not know it's there, as it does, not on many occasions, give any warning signs.

The operational definition of *health*, therefore, as it relates to the subject at hand—the health system—and in this context means that it is when an individual is able to maximize the use of biological, physical, emotional indicators and performs the assigned average everyday roles with no problems.[3]

The health field is such a wide area which encompasses a wide variety of professions and occupations that Wilner, Walkley, and Goerke (1973) make the following observation:

The health field provides an extraordinary arena for employment of men and women in the United States. Most familiar are doubtless those jobs involved indirect service in the management of institutions and organizations rendering health care. The hospital and private office work selling call to mind nurses, doctors, dentist, practical nurses and aides, technicians in various specialties, nutritionist and pharmacists. Less visible but equally integral are personnel in clinical laboratory and radiologic services; these are normally involved in patient assessment and treatment along with health records and social work staff Rehabilitation staff are also employed, involving various therapies, physical, occupational speech, psychology, occupational, and others.

Then there are the health and hospital administrators, the environmental health personnel at all levels, statisticians and data-processing personnel, and others. All these and more constitute the civilian health labor force.[4]

Neither time nor space will permit a detailed discussion of every health profession and the training programs involved in each of these areas. However, an attempt will be made to provide a brief description of some of the professions, occupations and a summary of education and information that is not only pertinent but also necessary for some, including medicine, nursing, and pharmacy. This should shed some light and understanding as to the background of some of these professions.

Before starting with the medical profession, one of the oldest and perhaps the main driving force behind all health care endeavors and, most certainly, in scientific quest for modernizing health care,[5] we will first begin with the definition of *profession* and the criteria or conditions that are necessary to transform an occupation into a profession.

2. DEFINITION AND CRITERIA OF A PROFESSION

The simple definition of any profession is simply meeting a list of requirements that include an advanced educational degree and having a body of people or guild that is involved in safeguarding the interests of the occupation.[6] This is an open declaration, a public affirmation to the knowledge and skills in that particular field of practice by the group of people making such claims and by meeting the standards of the professed profession.[7] A profession, therefore, is an embodiment of education, training in technical and clinical skills, and practice expressed through the knowledge so gained in the particular area of expertise of the occupation.

Within a profession, there may be occupations with technical jobs, such as in the case of laboratory technician or attendant, radiology technician or attendant, the physician or physician's assistant, and nursing—the registered nurse (non-baccalaureate-degree nurse), vocational nurse, or nursing attendant, etc. There are vocations—such as community, public, psychiatric, or pediatric nursing—and an internist versus an ENT surgeon in medicine and so on. These are all part of the health profession that have been fragmentized into different specialties and subspecialties. For instance, there are over thirty different specialties in just the medical profession alone, some of which have been mentioned in the preceding segments of this section. On the other hand, there are a lot fewer nursing specialties and subspecialties, than there are in medicine.

The criteria which stipulate as to what the standards for a profession should be were given by Abraham Flexner in the Flexner report on medical education released in 1910.[8] The five areas identified were the following:

1. A basic level of requirements for entering the profession, for example graduation from a college, a university education or training.
2. The size of faculty and its background training.
3. Endowment funds and fees for the professional institution. Endowments are a permanent source of funds for an institution faculty, supporting fees such as fees charged for membership and tuition, for such training.

4. Adequate and good quality laboratory for training, in the first two years. This means having all the required and approved instruments for clinical and practical purposes as well as an approved setting for such training for the would be professionals, and

5. A good working relationship between the academics with those in the practical settings in institutional training areas for the field and freedom of access to the clinicians in clinical settings students in the field.[9]

In addition to the 1910 report and recommendations for clinical training for the medical professional, Flexner (1910) made the following observations about the deplorable state of the medical training of physicians in the United States at the time:

That the school cannot much longer continue in its present stage is clear: for with the requirement of two years of college work for entrance in 1910, it takes a student to spend six years to get a degree in medicine, in attaining which he can enjoy only a very limited opportunity to learn internal medicine. It is safe to predict that on that basis the present facilities will not hold the student body together during the third and fourth years.[10]

3. THE MEDICAL PROFESSIONS

Medicine

1. Medicine and Physicians
The history of medical occupation in Britain and the United States, prior to its development and evolvement into a profession, is an interesting one. Before the advent of care in hospitals, Raffael and Raffael (1959) indicate that the sick were cared for at home by women who used home remedies like herbs, elderly advise from the old and the wise in the neighborhood, methods that were in vogue at the time. [11] Ruth M. French also indicates that "at the most primitive cultural level, the sick person was left to fend for himself or die. The well had not obligation to assist him."[12]

Before and during this period, physician training was by apprenticeship, which meant that a doctor could learn how to become a doctor by attaching him/herself to an already established doctor, who himself learned the art in a similar way. This is an exact manner in which carpentry or auto mechanics training are trained in present-day Nigeria. There are, however, technical schools for these occupations, just as there are school and institutions for training doctors and other similar vocations in the country.

There were no standards set for the testing of physicians, no examinations for licensing, or induction into the profession before the Flexner report in 1910. Once the period of the apprenticeship was completed, the graduating student received a testimonial of proficiency from his teacher and went off to practice medicine, and that was it! While this history of medical evolution differs from that of the development of the medical profession in Nigeria, as trained professional from full-fledged and developed profession, modern medical care was introduced to the Nigerian society. Physicians had attended formal education and training in colleges and universities and registered as medical practitioners in either Europe or North America before going to Nigeria. This was the case under the colonial rule, following it, and even administrations after in 1960.

The first faculty of medicine in the country was established at the Ibadan College University in 1948. Nigerian nationals trained as physicians, however, were not allowed to treat expatriates, and so forbidden from practicing medicine in colonial government hospitals, unless, of course, their subjects were Nigerians or other African natives, a racist arrangement to say the very least.

While the Flexner recommendations did not help establish the medical profession in the United States, as the profession already existed, it only help improve and upgrade it and its training program from a poorly organized occupation into a profession. However, by extension, it helped and benefited the Nigerians because the missionary doctors who had come from America were trained after the reorganized medical system for physicians training or education, they worked in mission hospitals in Nigeria.

b. Medical Education

A career in medicine usually begins in high or secondary school. During high school years, a student with interest in science subjects like biology chemistry, physics, and the like could, after completion, pursue similar subjects in college or university as a premedical student. In Nigeria or Britain, this commences during the secondary education period, culminating with either a general certificate of education (GCE) or West African Examination Council (WAEC) with passes in five ordinary level subjects.

To be a physician, it takes more than education and skills acquired during the years that lead to medical school. It requires, in addition to the intellectual stamina, physical and emotional stability as well as the ability to adjust to every imaginable hurdle. It also requires the ability to use common sense, logical thinking, a proper and an adequate financial preparation or backing, and the ability to work with all kinds of people.[13]

c. The Basic Medical Sciences
Methods of teaching include all avenues of learning, from lectures and group discussions to laboratory training program, which may include slide presentations with specimens study under the microscope experimentations. Subjects covered during this period include anatomy and physiology, biochemistry, microbiology, immunology, and soon. Refer to the brochure of any medical school for a medical curriculum for a model of the basic sciences of medical studies. This period may last from two to three calendar years divided in trimesters of four-month quarters.

d. The Clinical Phase
The following is the clinical phase, which may last for another two to three years, depending on the school's schedule, which are also divided into trimesters. During this phase, the medical student undergoes a variety of clinical rotations in internal medicine, surgery, and their subspecialties: pediatrics, obstetrics-gynecology, and psychiatry.[14] However, regardless of approach, the focus is on the organ systems of the body by nature of anatomy and physiology, microbiology, biochemistry, pharmacology, pathology, early contact with clinical situations, and some aspect of biostatistics and epidemiology.

The remaining time left in clinical rotation, which may range from one to two years, are devoted to clinical experience with emphasis with hands-on practical experience—this is to ensure that the students acquire the much-desired patient contact, develop relationship with other members of the health professions, practice history taking and physical examination. This affords the soon-to-be physician an invaluable experience, appreciation, and understanding of patients in the clinical setting, a much-needed sense of professionalism, and some level of maturity.

e. Graduation and Licensure

Every medical school is responsible for evaluating the performance, promotion, and graduation of its medical students through the following:

1. A combination of direct observation, oral and written examinations, methods used in assessing the ability of student to successfully complete the medical program. At the very end, some form of a comprehensive examination is usually given.
2. A thee-step licensing examination called the United States Medical Licensing Examination (USMLE—in the United States) is a requirement for graduation for many schools. If the prospective physician wants to practice in the United States, passing the first and second parts of this examination, and a similar body in Britain, is a must before any residency program post-graduation.

4. NURSING

Nursing is the biggest section with the largest number *of* employees in the health system, especially when it is combined with para-nursing personnel.[15] Therefore, in this context then, let us first briefly examine the history of nursing and how it got to this point. Nursing, in its traditional dates, goes immemorially back to antiquity.

Nursing, like the medical professional, has equally been a part of human caring activity since man started getting sick. It began as a helping occupation alongside medicine with its training programs associated with the bedside practical aspects of medical care in hospitals.[16] It was very lately, however, actually after the war second world, that nursing started moving out of the occupation domain or category and into the professional arena and looking more like a profession.[17] It is also noteworthy to point out how nursing the sick was mainly the domain of women and especially of the young when they were born,[18] just as the defense of the family and food provision were male domain of activities in the so-called early human communities or the primitive human society. However, nursing remained ill-developed and undeveloped all through the early periods up to the Christian era, when monasteries sprang up and the care of the sick moved somewhat from the home into religious institutions and become a religious activity.[19] The inborn tendency to self-preserve vis-à-vis adversities and all kinds of odds and the constant struggle to preserve life is an instinct always present in people everywhere, regardless of intelligence, location, or the level of development.[20]

By the time of Hippocrates, medicine had moved from the domains of mythology to become a science. In fact, Hippocrates is credited with moving medicine into the scientific arena.[24] However, nursing continued to lag behind other areas of human attitudes and endeavors to improve, until the mid-nineteenth century when it started gaining recognition with the untiring efforts of Florence Nightingale during and after the Crimean.

Some religious orders like the Catholic and Protestant have existed and practiced the art of nursing for centuries;[21] some of these religious groups had organizations and formal training for nurses, even before Florence Nightingale, who is credited as being the founder of nursing.[22] At any rate, Miss Nightingale catapulted nursing on the road to professional status through her reforms, during and after the Crimean War in Europe. She instituted both the nursing education by training and skills instructions and so pushed nursing squarely into the center of medical care efforts, a necessary part of the hospital organization.[23]

The term *nurse*, its role and functions, is derived from the Latin word *nutricius*,[24] meaning, to protect, nourish, conserve energy, to foster. Just when this term or title was conferred on those caring for the sick is still not very certain, but it may date back to the time of Christ.[25] By definition, occupation stands for devotion to the care of the sick.[26] Mothers are the first practitioners of this noble profession and art who, by nature of their motherly instincts and for whatever other reasons, care for children, sick people, the aged, and are involved with nursing in many forms. This calling is heavily laden with sympathy, a very difficult prerequisite, but nevertheless, an innate part of most human beings.

It further requires knowledge and skills, as at this juncture starts the professional aspect of nursing. The philosophical basis for nursing today is to enable people, both the sick and the well, to attain health and to maintain it.[27] rounding these two principles, perhaps, hangs and revolves all other nursing activities. If a society is to attain health, it has to deal with those who are sick with especially concerted effort by one and all, to be directed at returning the sick to a healthy status. Maintaining health, therefore, must, as matter of fact and necessity, deal with the preventive aspect.

The Flexner report for a profession makes clear that for an occupation to become a profession, it has to be based on a scientific body of knowledge, specialized training for practitioners, necessary skills, and the ethical basis (altruistic) for the services provided. [28]

The specifics of the set criteria for a profession include services for specific social needs based on socially established and accepted scientific principles; there must be an entry level of knowledge, a standard training program, skills, and accompanying scientific techniques of performance. There must also be a requirement for exercising discretion or judgment; group consciousness designed as an extension of scientific knowledge; a peculiar jargon; the ability to monitor and discipline members, an ethnical code of conduct; clearly stated obligation to society bound by ethical codes.[29]

The basic features of nursing that have evolved over the years to its present professional status include the following:

1. Basic principles and techniques that are based on adopted sciences peculiar to nursing.
2. A legal code that mandates care for the physically and mentally ill in procuring comfort through remedial measures, under the supervision of a licensed physician.
3. A body of knowledge, skills, training, and an entry level required prior to licensure.

As a science, nursing commands and demands a broad, yet sound education, with thorough knowledge of the human nature in all stages and processes of development, as there is hardly any field in the sciences that does not have some application in nursing.

The nursing curriculum generally covers four basic areas, namely, the biological, physical, social, medical, pharmaceutical, and nursing sciences as well as other allied arts and sciences. The biological and physical sciences include anatomy and physiology, microbiology, physics, and chemistry. Anatomy deals with the physical structures of the body while physiology deals with the functional nature of these structural components. These form the primary bases of therapy. Microbiology, on the other hand, deals with the causative nature of disease and illness and the particular conditions that govern the agents responsible for disease and how to control them. This approach takes the form of disinfection, antisepsis, and/or treatment with microbial agents like antibiotics and others.

Understanding chemistry, especially organic chemistry, enables one to understand some chemical processes of physiology and the physiology of the body. It is important to understand the effects of chemicals and their interaction with acids, acid bases, alkaline, hormones, and how they affect the physical constitution of the body.

Biochemistry and physics, on the other hand, explain the current understanding of the general laws of motion within the body. These principles relate to agents and other remedial properties in the body. They also shed light on issues like specific gravity, heat, pressure, light, weight, and friction in the body.

The social sciences deal with the interaction and processes of the whole person in his/her immediate social environment: the family, community, and ultimately the society at large.

Psychology, for example, enables the nurse to understand the dispositions of human behavior in different social settings by nature of mood displayed by emotions and a necessary part for effective nursing care. Sociology, on the other hand, deals with cultural knowledge as applied in dealing with groups of people and the meaning based on differences in customs and traditional practices that influence health behaviors, which enables the nurses to help patients with different backgrounds.

Medicine and medical sciences portray facts about known diseases and maladies with their treatment modalities, while nursing and other applied arts enable the nurse to apply scientific knowledge in the care of individuals, the sick and the well alike, in a holistic manner.

Therefore, to enter the educational training setup for nurses, the student must complete or finish secondary school or its equivalent, with a West African School Certificate (WASC) or general certificate of education diploma (GCE) prior to admission. Following the completion of the nursing training program, the graduate nurse must then take a licensure examination to qualify as a Nigerian Registered Nurse (NRN).

In United States, nurses trained in other countries must take the qualifying licensing examination also before they are eligible to practice nursing as professional nurses in any of the fifty states of the United States. This examination is conducted by all states through nursing boards or State's Boards of Examiners.

In Britain, the British Council of Registered Nurses for Britain and Wales determines the eligibility of a nurse from other countries with the intention to practice nursing in England. When a nurse is qualified by meeting the set standard, he or she is given the license after passing a licensure examination.

The Nigerian Council for Nurses, a similar body to the one in Britain, makes this determination, but without the benefit of an examination for overseas graduates; however, this might have changed in recent years, which I am not aware of at this point.

Finally, after the four-year university program, nurses graduate with a baccalaureate degree in the areas enumerated above that include a public health nursing component.[30] The four-year university programs was first introduced in the early 1960s at the Ibadan University, then Lagos University, Ahmadu Bello University, subsequently; and now almost all other universities in the country have a baccalaureate degree program in nursing.

These graduates are prepared for leadership roles in hospitals and other health care institutions. However, before the mid-1970s, admission requirements to nursing programs in Nigeria were changed or upgraded—seventh grade or higher or lower were admitted into the nursing programs.

The role of nursing in Nigeria is similar to the one in other developing nations, but oftentimes, it is more than that. While the preparation of nurses is adequate for the typical nursing role that nurses fill in Britain and United States, this role in Nigeria has expanded to encompass some of the duties and role of the physician. However, that is without the commensurate required training or pay, even though to the rest of the Nigerian workforce, nurses are a very well-paid group.

The role of the nurse includes diagnosis, ordering of laboratory tests, the interpretation of test results, and ordering of treatments or minor surgeries—all included within the scope of medical practice, which Nigerian nurses dabble with.

5. PHARMACY

This profession, like the medical and nursing professions, from its primordial form, dates back to antiquity, some aspects of which are still observed in some underdeveloped societies today. Roots and leaves concoctions and sometimes other naturally occurring elements were and are still being used.

From the Middle Ages on and up to the present, this practice was known as alchemy—a rather dangerous occupation, which was a great improvement from the primordial form that have led to the modern-era pharmacy, as we now know it.

During the seventeenth century, English pharmacists were known as apothecaries, who operated drugstores composed of many drug compounds and different medications.[31] The primary function of a pharmacist is to procure, store, and dispense of drugs or other chemical products for medicinal purposes. The pharmacist specializes in the science of drugs and medicines, their physical properties compositions and their effect impact on people. As a profession, pharmacy meets the standard required of a profession. Like medicine and nursing, it also demands graduation from an accredited college, with a degree program in pharmacy science, leading to a baccalaureate science degree.

Following graduation, a one-year internship is required and passing a state board examination prior to licensure. A pharmacist is therefore able to make informed decisions and recommendations on drugs to both the doctor and patient. In the hospital setting, the pharmacist performs, in addition to functions already described above, the control the traffic of drugs within the organization. He or she ensures that patients receive not only the correct and appropriate medication but the correct doses with the right instructions for taking the medication.

Pharmacy is believed to the third largest health profession in the United States besides the nursing and medical professions. To some extent, nurses and especially dispensary attendants also assume some roles of the pharmacist in the Nigerian health care system. This is also blamed on the shortage of pharmacists.

6. DENTISTY

With the prevalent dental problem of a population, dental health needs are among major national health priorities. There is no question as to the importance of dental health in the ranking of this nation's health issues. Knutson and Klein have this observation on the matter:

> In as much as the etiology of dental carries is unknown, prevention of the disease causing these defects is still in the experimental state. It is, generally by knowledge, however that the treatment of early carious lesions by the proper placement of chemically and physically terminating stable filling materials will largely prevent carious teeth from tooth loss or tooth mortality. The primary purpose of dental health program becomes, therefore, the promulgation of procedures whereby the early detection and treatment of carious teeth is accomplished and tooth mortality thereby prevented.[32]

The need for dental health cannot be stated any better than what is stated in the above quotation, even though this article is policy oriented and for a specific population, i.e., elementary school children's screening, etc.

While this is the case, it still addresses a very subtle and, yet not so clear truth. It addresses the need for early defection and treatment of dental problems in children, as the solution for adults with dental problem-free in later years. The heavy sugar-laden diet and snacks in developed countries, besides being precursors for other health problems, are definitely shortcuts to dental cares. In the underdeveloped world, besides the attendant's poor dental hygiene, the high carbohydrate content in diet, which often is converted to fat in the body, affects the body in the similar manner as is the case in developed countries, even if the results of such an affect may differ.

The dental profession usually comprises the following subspecialties: orthodontics, which involves the strengthening of teeth; endodontics, the treating of diseased and injured pulp and tissues around teeth; prosthodontics, the making of artificial teeth and dentures; periodontics, the treating of gum and underlying bone diseases; pedodontics, dealing with children's dental problems; oral pathology, dealing with diseases of the mouth; and public health dentistry, which deals with such public health issues as fluoridation and the treatment of water to prevent dental problems.

Before entering a dental school in the United States or in most other countries, the prospective dental student must also finish high school or the equivalent of secondary education and earn a college degree measuring in any of the sciences required for medical school admission. After admission into an approved dental school, the student must then pass a licensing examination, both written and practical, after graduation. To become a certified specialist, after receiving the doctor of dental medicine (DDM) or doctor of denial surgery (DDS), the dental doctor then spends another two or three years in oral and/or maxillary surgery, plus another three to four years of certification.[33, 34] Currently, all dentists in Nigeria are trained abroad. Dental practice by practitioners of the profession is either in a private office or in public health facilities in the Nigerian society.

7. VETERINARY MEDICINE

In veterinary medicine, treatment and prevention of disease and injury to animals is the main focus. There is, therefore, no question as to the importance of this profession in the human health efforts. In addition to above activities, the veterinarian is a resource person in breeding animals, as well as the control of animal (zoonotic) disease epidemics.

The veterinary doctor physically examines, tests, and vaccinates animals. Thus, the veterinarian helps immensely in preventing meat contamination, food poisoning, and humans contracting such zoonotic diseases such as bovine tuberculosis, rabies, brucellosis, salmonellosis, and a lot more.

Like the medical profession, before entering an approved veterinary medical school, a prospective student must have completed high or secondary school or an equivalent qualification. He or she must also graduate from college majoring in one of the biological sciences. Upon completing five to six years in veterinary medical school earning the doctor of veterinary medicine degrees (DVM) and passing the licensing examination, the veterinary doctor then qualifies to practice veterinary medicine. Most universities with medical schools offer veterinary training in Nigeria.

Most veterinary doctors in Nigeria work for the government and are involved directly in regulation of public health policies and research. Very few used to engage in private practice of treating domestic animals, but this situation has changed as many veterinary doctors now have solo practice.

8. NUTRITION AND DIETARY

The nutritionist engages in the investigation and solving problems that relate to human nutrition for the purpose of health promotion. The subject of nutrition essentially involves the sum total of all the processes of taking in what should and needs to be taken as food and the avoidance of what should not be taken by measuring and using nutriments appropriately. Nutritionists are involved in educational programs of preparing other health professionals in the health field for preserving human health.

On the other hand, the role of the dietician, fundamentally, is to guide others in the application of principles of nutrition in food preparation. This includes food selection, its preparation, the service of balanced and nutritional meals to groups and individuals alike.[35] The profession measures up to the criteria set forth by the Flexner report for a profession or for an occupation to qualify as a profession. Prospective nutritionists have to graduate with at least a bachelor's degree from college or university majoring in nutrition or biochemistry to work in the occupation and use the nutritionist designation and a masters or doctoral degree to qualify as a nutritionist or dietician. Furthermore, this service is altruistic since it is tied to many health institutions in both private and public places. A proper nutrition or food intake and/or lack of it is implicated in a wide range of health issues and social programs that affects public health.[15]

9. HEALTH ADMINISTRATION

The health field is so wide that it requires a wide range of well-trained personnel as well as money to operate properly, even in developing nations like Nigeria. By implication, this occupation also requires properly trained administrators who are both skilled and responsible in the running of health facilities, a point that is particularly salient to the running of health facilities in Nigeria.

The successful running of a health facility simply boils down to, in addition to good training and dedication, proper planning, securing, or the assemblage of appropriate resources, then in a meticulous manner planned execution of programs and the organizational policies responsibly. The proper planning and use of the resources for the smooth running of a health facility should, if done right, ensure a good quality of patient care as the end product, which points to the quality and capability of administration.

Historically, the administrative position in the hospital, at least in Nigeria, has always been the domain of the chief medical officers and matrons, some of whom came up through the rank by promotion and have had no prior administrative training or experience. Some of the chief medical officers also come to this important position by accident and, in a similar manner as that of the matrons, without training, experience, or both. Like nurses, the role was foisted on them, and so many have floundered, leaving trails of disaster in almost every instance.

10. OTHER HEALTH PROFESSIONS AND OCCUPATIONS

There are other professional areas like eye and vision, podiatry, chiropractic, and so on. Those that pertain to eye and vision are also part of the Nigerian health system and care delivery scenario and will also be mentioned in brief here too.

a. **VISION:** Visual services and eye care employ a few professionals and that requires some level of discussion.

121

1. **OPHTHALMOLOGY:** Ophthalmology is a specialty in medicine and a subspecialty of surgery. An ophthalmologist is a physician who specializes in the medical and surgical care of the eye and able to prescribe eye treatment, including lenses and other prescriptions. The educational training of ophthalmologists follows the same path as that of other physicians.

   a. **Optometry.** It deals primarily with the eye, vision care, diagnosis, treatment, and prevention of associated disorders. The optometrist specializes in this area of care so as to improve vision through the prescription of eyeglasses and other optical or pharmaceutical means permitted by law. To be an optometrist, after college degree, one must spend six years in an accredited school of optometry and graduate with a doctor of optometry (OD) and pass a state board examination before engaging in the professional practice of optometry.

   b. **Opticianary**: The field of opticianry deals with fitting and adjusting eyeglasses as prescribed by an ophthalmologist or an optometrist, but an optician does not examine or treat eye disease problems.

   c. **Optical Technicians:** These are the ones who grind and polish lenses, while the optician only fits them properly on the patient.

2. **RADIOLOGY**: Radiology is a branch of medicine, a health science that deals with radioactivity, i.e., radiant energy that is used in the diagnosis and treatment of diseases, with x-rays and/or ultrasound radiation.

   The radiologist is a physician who specializes in radiology by training, for three to four years after formal medical education. Radiologists make diagnosis by reading x-rays.

3. **LABORATORY TECHNOLOGY:** The clinical or medical laboratory plays a crucial as well as central role in health services through testing and the analysis of medical specimens in the diagnosis, treatment, prevention, and control of diseases. A medical laboratory may exist in any setting, including the practitioner's office. In proprietary settings, laboratories exist solely for commercial purposes, and that

is to perform services for a fee to health care facilities, physician group practices, solo practitioners, or other industrial facilities.

Testing services areas include blood and chemical analysis, WBC, microbiologic and immunologic tests, etc. In the hospital setting, the laboratory requires a set of well-trained technicians headed by a medical technologist.

a. **Medical Laboratory Technologist:** This is a physician who specialized in both the technical aspect of the laboratory as well as the pathology of the different medical conditions (biology, microbiology, and other chemical expertise). A laboratory technologist is a physician who, after medical education, specializes in tests and analytical work of medical laboratory.

b. **Medical Laboratory Technician**: A laboratory technician is not a physician, but someone thoroughly trained in laboratory technical procedures, instruments, and test procedures, but cannot diagnose or interpret test results.

The health professions described above have expanders, i.e., assistants and other occupational categories that are used either to assist or to perform some of the different occupations that fall under the umbrella of these specialties. The only exception to the above classifications on technical basis is that, in Nigeria, the medical profession has no physician assistants, as nurses fit that role perfectly. Furthermore, for the sake of parsimony and brevity, not every subspecialty in medicine or other health professions have fully been described in the foregoing discussions, as a number of these subspecialties are either absent or insignificant in the context of the Nigerian health system.

REVIEW OF LITERATURE

Institutions and schools that train health care professions have different programs and goals of training each for professional area listed in previous sections of this chapter. As it is apparent, these different schools of training professionals may differ in the objectives while the overall goal and mission are the same. In practice, each profession addresses or emphasizes some particular area of health, but the basic philosophy for health dominant in these institutions remains the same. The medical and paramedical professions, for example, generally are "cure" oriented as this is what drives most of their activities. Their aim is to ensure that the sick get treated; on the other hand, preventive measures are directed toward the well and healthy people. Other health professions have a focused attention on activities that support some other aspect of health endeavor.

A review of both the American and British medical histories is germane to the medical history of Nigeria and indeed of the world as these two societies have champion research work not only on health issues but the sciences in general. They review the development of specially boards, the Flexner report, and the Mills Commission which revolutionized the medical profession as well as other health care areas. They summarize the training, practical aspects, and the licensing requirements prior to the professional practice of all health professions.

Helen Metz (editor, 1990), in *Area Handbook Series*, describes the general health system in Nigeria with some historical background, distribution, training, and staffing problems found in health care facilities.[36]

The Association of American Medical Colleges (1994) has a detailed description of how to prepare for enrolment in medical schools and the conditions that govern studies in medical education in a brochure titled *Medical School Admission Requirements in the U.S. and Canada*.[37, 38]

Abraham Flexner (1943, 1966), in his report on medical education in United States and Canada in 1910, recommended specific steps needed to improve the unorganized medical education in the respective societies whose standard of medical practice was not up to par.[39, 40, 41]

Puschman (1994) discusses the need for changes in medical education continually in *A History of Medical Education* as a result of constant changes wrought by new discoveries in the medical science, but especially in the United States. His discussion starts with the historical perspective right from the ancient times leading up to modern periods with an avalanche of accumulated medical knowledge right from the very beginning.[42] Johnson (1953) describes the characteristics of medical students in *Physician in the Making*. Although in the past fifty years in the

United States students in all medical schools have had a lot in common, he however indicates that the characterization is universal in nature and how medical schools nowadays select prospective students.[43]

Heidgerken (1965) advocates a new look at the teaching approach of nursing education by making changes in nursing curricula and making it lot more dynamic in the preparation of nurses. She suggests the integration of inter—or multidisciplinary approach in teaching nurses in all nursing school programs and the incorporation of new advances in medical sciences. She also suggests methods of developing, planning, and implementing more effective curricula for nursing programs.[44]

Cohn (1967) and Griffin and Griffin (1969) independently discuss the historical background and significance of nursing, medical and other health sciences, drawing distinctions between modern nursing from the original practice, its impact on nursing education and the student.[45,46] Spalding and Notter (1970), Conley (1973), and Lambertsen (1958) discuss trends and problems facing nursing from a historical-political viewpoint with the socio-economical perspectives that require changes in nursing programs, from the curriculum perspective that is based on available scientific information and professional nursing principle that identifies the educational need and the promotional incentives for nurses in leadership positions.[47, 48, 49]

Soran (1977), in *Nursing in the World*, presents in the thirtieth chapter the social background and basic midwifery nursing education, training, and regulation in Nigeria.[60] It could very well be that all these recommendations for change to improve nursing had the Nigerian nurse in mind.
Knokpe and Dicklemann, (editors, 1981) discuss the approaches to organization and education for primary health personnel. They suggest practical and effective ways of teaching and training programs for these groups of health care workers.

Levey and Loomba, in the first chapter of *Health Care Administration: A Managerial Perspective*, describe the concepts and domains of the three health perspectives, namely, individual, professional, and the care manager. They delve into the nature of the health industry, its competitive nature, regulatory aspects, and future prospects.

Carl Willgoose (1982), in *Health Teaching in Secondary School*, 3rd edition, acknowledges the multifactorial, multidimensional complex nature of health care in the modern society. He outlines the implications and some of the ramifications of individual health decision-making as they affect every member of the society and especially the adolescents. The book also deals with curriculum development and some practical means of implementing comprehensive health programs by research in health learning institutions through the use of teaching aids.

NOTES

1. *Anatomica's Body Atlas* (San Diego, CA: The Thunder Bay Press, 2007) 44.
2. F. F. Heidgerken, *Teaching and Learning in School of Nursing: Principles and Methods* (Philadelphia: J. B. Lippincott Co., 1965).
3. *The Random House Dictionary* (New York:, Random Houses, 1989) 701.
4. D. M. Wilner, R. P. Walkley, and L. S. Goerke, *Introduction to Public Health*, 6th ed. (New York: MacMillan Pub. Co. Inc., 1973) 71.
5. E. Ginzberg, ed., *Health Services Research: Key to Health Policy* (Cambridge, MA: Harvard Univ. Press, 1991) 287.
6. *The Century Dictionary: An Encyclopedia Lexicon of the English Language*, vol. 6 (New York: The Century Co., 1995) 47—55.
7. *The American Heritage Dictionary of the English Language* (Boston: Houghton Miffin Co., 1976) 1044-1045.
8. A. I. Flexner, *Remember* (New York: Simon & Schuster, 1940) 120-122.
9. M. W. Raffael and N. K. Raffael, *The U.S. Health System: Origin and Functions*, 3rd ed. (Albany, NY: Delmar Pub. Inc., 1989) 11.
10. A. Flexner, *Medical Education in the United States and Canada*, Bulletin 4, (New York: The Carnegie Foundation for the Medicament of Teaching, 1910) 264-265.
11. M. W. Raffael and N. K. Raffael, *The U.S. Health System: Origins and Functions*, 3rd ed. (Albany, NY: Delmar Pub. Inc., 1989) 182.
12. H. M. French, *Dynamics of Health Care*, 3rd ed. (New York: McGraw-Hill Book Co., 1979) 21.
13. *Medical School Admission Requirements 1995-1996 U.S. & Canada*, 45th ed. (Washington, D.C.: Association of American Medical Colleges, 1994) 17.
14. Spartan Health Science Univ. School of Medicine Brochure (1990) 17.
15. D. M. Wilner, R. P. Walkley, and L. S. Goerke, *Introduction Public Health*, 6th ed. (New York: MacMillan Pub. Inc., 1973) 72, 74, 75, and 77.
16. M. W. Raffael and N. K. Raffael, *The U.S. Health System: Origin and Functions*, 3rd ed. (Albany, NY: Delmar Pub. Inc., 1989) 41.
17. Ibid., 43.
18. J. A. Dolan, *History of Nursing*, 12th ed. (Philadelphia: W. B. Sounders Co., 1965) 2.
19. G. J. Griffin and J. K. Griffin, *Jenden's History and Trends of Professional Nursing*, 6th ed. (St. Louis: The C. V. Mosby Co., 1981) 9-10.

20. J. A. Dolan, *Goodnow's History of Nursing*, 11th ed. (Philadelphia: W. B. Sounders Co., 1960) 44.

21. E. K. Spalding and I. E. Notter: *Professional Nursing*, 8th ed. (Philadelphia: J. B. Lippincott Co., 1970).

22. G. J. Griffin and I. K. Griffin: *Jenses' History of Trend of Professional Nursing*, 6th ed. (St. Louis: The C. V. Mosby Co., 1966) 65.

23. Ibid., 65-79.

24. M. E. McClain and S. H. Gragg, *Scientific Principles in Nursing*, 5th ed. (St. Louis: The C. V. Mosby Co., 1996) 14.

25. O. E. Orem and K. S. Parker, eds., *Nursing Content Interservice Nursing Curriculums* (Washington, D.C.: The Catholic Univ. of Am. Press, 1964) 14.

26. Ibid., 15.

27. M. F. McClain and S. M. Gragg, *Scientific Principles in Nursing*, 5th ed. (St. Louis: The C. V. Mosby Co., 1966) 3.

28. E. K. Spalding, *Professional Nursing: Trends, Responsibilities and Relationship*, 6th ed. (Philadelphia: J. B. Lippincott Co., 1959) 24.

29. Ibid., 24-25.

30. M. W. Raffael and N. K. Raffael, *The U.S. Health System: Origins and Functions*, 3rd ed. (Albany, NY: Delmar Pub. Inc., 1989).

31. Ibid., 115.

32. D. M. Wilner, R. P. Walkley, and L. S. Goerke, *Introduction to Public Health*, 6th ed. (New York: MacMillan Pub. Co. Inc., 1973) 85-86.

33. J. Knutson and H. Klein, "Tooth Mortality in Elementary School Children," *Pub. Health Rep.* 53 (June 1938): 1021.

34. M. W. Raffael and N. K. Raffael, *The U.S. Health System: Origins and Functions* (Albany, New York: Delmar Pub. Inc., 1989) 116-117.

35. N. Scrimshaw, C. Tylor and J. Gordon, "Internationals of Nutrition and Infection," *WHO Chronicle* 23 (1969): 369-74.

36. H. G. Metz, *Nigeria: A Country Study* (Washington, D.C.: Library of Congress, Fed. Research Div., 1992).

37. Medical School Admission Requirements, AAMC 45th ed., (Washington, D.C., 1994).

38. Ibid., 23rd ed.

39. Abraham Flexner, *Medical Education in the United State and Canada: A Report to the Carnegie Foundation for the Advancement of Teaching* (Washington, D.C.: Science and Health Pub., 1973).

40. D. M. Wilner, R. P. Walkley, and L. S. Goerke, *Introduction to Public Health*, 6th ed. (New York: MacMillan Pub. Inc., 1973).

41. B. Bullough and V. Bullough, eds., *Issues in Nursing* (New York: Springer Pub. Co. Inc., 1966).

42. A. Puschmann, *History of Medical Education* (1994).

43. D. G. Johnson, *Physician in the Making* (San Francisco: Jessey-Bass Pub., 1983).

44. F. F. Heidgerken, *Teaching and Learning in School of Nursing: Principles and Methods* (Philadelphia: J. B. Lippincott Co., 1965).

45. J. A. Dolan, *Goodnow's History of Nursing* (Philadelphia: W. B. Sounders Co., 1963).

46. G. J. Griffin and J. K. Griffin, *Jensen's History and Trends of Professional Nursing*, 6th ed. (St. Louis: The C. V. Mosby C., 1960).

47. E. K. Spalding and I. E. Notter, *Professional Nursing Foundations: Perspectives and Relationships* (Philadelphia: J. B. Lippincott Co., 1970).

48. V. Conley, *Curriculum and Instruction in Nursing* (Boston: Little Brown & Co., 1973).

49. E. C. Lambersen, *Education for Nursing Leadership* (Philadelphia: J. B. Lippincott Co., 1958).

50. Kango K. Soran, *Nursing in the World: The Needs of Individual Countries and Their Programmes* (BINF, 1977).

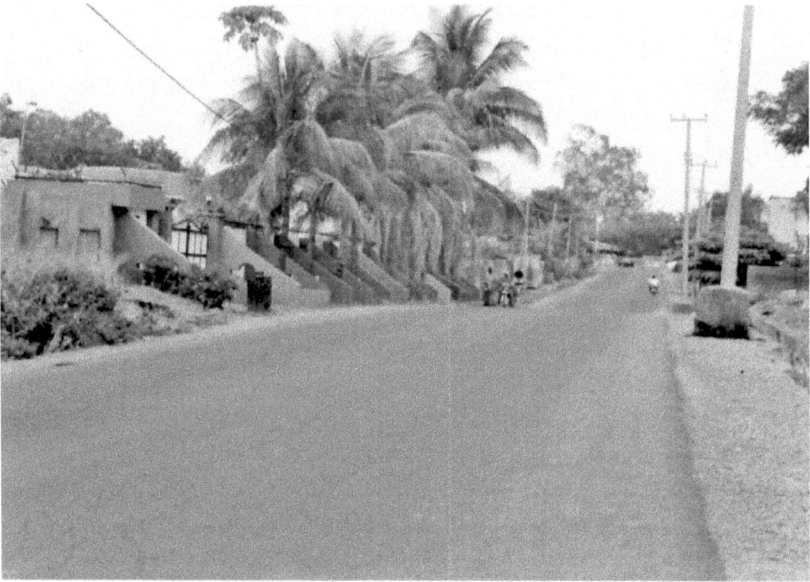

This is the well fortified residential house of General Mohammed Buhari, former Head of State during the Buhari-Idiagbon military regime or administration. General Buhari later on served as the Head of PTF that was responsible for road's constructions during the tenure of the 2nd President Olusegun Obasanjo Administration, (1999—2007). General Buhari had made unsuccessful in presidential politics and displayed behaviors that raised a lot of eyebrows but that are typical behavior of most Moslems, by showing extreme partiality in making sure that good and well built road pervaded most Islamic communities in Kaduna States. However, he showed little interest or concern for that matter, but perhaps antipathy and total disregard to the road conditions in non-Islamic communities.

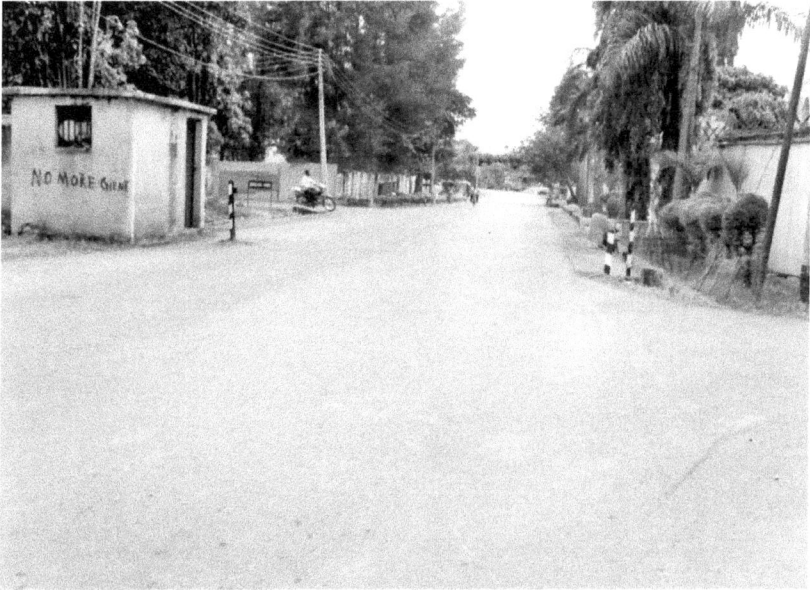

Extremely well-built and spaciously tarred roads in Islamic communities are facts that are indisputable in the daily lives of most Nigerians.

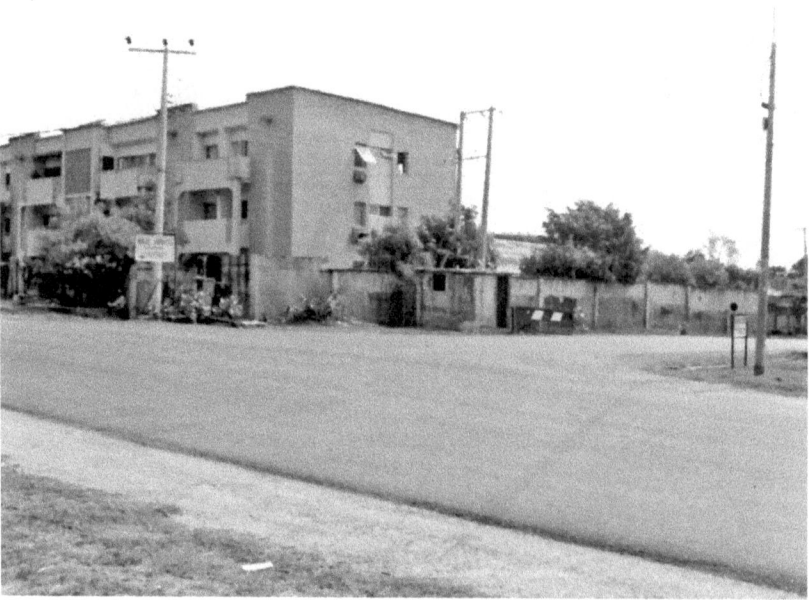

A clear picture of Dahiru Dan Toro Close road junction, one of the highly privileged sections of the City of Kaduna where one of the fortified houses of the former Head of State, General Mohammed Buhari is located. The system of road networks in such areas is typical in Moslem communities of this Moslems' dominated capital of Kaduna State and everywhere else in the state.

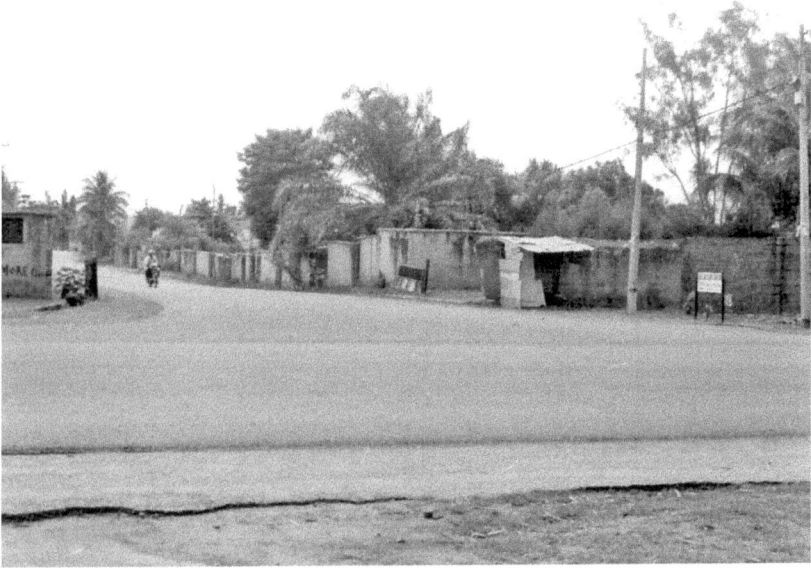

Another example of a good and well maintained road in a Moslem section like this one abound in Kaduna City, Kaduna State and many other states of the Nigerian nation. The idea and claim that Moslems have a clear majority in Nigeria is not only patently false, but also peposterous.

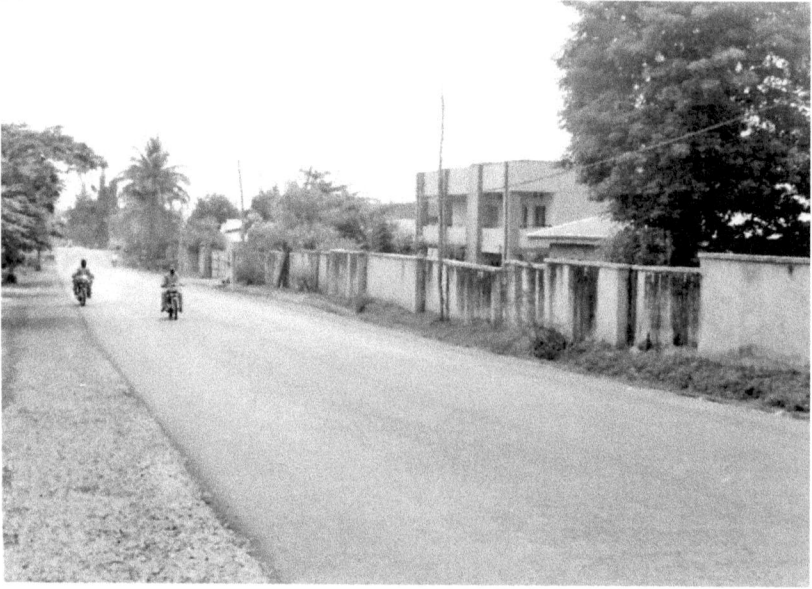

Examples of a good road network like this one are never in short supply. Roads like this are duplicated in every nook and cranny of the nation. Wherever and whenever members from these dominant groups in any of the communities that belong to this unholy triad (Islamic-Hausa-Fulani) live in Nigeria.

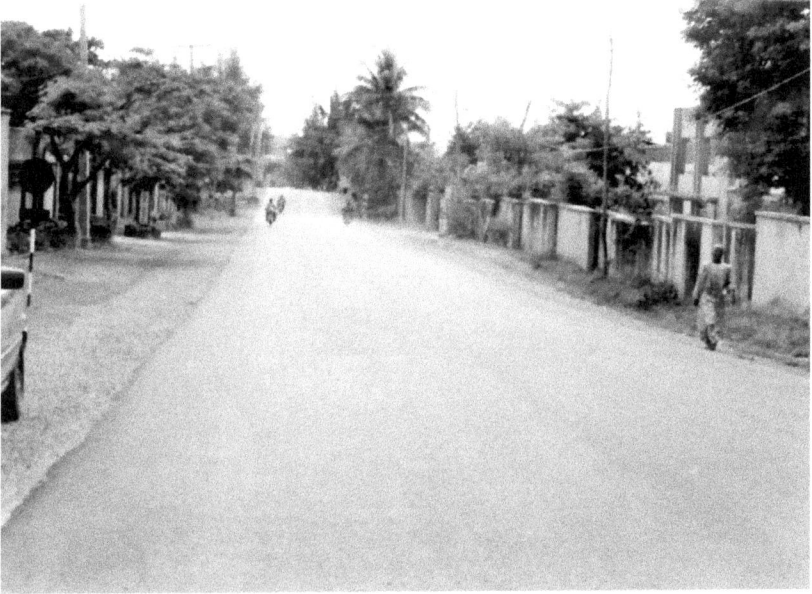

This picture is symbolic of one of the many things that are terribly wrong in the Nigerian society ever since Independence on October 1st, 1960 when autonomy was granted to its nationals to run the county's affairs. Again this particular picture was taken in the vicinity of of the house of General Mohammed Buhari, a one time Head of State (1983-1985). This particular street/road, in certain quarters (such as in some undeveloped nations, which Nigeria is certainly a perannial member, eventhough it dubs itself as the "Giant of Africa"), simply qualifies as an airstip, where minor aeroplanes are able to land and take-off with aboundant space and comfort and no danger or problem whatsoever!

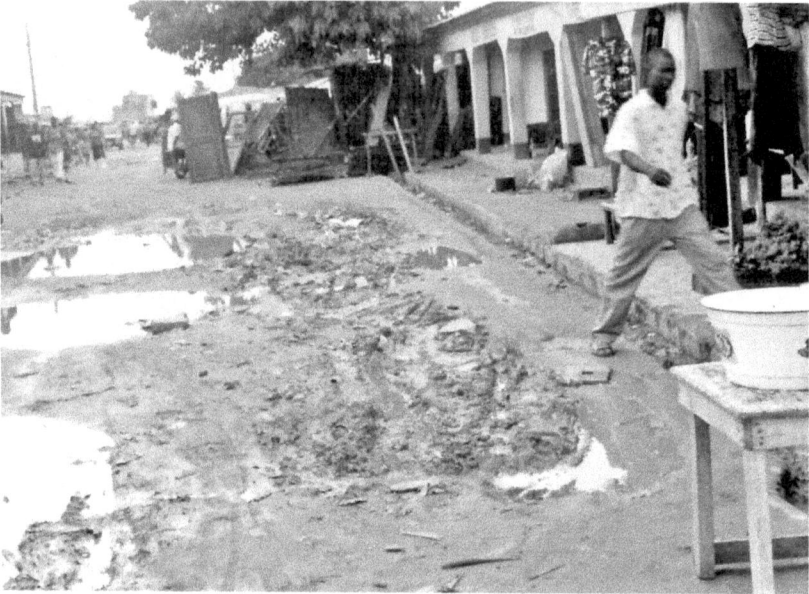

The above picture was taken of one of the main roads in Ungwar Sunday; his is another section of Kaduna City where the population is non-Moslem. Damaged roads with pot holes interspersed with mud, water pools and islands of marsh, all serve as havens for mosquitoes, flies and other unholy creeping characters as road gutters are filled with stagnant and repugnant smelling water pools in this and many similar "arna" and or "kafirs/kafirai" areas, pejorative or derogatory terms used for anyone that is not a Moslems. During the rainy seasons pedestrians, as it is clearly exemplified above, constantly struggle to find dry spots that would serve as paths to walk.

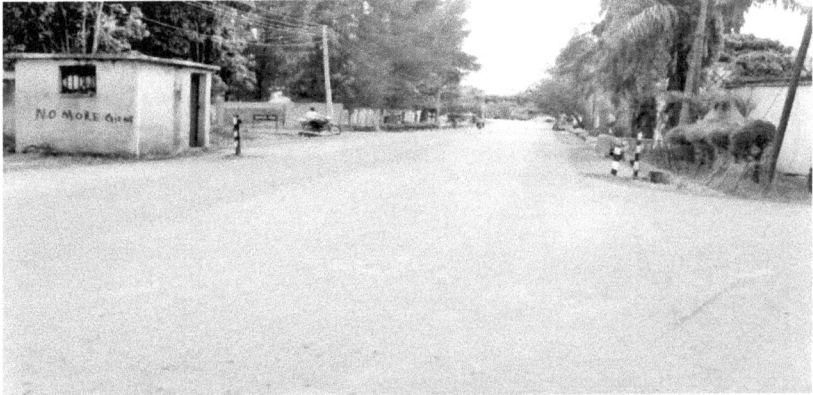

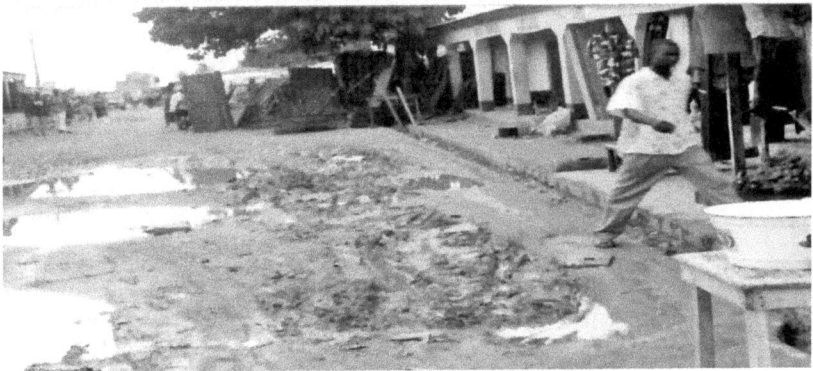

There is a sharp contrast between Moslem and non-Moslem
residential areas as the above pictures clearly depict. Top:
picture was taken from a Moslem residential area: smooth
streets and fortified homes and Moslems. Bottom: picture was
taken in non-Moslem residential areas with open streets with
pedestrians struggling to find dry areas to

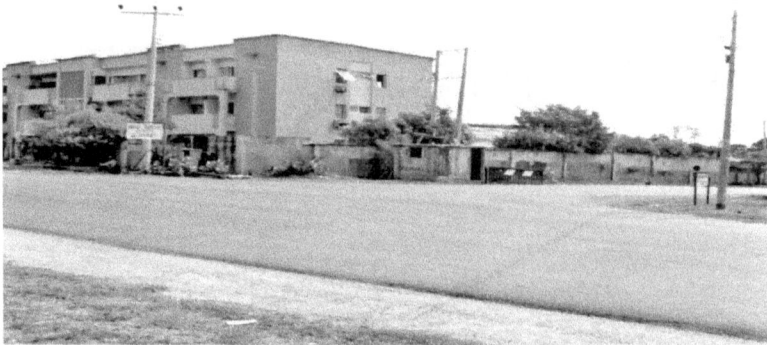

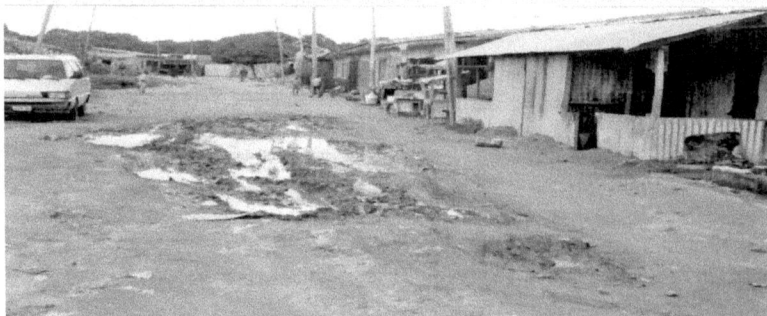

Another glaring example of the differences between of Islamic communities in Nigeria and the non-Islamic ones; a sort of social apartheid, if you will. The two pictures above do not even begin to tell the entire narrative as to the tale of woes that the minorities in the Nigerian society suffer and endure. The naïve mind may accuse me of sensationalizing this condition of misery and might think that this is all there is or the extent of it; but that is not the case, as this might even be laughable were this not such a serious issue. This manner of social segregation extends into all other aspects of the every day living arrangements in today's Nigerian society. Not only are the streets in Islamic communities better, so are all other forms of socially services like electricity, piped and running water, medical and all forms of health facilities and services, etc. which are all in contant supply to the dominant groups residential areas.

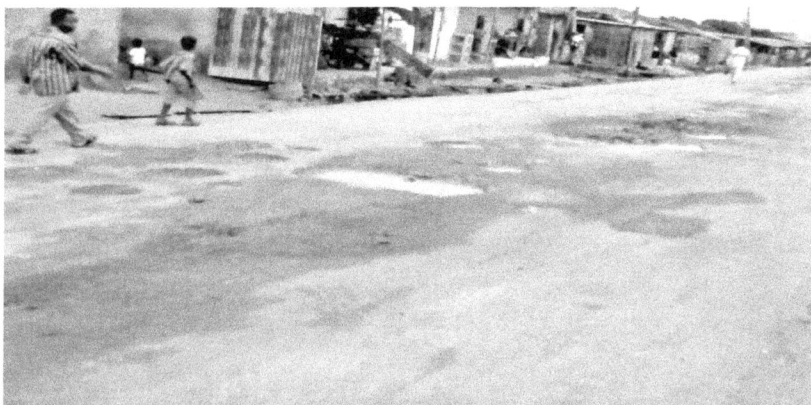

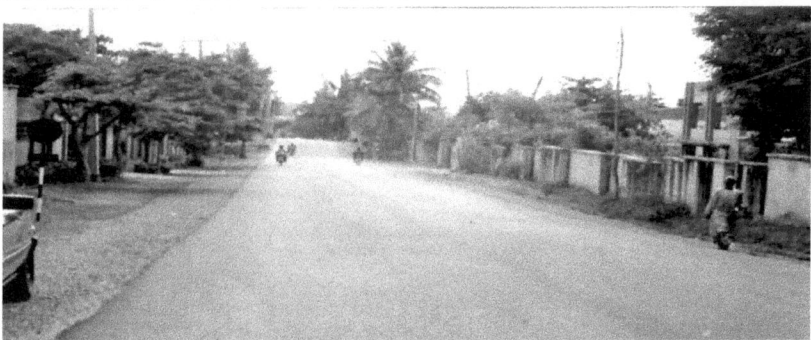

The juxtapositioning of these pictures is merely to provide another angle or contrast to the differences in the living arrangements and conditions of the under-priviledged non-Moslem population in Nigerian people in the same society. While they may have the same government and yet have such a difference in their living conditions or arrangements, with no one in the authority seeming to care or giving a hoot. The only reasons are ethno-centricism and the intolerant hatred of Islam as it is practiced by its religious or perhaps irreligious adherent and bigots. Hatred and intolerance are neither taught nor condoned in Christianity nor are they practiced by true adherent to the tenets of Christianity.

Bottom: This picture contrasts sharply to the top one. It is the major roads in Television Village, a heavily populated non-Moslem section in the City of Kaduna, in Kaduna State. This portrays and clearly shows the deplorable state of the only road in one community (non-Moslems) from a well developed and maintained, one of many roads in another (Moslem).

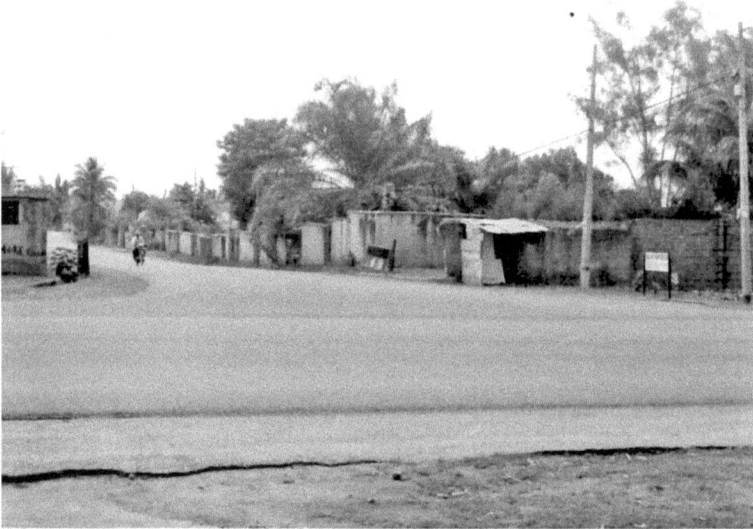

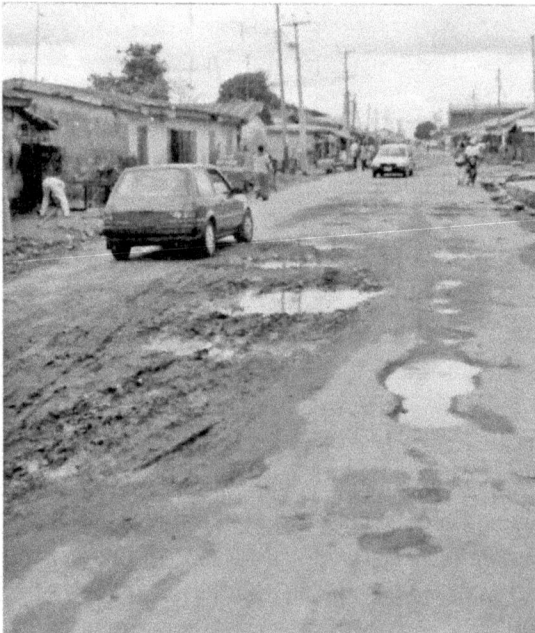

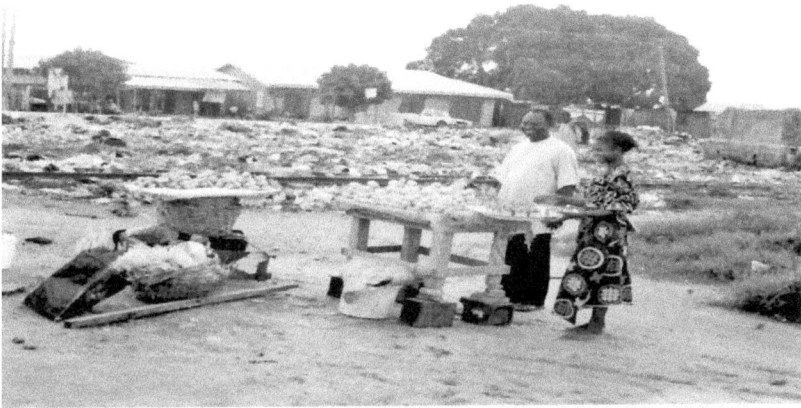

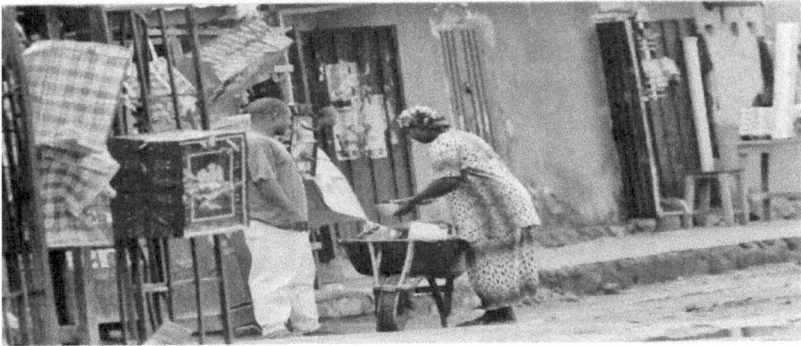

Top: This is a picture of a road side mini-food market, as desperate people will do desperate things when their very survival comes into question. Desperate women, in Nigeria, a land of plenty—in this so-called "Giant (giantess) of Africa"—set-up shop just about anywhere and everywhere, including near a refuse dumping grounds. They sell food products including cooked food meant for human consumption that is ready to be eaten. This dumping area starts from the rail-tract, seen to the right of the two people standing besides the tables with food stuffs.

Bottom: This is another road side shopping center in one of the congested residential areas of a non-Moslem area.

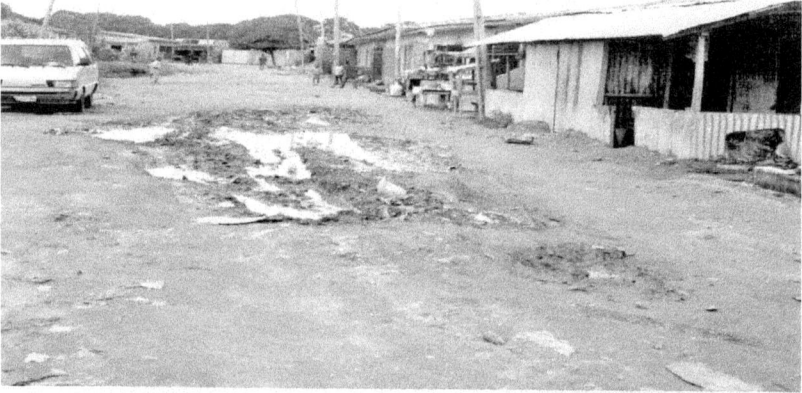

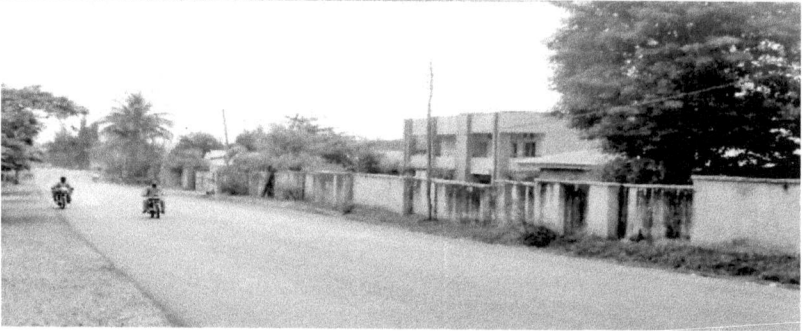

The contrast as presented in the discrepancy of the two types of roads above. While palpably glaring, these are by no means an exaggeration, as they are very real!

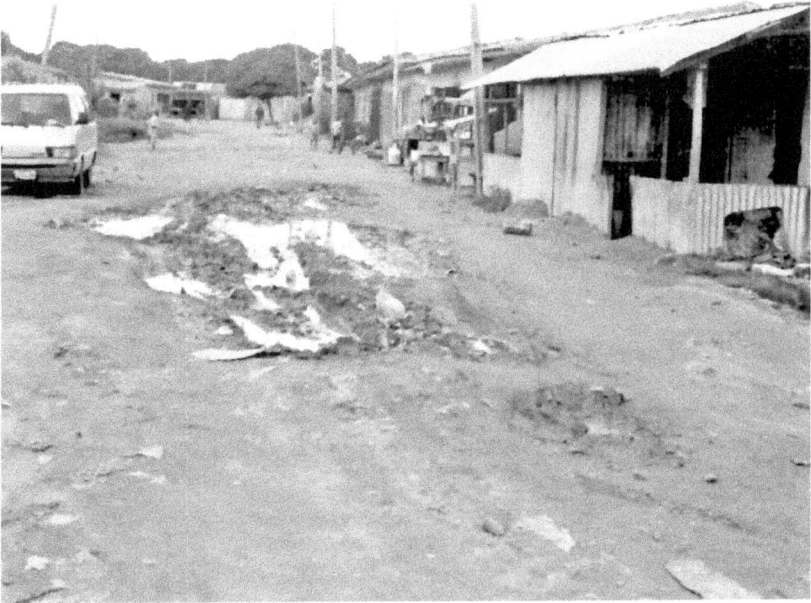

This damaged road is one of the main streets in Ungwar Sunday,
a section of Kaduna City that is populated by non-Moslems.

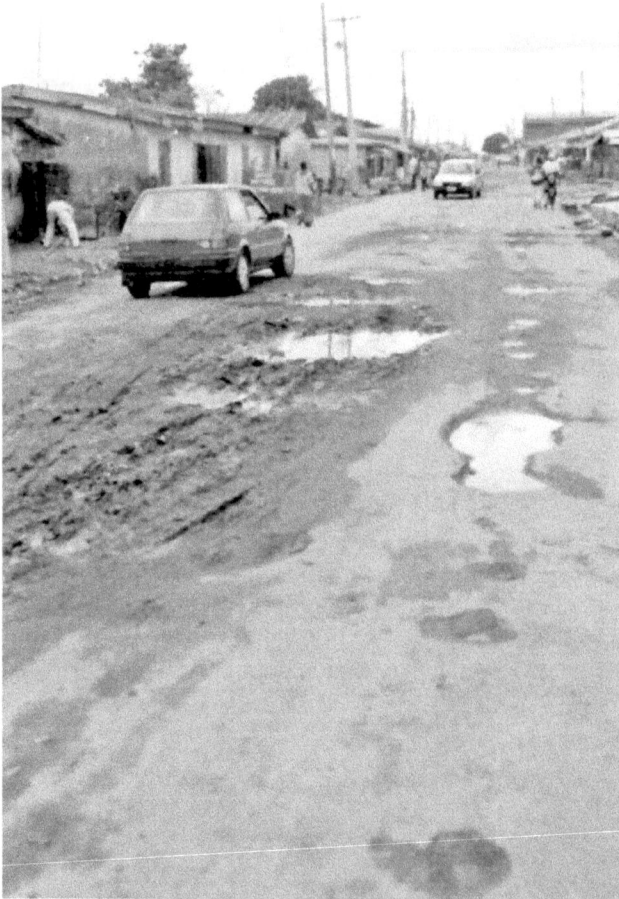

This is both an unedited picture, as well as unadulterated; it is one of the only major tarred road in Television Village, another section of Kaduna City, the capital of Kaduna State in Nigeria.
Picture by Allover Photos, U/Sunday, Kaduna, August, 2004.

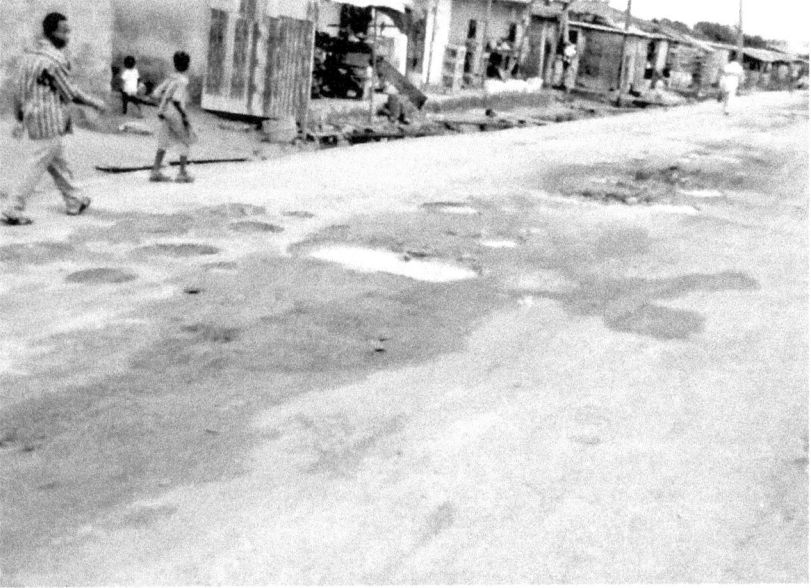

This picture, too, is of other portions of the same major road in Television Village in Kaduna City. However, what these pictures are incapable of portraying in these settings are the swampy gutters teaming with hoards of flies, (the day-time missionaries and distributers of dysentery, the killer typhoid fever and hepatitis-A, etc) mosquitoes, (the slender nightmare and night-merchants of malaria, dengue fever, etc). In dry seasons, these marshy streets turned into dry beds of ground dust powder that harbor the dangerous agent of meningitis, tuberculosis and many other deadly diseases.

The following photographs are short but also brief pictorial descriptions and or summations of the horrific life of not only most non-Moslems in Nigeria, but also some Moslems in Moslem dominated North live, day in and day out. Some of these pictures vividly capture a tale of woes that have come to symbolize and, also has become the daily portion of teaming millions of ordinary non-Moslem Nigerians.

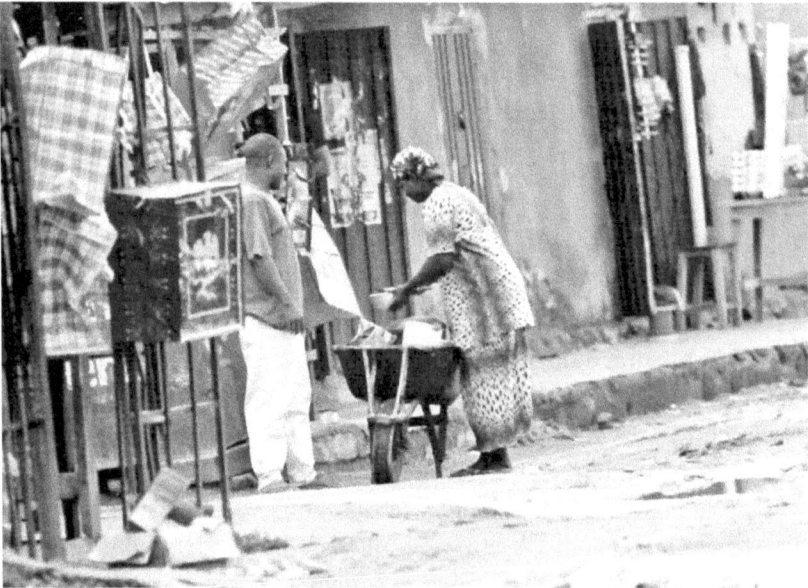

This is a side-street shopping center. Note the some of the opened shops and their wares, of all sorts, on display and for sale.

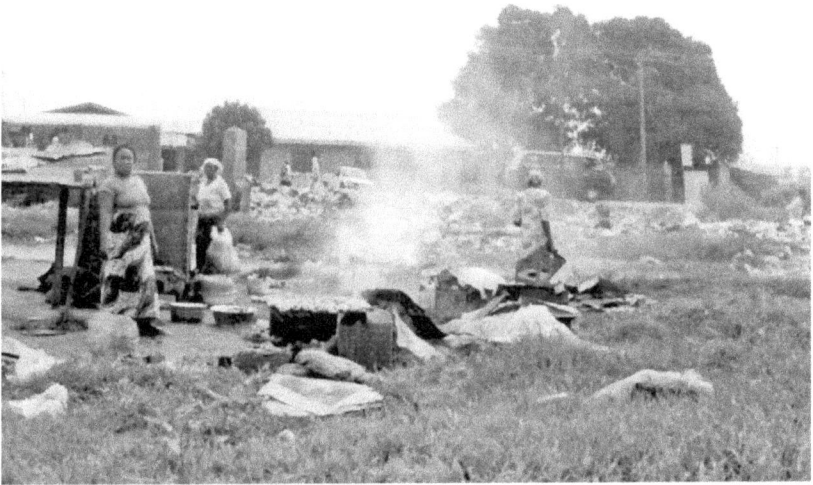

In the middle of this picture are some women getting ready, or have even started, cooking food that would be sold to the the hungry, unwary public. This food is being cooked near opened gutters and a marshy areas, that are both eye sores, are right next to a dumping ground heaving with human wastes and garbage of every imaginable variety. This time of the day, between 8 & 9 AM, catories of swarming flies are already busy investigating, sampling by trying to taste every available food sample in opened pots that contain cooked food. During the day time most mosquitoes are either in recess or in bed with wimpy brittle legs tugged under their flimsy brittle little tow-like-blade wings, as they are incapable of withstandind neither heat nor smoke from the aundant fire from these opened-air kitchens or wind; so they can only come out at night.

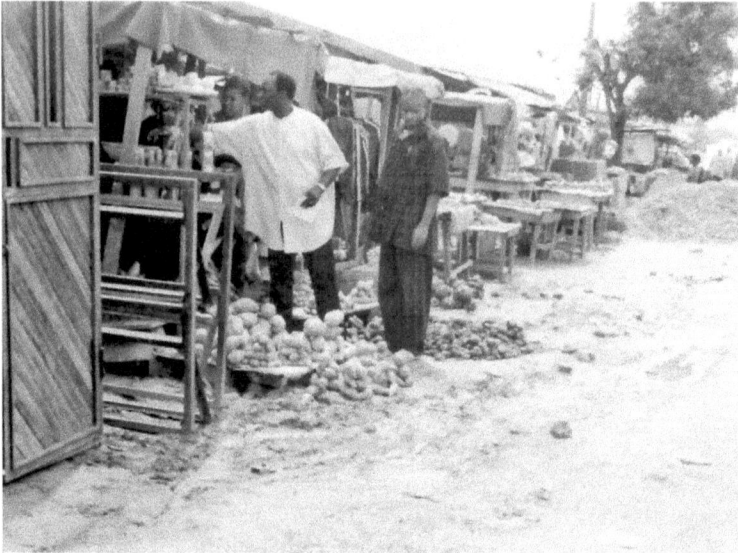

Some food racks with raw food stuffs on them and some on the ground. If not properly cooked, food prepared from this raw food stuff can easily send its consumers to hospital with a variety of illnesses including typhoid fever.

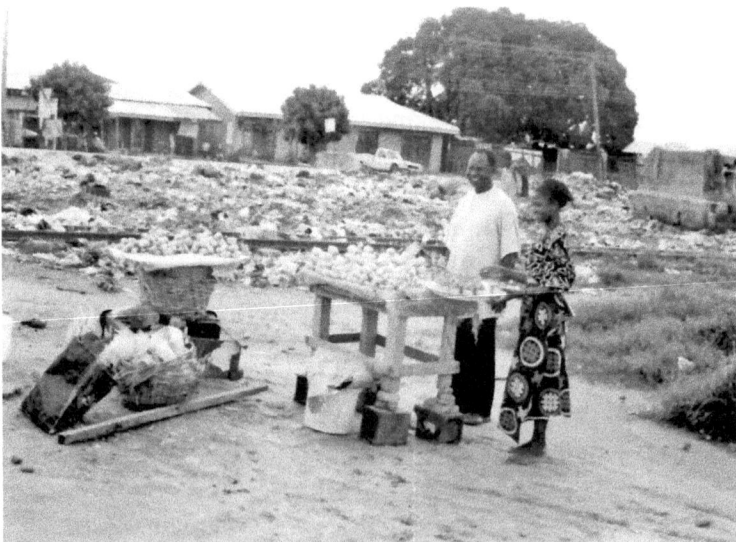

More of the same of some of these food items: fruits and tubers on sale. Some of the food stuffs will need to be Pasteurized and not just mere boiling before they are fit for human consumption by the very fact of their propinquity to the seeping dumping ground.

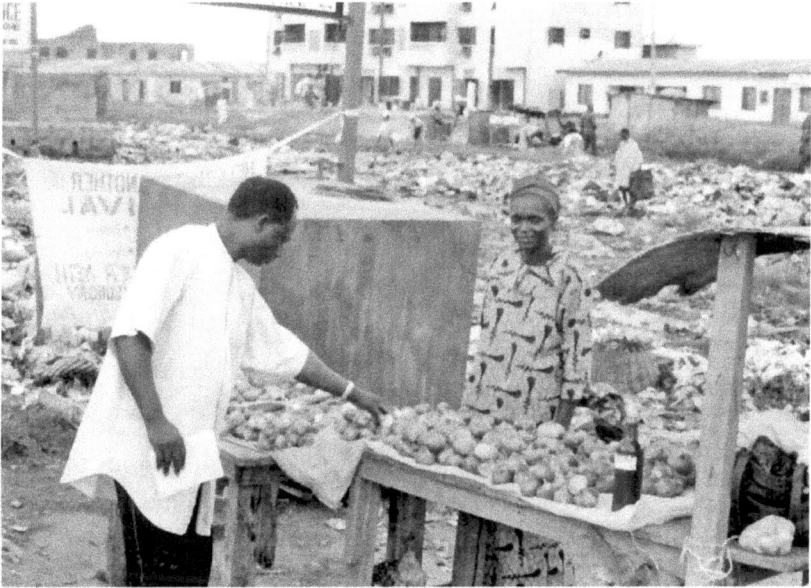

This mini-store stall and its owner (lady in the yellow dress) specializes in selling onions and, onions only, nothing else!

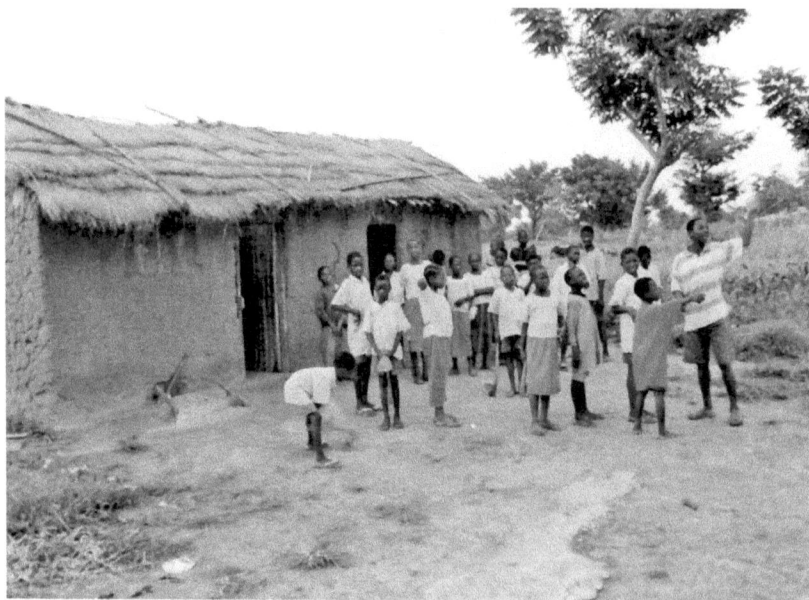

This is supposed to be an elementary school (with all the Nigerian style of an elementary-school-area trappings) in one of the villages in the outskirts on Kaduna City in Kaduna State, Nigeria—the "Giant of Africa".

In the above picture, the building with a grass-thatched roof is an elementary school building with some of the pupils out in the open field on break. In front of this school building is the play ground, but beyond it and its surroundings, are maize farms and other crops being grown; however, hidden behind the bushes and trees are village houses from which some the school pupils hail.

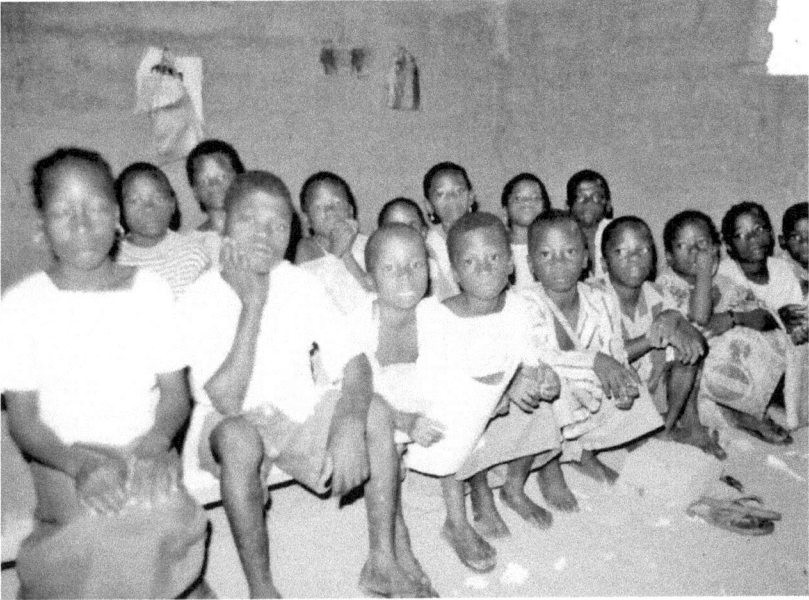

This looks classroom sitting arrangement like sardine menu, e.g. call the setting what you may, but some of the students are sharing a rough surfaced (unplaned) long plank, which serves as a "community chair" from which pupils are supposed to sit and do school work including learning! A few of these pupils are not so lucky to find a spot to sit on, so they end up sitting on the dirt floor. At the top and to the far right, on the wall is an opening that serves as a window; together with the opened door, both serve as the sources of light into the classroom and, of course ventilation for everybody!

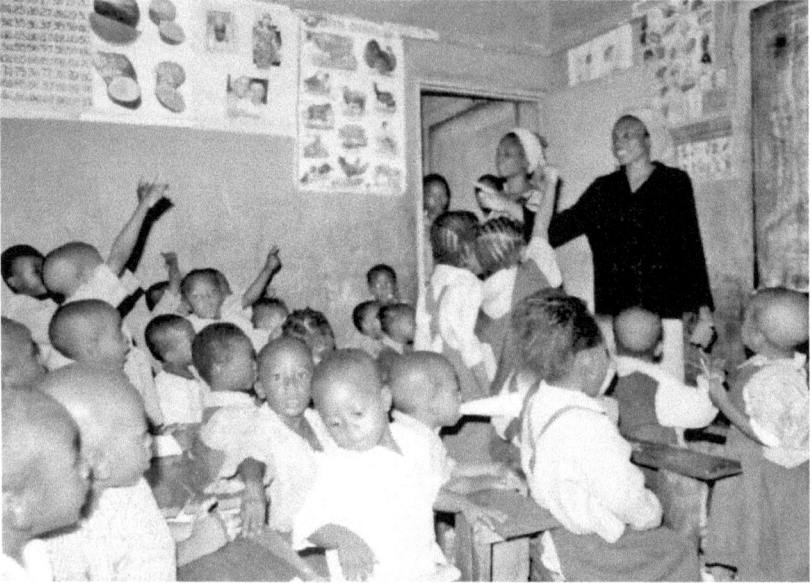

This is another angle to view this "sardine arrangement" for a school classroom. Many hands are up in the frantic attempt to try to give the correct answer to the question that the teacher has asked. Some of these bright pupils are having a heart-to-heart conversation and not giving a hoot as to what the teacher is saying. Others are in such pensive ruminations, while yet a few other are wondering: "Who's this guy and what's he doing, taking our pictures and, without our permission!"

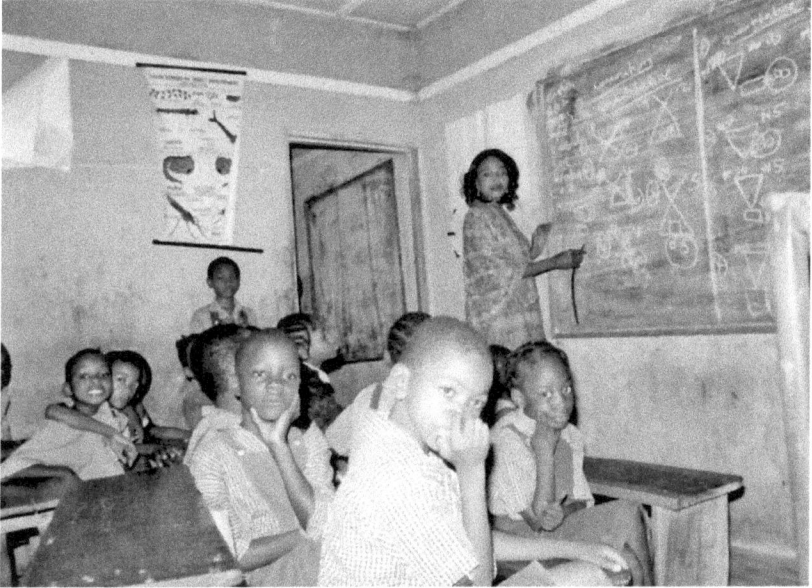

This is another classroom in the same elementary scool. This classroom is not as packed as the others within the same complex school. However, most of these pupils are more interested in the "invading photographer" than in their lesson! So is the teacher too! Incidentally!

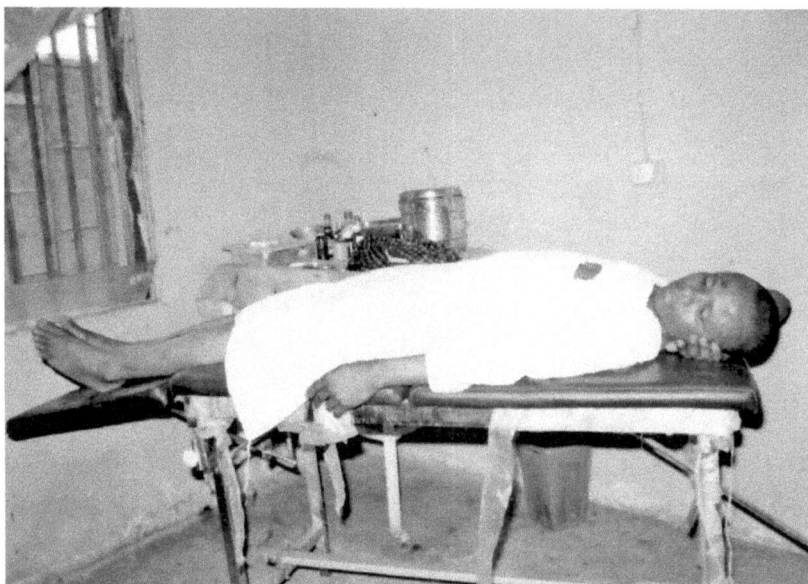

Another tale of woe! Health care and services in Nigeria are a joke!

This is a sick patient on a so-called examination table or couch. The couch is virtually an arrangement of some broken chairs thrown together with no top and a flat part of a legless or broken gurney; this was thrown together, apparently in haste, perhaps to form what now looks or resembles an examination table.

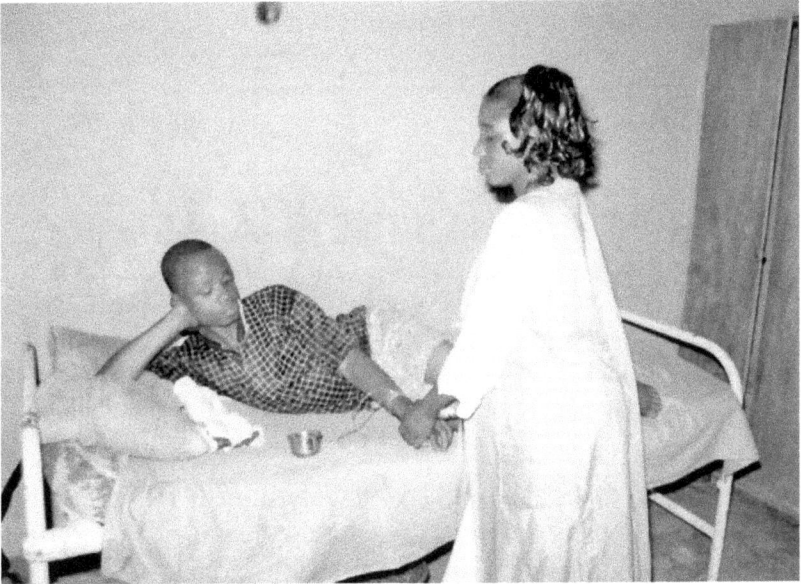

This picture is of another patient (lying in bed with his pulse being checked by) a nurse (standing at bedside). This picture was taken from one of a very few good private clinics in the City of Kaduna. However, take note of the wear and tear on the wall behind patient's bed; the many colors of the wall as a result of pilled-off paint as well as the broken-off door-frame leaning on its side.

CHAPTER SIX

HEALTH FACILITIES AND DISTRIBUTION

INTRODUCTION

There are various approaches on how to determine health needs and the direction of any society and how to adapt the health system to fit those needs, which can and should include preventive, curative approach, or a combination of the two and environmental health issues—approaches to fit patient care needs. Of extreme importance also are the issues of accessibility, affordability, since a health service that is inaccessible is also not affordable. It is based on these determinations that the model for the health system is made.

The Nigerian health system is an amalgam of all different approaches in the manner in which health care services are delivered to the Nigerian populace. However, while there have been so many changes in the health system in general, at least in some of the areas, that approach or line of argument is no longer an issue as health facilities are available, as every nook and cranny of the vast expanse of the country now has access to a health clinic of some sort.

The other two areas are environmental health and affordability, both of which remain intractably recalcitrant issues, and to deal with these effectively, stringent approaches must be applied, with diligence to both. An unhealthy environment will not go away, nor will it disappear in difference to the careless attitudes and filthy living conditions of the people who live in it. A clear example is the fact that if any environment policy exists, it is only a symbol as sanitation, and environmental practices have been reduced to mere tokenism, because there are no signs of any effort in that direction.

Similarly and with regard to the ability to afford the cost of health care services, there is no magic wand, the waving of which is able to make corruption in the health system itself go away. That ain't possible! The people that live in such an environment must show concern and then make effort to change their views, attitudes, and approaches to money and the material world.

DISTRIBUTION

Nigeria is rich with a vast array of natural resources with which it can and should be able to comfortably feed and take care of all its health and development needs of its people, but unfortunately, this is not the case. Helen Metz (1992) seems to capture this rather well in the following statement,

> In a comparison to the distribution of hospitals between urban and rural areas in 1989, Denis Ityanyar found that whereas approximately 80 per cent of the population of those states lived in rural regions only 42 per cent of hospitals were located in those areas. The mal-distribution of physicians was even more marked because four of the trained doctors who had a choice did not want to live in rural areas. Many of the doctors who did work in rural areas were there as part of required service in National Youth Service Corps, established in 1973. Few, however, remained in remote areas beyond their required terms.[1]

There are, however, two issues that Metz did not make any attempt to raise, and these are the issues of ethnocentrisms and religious bigotry, as indicated in our previous discussions. Metz may be ignorant of these two points, as they play immense roles in Nigerian politics, because she is a foreigner, a non-African, and perhaps astute in observing what she wants to observe and make notation, but not very aware of social differences that exist among Africans. According to the above excerpts, only 40 percent of doctors graduating from medical schools each year stay in the rural areas and only as part of a requirement for them to do so. This then means that 60 percent of physicians work in the cities and the surrounding suburbs, but for the government-owned health facilities in the rural areas, the government has to use incentives to improve the staffing conditions of the health care facilities in those same areas.

It has already been mentioned earlier in this chapter that the amount of money spent by the states and federal governments of Nigeria is a lot less than what the ideal should be. It is, however, adequate enough to ensure that every nook and corner of the country has a health care facility. This statement is made under the assumption of proper planning with careful evaluation, but minus factors like tribalism (ethnocentrisms), religious bigotry, and corruption as part of the consideration.

Finally, Nanguang (1980) has also made the same assertion by listing six points as areas of problems or concerns for Nigeria's health system that were identified by the Basic Health Service Scheme Manifesto in the mid-1970s. Some of the points included inadequate health facilities due to mal-distribution and poor or inadequate physician-nurse coverage of health care facilities which results in poor services to targeted populations. He also points out how the rural areas are greatly affected as a result of poor health services even though they have the highest number of the population.[2]

ROLE OF ECONOMICS

Economics plays a big part in deciding the locations of hospitals and other health service facilities in districts and localities. Economically, putting a hospital in an area with a very low population, and where its full utilization would be severely limited, is a waste of a valuable resource—qualified medical staff and other resources—that could be put to better use elsewhere and would be wasted in an area of poor utilization. Furthermore, many people in rural areas have no income and so can ill afford payment for services they are not able to pay. The cost in human suffering and lost of life is so enormously high as a consequence of poor planning and such decisions.

However, while it is clear that some of the health facilities should be built in rural areas to stave off some of these problems, yet only the facilities that are cost-effective and can meet the needs in such areas, while due diligence is applied to ensure that they are both equipped and well supplied.

Let us remember that no matter how good an idea is and no that matter how good and beneficial the outcome of such an idea, if that is racist or based on racist intentions, it is not nature that is "good enough" and, therefore, unjustified regardless of the rationale behind it.

This has been so since independence because regardless of qualification, a lopsided majority of office holders hail from certain ethnic groups (the Hausa/Fulani dyad). It is amazing that since the installation of this diabolic concept, some dominant groups have forayed savagely on the public treasury without any regard or its effects on the essential services of this country and especially the basic among which health facilities rank very high.

Helen Metz (1992), in her book *Nigeria: A Country Study*, has this to say on the distribution of health facilities in the country:

> The 1946 health plan established the Ministry of Health to co-ordinate health services throughout the country, including those provided by the government, by private companies, and by the missions. The plan also budgeted funds for hospitals and clinics, most of which were concentrated in the main cities, little funding was allocated for rural health centers.3

> There was also a strong imbalance between the appropriations of facilities to southern areas, compared with those in the north. The problems of geographic mal-distribution of medical facilities among the regions and of the inadequacy of rural facilities persisted. There were also significant disparities within each of the regions. For example in 1980, there were an estimated 2,600 people per physician in Lagos State, compared with 38,000 per physician in the much more rural Ondo State.[4]

LESS URBANIZED AND RURAL AREAS.

Metz's observation is not complete as she ignores or withholds her commentary, deliberate or otherwise, on the past legacy and policies that led to the mediocre results that we are today witnessing. Nor does she comment on the monstrosity of ethnic intolerance, bigotry, and prejudice that are tearing the country viciously apart.

STATISTICAL FIGURES

Hospitals Qualified Health Care Personnel

In the early 1950s, there were about 562 general hospitals, *16 *maternity, and/or pediatric hospitals, 11 military hospitals, 6 teaching hospitals, and 3 prison hospitals with about 44,600 capacities mostly in the Hausa-Fulani-Yoruba-Igbo (the quadruple unholy alliance of dominators) dominated areas. However, by 1987, there were about 517 hospitals, 7,910 other health facilities with 95,776 beds combined capacity,[3] all concentrated in cities and urban metropolis of the dominant tribal areas, with just token facilities and services to other areas where the major portion of the population resided at that same time period.

While the policy of maldistribution remains fairly unchanged, it is very clear from the above figures that the trends of disparity in the number of health facilities and number of hospital beds continue to increase in favored urbanized areas of the dominant tribes, which already have, at saturation levels, hospitals another categories of health facilities. Metz, conveniently, has no figures on the number of health facility distribution to rural areas, but a figure of 38,000 people per physician in rural Ondo. This is not a number anyone should be proud to report about a country with such a vast expanse as Nigeria, but just imagine that number and just quadruple it. When you do, the figure that you come up with (about 152,000) and perhaps more should, in all fairness, represent any of many rural areas in the Middle Belt section of the north per one physician at the same time period.

The issue of health care personnel is another area of mal-distribution that requires some attention here. Based on the clustering of health facilities in certain areas, which helps in understanding this situation better, is that while other areas have, from few or none, the normal expectation is that with an increase in the number of health care facilities, so is also a commensurate increase in the number of health care workers to these locations. John Bryant (1969) has this to say about it:

Most of Nigerian doctors have been clustered about the academic centers of Lagos and Ibadan. Beyond, in the far-reaching expanse of the country, a handful has tried to provide medical care. *The Northern Region, for example, a vast area with a population of about 30 million, has the thinnest of health resources: 120 doctors in the government service, 55 doctors in missions, a ratio of " . . . 1to170,000 and an annual government expenditures of cents per person."*[5] (Emphasis added).

And

in the year 1965-1966, the Northern Region of Nigeria spent approximately $14.5 million on health—about fifty cents per person. It is difficult to guess what Nigeria's expenditure on health might be in 1980. One way of arriving at it is to use the mid 1960 rate of increase in per capital expenditure of about sixty cents. Assuming the population of the Northern Region to be 44 million in 1980, the health budget would be about $26 million.[6]

Well, we now know that this estimate is wrong since it was based on the population of the 1960s. We also now know that the estimates of Nigeria's population in the 1980 were at least 80 million (*Sunday Time* newspaper, September 25, 1986), if not more. These figures, then, do negatively skew the estimated expenditure at the time, some thirty-three cents on the dollar lower, instead of sixty cents that was projected, thus making the allocated amount insufficient to spend on health programs in the 1980s and, even much less so, in the 1990s. This, of course, does not help an already bad situation as the health system is severely understaffed and also underfunded.

However, Bryant also projected that with good economic growth, the health expenditure would increase from fifty cents to one dollar.[7] But then, even with a fifty percent increase, that projected amount is instead $26 million, and the amount would be about 3.12 million naira only at rate of exchange at the time of estimate. This is still pathetically, dismally miniscule as judged by today's standards of health demands and budgets and at the same rate of exchange, and I have not yet even factored in the corruption or embezzlement factor that government officials demand. So even with this 50 percent projected increase in health budget, it remains terribly insufficient.

Based on these records and many others, it seems that health care activities—including health facilities, to the rural populations, a major section of the society by the way—have been reduced to rudiments and sketches only. Most, if not all, are unequipped and badly understaffed. Similarly, health care activities have been reduced to basics and, sometimes, not even that. No spare parts for equipments that break down; no drugs or medications are available for treatment in facilities' pharmacies, with inpatients having to buy medications outside the hospitals to be treated inside these hospitals. These are just a few of the problems of this health system.

DESCRIPTION OF THE DIFFERENT HEALTH FACILITIES IN NIGERIA

1. THE GENERAL HOSPITAL

The general hospital represents the largest segment of all health facilities, with the largest number of health workers and professionals of the entire health system. This is the case because it is in the hospital that complex procedures and all sorts of activities take place daily. The operating theater, for example, where complex procedures like brain surgeries, hip replacements, caesarian sections, deliveries, and many more procedures are done.

However, a general hospital is an exact opposite of a specialized hospital where only special procedures are done daily. For example, special eye surgeries are done in specialized eye hospital, and so are orthopedic (bone) hospitals for orthopedic conditions. On many occasions, some of these special procedures are done in general hospitals, as it is not the intention to give the impression that no special surgeries are done in the operating rooms of general hospitals and vice versa.

As a component of a health system,[9] most of the activities in the hospital are geared toward acute care, its central aim and prevention as secondary. It is not my intention to suggest that other forms of health activities do not take place in hospitals, as they very well do. However, curative activities are the main courses and the primary focus of hospitals.[8] Specialized or otherwise, other distinctions, as to the type of the hospital, include the number of beds in the hospital, its status—a teaching or nonteaching hospital, etc.

Brown and Lewis[10] have the following classification for the hospital system, i.e., whether it is a "governmental," "nongovernmental," "for profit," and "local" such as city, county, region, or multistate owned. This variety is not reflected in the Nigerian health care system and especially from the state level and below.

Of course, the state system has changed this nomenclature slightly as cities do not own or run hospital services, while local governments do and finance hospitals, as federal and state governments do, as it is reflected in chapter four of this book. In United States, for example, state and local governments control about one-third of all hospitals while the federal government operates only about 6 percent[11] of the total number of hospitals in the United States.

A hospital, therefore, can be described as a place in which medical care, social, educational, and other health care activities take place. As such, a hospital is an instrument for community health. Its functions include medical care for the sick, for all kinds of therapies: rehabilitation, education, diagnosis, prevention,[12] and research for better ways to improve health activities. It is the center of activity for the entire health system and represents the core area for medical technology trial, as it is an ideal environment to try of all such new inventions and innovation in medical technology. It also presents the doctors' ideal workshop or workplace.[13]

2. ABMULATORY CARE SERVICES

a. The Health Center
The health center and dispensary play a crucial role and very busy areas, one might add, in health activities in communities. One of the central goals of a health center is community services by nature of health care services rendered to the sick and diseased for the promotion of the general health and welfare of the public. The Milbank Memorial Fund Commission on Higher Education for Public Health succinctly captures this same sentiment by reflecting on the primary objectives in the following excerpt:

the effort organized by society to protect, promote and restore the people's health. The programs, services and institutions involved emphasize the prevention of disease and health needs of the population as a whole. Public health activities change with changing technology and social values but the goals remain the same to reduce the amount of disease, premature deaths and disease-produced discomfort and disability.[14]

Historically, the focus of public health has mainly been the control of infectious diseases with accentuated emphasis on prevention—primary prevention, that is, at both personal and communal levels. Community health services include the control of the following:

1. Communicable diseases, family and dental health services, good nutrition, and accident prevention.
2. Environmental services, including food and drinking water protection, proper waste disposal and sanitation, pest control and rehabilitation services.
3. Mental health services, including prevention, diagnosis and treatment (short-term and long-term), and hospitalization.
4. i. Personal health, which deals with the role of individuals: doing and taking responsibility for one's personal health issues, such as hygiene, diet, etc., and
   ii. Health care services, which are provided where and when individuals are incapable of doing so themselves.[15]

This particular area (as stated in 4ii) is not a plan of care for health services in Nigeria, as this has been relegated to family members and relatives or local communities as well as self-help projects.

The health center is essentially an ambulatory service program, where patients come at set periods of the day and receive care then return home. Preventive services like immunization, antenatal, pediatric and care, or maternal care services are provided. In certain settings, a few beds are available for inpatient care on a twenty-four-hour basis. However, in Nigeria, the primary focus of the health center is to improve the quality of life through primary care given by nurses and other health care auxiliaries. Infrequently, this effort may employ the services of physicians into such settings.

b. Dispensary Services

The dispensary is similar to the health center and is an extension of medical services to the rural countryside or areas with the sole aim of broadening the medical care services to the rural population.[16] The purpose of dispensary, originally, was to serve as a mini or quasi-type of a hospital to the underserved areas, as it was "intended to function primarily as a poor copy of the hospital" in that it was mainly a center for "curative" medical care, despite the fact that one of its main purposes was a preventive approach to health care center.[18] However, some will argue that the dispensary functions also as a pharmacy,[19] even though it is by far more like a hospital clinic and, less so, a pharmacy. While it has not functioned or has been used as it was originally designed to be, yet it has been the only available source of medical help and has been of tremendous relief to countless millions of rural dwellers.

c. Clinics

A clinic in Nigeria is, functionally, a miniaturized hospital where patients come for treatment either as outpatients or inpatients on a twenty-four-hour basis. It is operated or administered by either a doctor or a nurse and staffed with other doctors, nurses, and other health-assisting personnel. It is quite dissimilar to the way the American medical clinic system operates.

d. Others

Other health care facilities include such places as drugstores, patent medicine store, quack dens, etcetera, whose impact on both the economy and the health of the nation is incalculable. However, it is almost impossible to detail all the effects of these areas on the lives and livelihood of Nigerians. The reader is advised to read the daily newspapers and other periodicals that tend to report on these aspects on almost daily basis.

i. NURSING HOME OR OLD FOLKS HOME

A network of such institutions may be owned by either nonprofit or profit organizations or governmental agency. Nursing homes or long-term care facilities cater to the needs of the elderly or for the rehabilitation of long-term conditions, such as strokes diabetes and other chronic but crippling, geriatric conditions. Home health care service settings and/or hospices do not exist in Nigeria, however; but in the Muslim-dominated north, community nurses do perform health care services in accordance with Islamic customs and traditions in locked homes or *gidajen kulle* of Muslims, where married women are ensconced or locked-up women (*matan kulle*) are forbidden to come out by day, as they are prevented to have any contact with men outside family circles. This is still in practice, even now.

Nursing homes are basically institutions widely used in the care of the elderly who are unable to care for themselves in the Western culture. This form of care is almost absent in most African countries, as the care of the elderly is considered, without a question, a part of family responsibility of family members and/or other relatives. This form of institutional care flourishes in Europe, the United States, and Canada as the customs and cultural practices of Western societies differs significantly, as they are centrifugal (gravitation force or pull that separates or pulls away from group dynamic into individualism) from the African culture, which tends to be predominantly centripetal (group gravitational pull toward group-mindedness toward the center).

ii. LEPROSARIUM
This is a hospital for the treatment of leprosy patients, which is not limited to just medical treatment, but also some special surgical procedures, as well as certain rehabilitative measures, are performed in it.

iii. LEPROSY TREATMENT POST
A leprosy treatment post is similar to a clinic program or center in many ways, except for the fact that it has no beds like either a health center or hospital. This arrangement is not meant to preclude the use of beds if and when such needs do arise, as a treatment post is similar, in many ways, to a leprosarium.

iv. LEPROSY CLINIC
This is a fixed treatment center but may vary from the type of services offered. Some leprosy clinics do have a limited number of beds while others do not.[20]

v. OUTPATIENT SERVICE
This is usually a part of general hospital; and a variety of clinic systems, i.e., medical, surgical, ENT (eye, nose, and throat), pediatric clinics, etc., may be part of the outpatient department in a general hospital.

These clinics usually feed the inpatient units of the different departments of the hospital with patients as they frequently serve as emergency units as well. They may have treatment and medication, an injection room, which are all attached to them as extension areas of treatment. Usually, this has a "minor theater" or a casualty unit, which is a small surgical unit with a few beds, where simple surgical emergency procedures such as stitching lacerations after road accidents, etc., and other minor surgical cases are treated and released within twenty-four hours.

3. THE MANAGERIAL PERSPECTIVE

Management is perhaps the most important aspect of all the other parts of the health systems, and so its effectiveness or lack of it determines the success of a health facility. Failure in any aspect of a system, as indicated in the general system theory, has a telling effect on the entire organization. Put differently, the wholesomeness of any system—be that system a human body, a hospital, or any other thing for that matter—is reflected in the quality of its products. A defect anywhere in the system, without equivocation, results in less than a wholesome end product. For example, a defective liver, kidney, heart, or any other organ of the body results in a sick body whereby the performance of the body is less than optimal and, consequently, the outcome will reflect the presence of such a defect. Similarly, a defective or broken-down x-ray machine or electric generator in a hospital results in the shutdown of services that depend on the x-ray machine or electric generator. The end result is poor quality of service or the lack of it altogether. However, improvisation is an alternative that is frequently employed, but the result is usually an inferior product quality. Although this is not always the case, nor does it always follow this pattern, because an administration improvises, as such, the result is bound to be inferior and thus those in charge are incompetent. Nevertheless, this is not always the case because it—for instance, resorting to improvisation—is as a result of lack of funds to buy proper equipment for operations and if there is an emergency, improvising might save a life. However, the quality of management employed in a health care system determines the success or failure of a particular health care effort. This recognition and the meticulous attention to its basic tenet can help shape activities within the organization toward a vibrant dynamism, expansion and growth, or decline and ultimate death if the administrative tenets are not observed as the case may be. The determination to make management a panacea rests, to some extent, with the administration and also ultimately with the public, who has to insist on nothing but the very best of quality for rendered services by a health care facility. This is because it is the public that supports all the health care facilities through taxes and other revenues generated from within the society and members of the society are the objects of all health activities. Furthermore, corrupt officials must be dealt with since no amount of dexterity or administrative savvy can succeed under irresponsible, unaccountable, and uncontrollable corrupt official. An important aspect of management includes human relations or interaction with people at the workplace. Also good organization management behaviors—like discipline, research, financial management, professional ethics, but above all, moral responsibility and accountability—are all very necessary ingredients that are germane to good organizational administration.

REVIEW OF LITERATURE

The open secret is this gaping schism of disparity which exists between the health systems of developed nations and the rest of the world and the developing nations, but especially the one in Nigeria. As we have already seen, there is little doubt that in Nigeria, health facilities are concentrated in metropolitan areas, but scanty, if any, in the suburbs and even less so in the rural areas, where in so many of them, no health facility exists. This disparity is startling in the north, where in the Hausa/Fulani districts, including the normally neglected rural areas, health care facilities both exist and health care services are available to rural dwellers because of their ethnicity with Islam as the religion that dominates the culture and tradition practices.

Literature is and newspaper reports are replete with factual information about the sentiments expressed above, as it is amazing to see the lopsidedness of such behavior in a group of people profess God in every other word of their conversation, yet so disdainful by mistreating their fellow human beings created by the same God whom they claim to revere! The point is that these non-Hausa/Fulani and non-Muslims are at a great disadvantage, and the cost for such level of intentional neglect, in terms of human suffering and loss of life, is enormously humongous!

Rosenthal and Frenkl (editors, 1992) portray the clinical practices of the health professionals in international settings of the various health systems. For example, they discuss the pros and cons of the British concept of a "health practitioner," from, both private and public points' of view and or perspective, as well as the effect these have on the health system. They present salutary recommendations and what should be the expected results.[21]

Raffael and Raffael (1989), on the other hand, point out the major disadvantages for such concentrations of health facilities in areas where they are misused. They seem to stress the importance of standardizing the educational preparation for health care professionals and the management of the public health facilities that has been entrusted to their care. They also suggest ways that could improve institutions that train health professionals and how to improve and regulate professional practice.[22] J. Bryant (1969) also discusses the economic impact that would result by the proper training of the health professional and other staff and the potential that exists for reducing the currently disparities that exist.[23]

M. A. King (1960) similarly points out some discrepancies in economic and educational planning of developed nations from underdeveloped ones, which inevitably shows in the effectiveness and the qualities of both types of systems. He also suggests ways to improve the available services and preventive strategies for the poorly served areas.[24] Similarly, Helen Metz (editor, 1992), in the case study book, *Nigeria: A Country Study*, describes the problem in this manner:

> The problem of geographic mat-distribution of medical facilities among the regions and of the inadequacy of rural facilities persisted. By 1980 the ratios were an estimated 3,800 people per hospital had in the north (Borno, Kaduna, Kano, Niger and Sokoto States), 2,200 per bed in the Middle Belt (Bauchi, Benue, Congola, Kwara arid Plateau Slates), 1,300 per bed in the south cast (Anambra, Cross River, Imo, and Rivers States) and 800 per bed in the south west (Bendel, Lagos, Ogun, Undo and Oyo States). There were also significant disparities within each of the regions. For example, in 1980 there were an estimated, 2,600 people per physician in Lagos, compared with 38,000 per physician in the much more rural Ondo State.[25]

The Europa World Year Book (1994) details the history and survey of Nigeria, which includes a lot of statistical figures and surveys with important information on health budgets and their effects on health facilities' distribution and services delivered.[26]

In "Health and Development in Africa" by Internationales, Interdisciplinares Symposium (1983), figures and tables presented an attempt to describe or show the per capita allocations between the years 1962 and 1972 of the health manpower of Nigeria.[27] Abu Saad (1992), in a similar line of thought, gives a brief description of the primary as well as the expanded roles of nurses in Nigeria, which by implication shows a desperate need for physicians, who concentrate more in urban areas, but to the disadvantage of the suburban and rural areas.[28] In response to this sad state of affairs, the then minister of health, the late Dr. Ransome Kuti, in October 1986, reprimanded Nigerian physicians for failing to provide medical care in rural areas at the appointment of two health officers for the new Federal Capital Territory (FCT) of Abuja. Abuja is in the Middle Belt area and inhabited by populations of many tribal groups numbering several millions, yet until recently, it had no hospitals or dispensaries properly equipped to meet the care and needs of its population. Only two doctors and two pharmacists were recruited for this large area with such a large population.[29, 30]

Recently, in a four-series presentation, the executive editor of the *African News Weekly*, a weekly newspaper based in North Carolina, USA, Helen Okpokowuruk[31] related her experience in the hospital in Cross River State, Nigeria.[32] She recounted two emergency situations that made it necessary for her to come to the hospital for help. Helen Okpokowuruk's chilling experience[33] is a reflection of what is generally obtained across the country in all the current thirty-six states, plus Abuja the Federal Capital Territory of Nigeria.

While the mal-distribution of health care facilities and of trained medical personnel are definitely major problem areas, the scarcity or absence of medical equipment, pharmaceutical products, and worse, the callous attitude of health workers further compound the problem irredeemably down a definitely wrong path. The above paradigm strongly supports some of the observations already made and other similar sentiments also expressed elsewhere.[34] This case, as many others with similar bent, are not only true as portrayed in news media on almost daily basis,[41] but in several other sources[35] as well have commented on the sad state of the health system and health care facilities in Nigeria. Stories of hardships abound, which confirm the pathetic health situation in Nigeria. Unfortunately, no one in the government seems to gives a hoot!

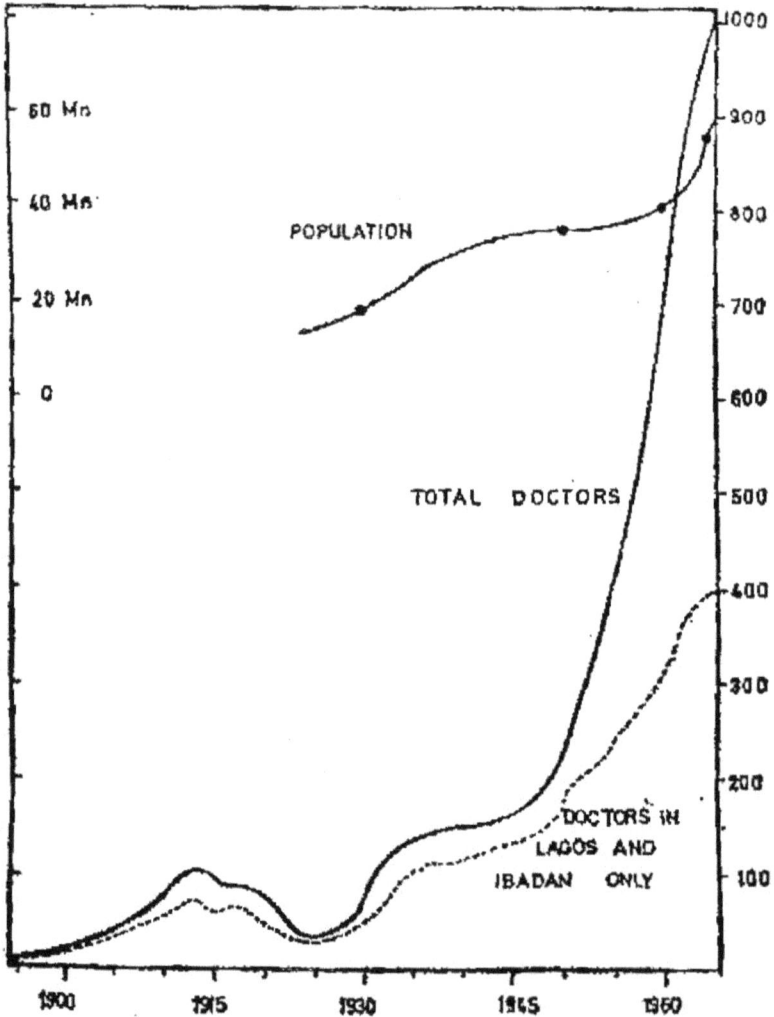

Graph: A growth in the number of doctors—adopted from Schram's *A History of the Nigerian Health Services*, published in 1971

Nigerian Health System: Efficient as Designed Or A Debacle in Shambles and Tatters?

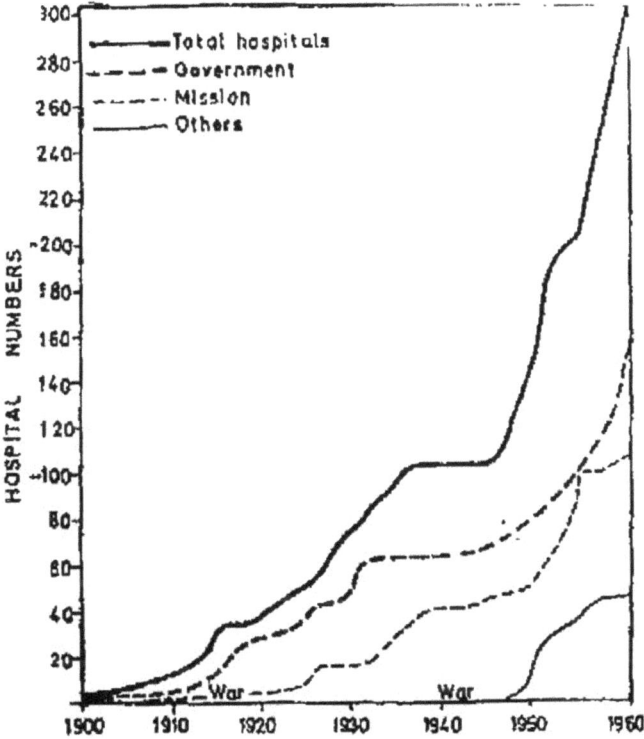

Adopted from Ralph Schram's *A History of the Nigerian Health Services*, published in 1971.

NOTES

1. D. M. Nanguang, *Causes of Problems for Nursing Administration in Nigeria* (New Orleans, Louisiana: South Western Univ., 1989), 29.
2. H. C. Metz, Nigeria: *A Country Study*, 5th ed. (Washington, D.C.: U.S. Government. Printing Office, 1992) 147-48.
3. Ibid.
4. Ibid.
5. J. Bryant, *Health and the Developing World* (Ithaca, NY: Carnell Univ. Press, 1969) 763.
6. Ibid.
7. Ibid.
8. Ibid., 262.
9. Ibid., 263.
10. Ibid.
11. M. Brown and H. L. Lewis, *Hospital Management System: Multi-Unit Organizations and Delivery of Health Care* (Germantown, MD: Aspen System Corp., 1976) 27-28.
12. S. R. McGibony, *Principles of Hospital Administration*, 2nd ed. (New York: G. P. Putnam's Sons, 1969) 6.
13. Ibid.
14. A. Kaluzny et al., *Management of Health Services* (Englewood Cliffs, NJ: Prentice-Hall Inc., 1982) 364.
15. Ibid., 339.
16. Ibid., 1-25.
17. Oscar Gish, *Planning the Health Doctor: The Tanzanian Experience* (London: Croom Helm, 1975) 14-15.
18. Ibid., 15.
19. Ralph Schram, *A History of the Nigerian Health Services* (Ibadan University Press, 1971) 349.
20. Ibid.
21. D. M. Wilner, R. P. Walkley, and L. S. Goerke, *Introduction to Public Health*, 6th ed. (New York: MacMillan Pub., 1973).
22. M.M. Rosenthal and M. Frankel, eds., *Health Care System and Their Patients: An International Perspective* (Boulder, Colorado: Westview Press, 1992).
23. M. W. Raffael and N. K. Raffael, *The U.S. Health System: Origins and Functions*, 3rd ed. (Albany, NY: Delmar Pub. Inc., 1980).

24. J. Braynt, *Health and the Developing World* (Ithaca, NY: Cornell Univ. Press, 1969).

25. M. King, *Medical Care in Developing Countries* (Lusaka, Nairobi: Oxford Univ. Press, 1996).

26. H. C. Metz, *Nigeria: A Country Study*, 5th ed. (Washington, D.C.: U.S. Government Printing Office, 1992) 1147.

27. *The Europa World Year Book* (Europa Publication Ltd., 1994).

28. "Health and Development in Africa, June 2-4, 1982" (International Interdisciplinares Symposium: Univ. Bayreuth, 1983).

29. H. Abu-Saad, *Nursing: A World View* (St. Louis: The C. V. Mosby Co., 1974).

30. F. Ramsone Kuti, "Doctors Attitude to Health Care," *Concord*, October 11, 1986.

31. H. A. Okpokowuruk, "Journey Home, Health Care in Nigeria: My Personal Experience," *African News Weekly*, vol. 5, no. 37 (October 28, 1997): 27.

32. *Today*, Saturday, August 1986, 2.

33. Ibid.

34. Ibid.

CHAPTER SEVEN

GENERAL PRINCIPLES OF ADMINISTRATION

INTRODUCTION

A good administrator with good quality of management style is the single most important person in any organization. Peter Drucker, (1974) makes this salient point on this idea when he indicates that, without management, there is no institution or organization because

> . . . management is the specific organ of the modern institution.
> It is the organ of which the performance and the survival of the
> institution depends.[1]

Good management and the effective running of a health care facility depend on the competence of its administration. In a similar manner, a facility that is successful because it provides good services, or the one that is deteriorating due to poor and inefficient services, is a reflection of good and an effective administration.

Granted all the occupations employed in the running of services are all important, but without competent administration, none of the service areas will have a real sense of direction or success in rendering the type of quality patient care that is required. Everyone in the organization must be a full participant; for that to happen, there must be a competent administration and an effective leadership style by a savvy management team (which includes middle management), or the organization, sooner or later, will fold up.

An effective administrative management that is able to control all the different parts (or occupations) of the organization to conform to organizational policies in performing tasks is able to make organization vibrant. This is usually accomplished through delegation of responsibility which is accompanied by accountability from all involved, and Raffael (1980) makes the following observation to that effect:

> . . . In practice, the hospital tends to function reasonably well, over the years accepted patterns of functioning have been agreed to so that each group knows what its role is, what its responsibilities are, and what its authority is. The medical staff, in particular, has delegated to it by the board certain professional responsibilities, and those are typically described by the medical staff by-laws, which the board had approved. *More importantly, however the smooth functioning can he attributed to improved quality of administration which come with the introduction of sound management practices and appropriately trained administrators.*[2] (Emphasis added)

Hodgetts and Cascio, (1995) agree by making this similar point in the following statement:

> . . . In modern society many jobs have become highly specialized. Large organizations are formed to produce a single product with combined efforts of thousands of workers, each with a particular skill. As a result, only as a team working together can they effectively produce a good quality product. This represents a high degree of specialization that characterizes efficient health care services. Specialized institutions are established solely for diagnosis or treatment of certain types of diseases. Some doctors specialize in the treatment diseases requiring surgery and internal medical doctors for medical situations, while others specialize in diagnostic services e.g. radiologists and pathologists etc. Many nurses specialize in a particular type of patient care such as pediatrics or intensive care. *Specialized departments within health care organization*

include x-ray respiratory therapy, physical therapy pharmacy, housekeeping, engineering and food services. Each department or specialization must have a manager to co-ordinate and direct its activities.

As you can see, management is necessary whenever there is a need to integrate, co-ordinate or direct the activities of more than one individual or group, in the health care field, many individual are in management positions and can profit from the study of health care management.[3] (Emphasis added)

Finally, John R. McGibony, (1969), in agreement with these assertions on the importance of this role in the health setting, cautions that

. . . the functions of the hospital administrator, for simplification can be roughly divided into executive, clinical and service activities. It is one of the most complex of all administrative endeavors. For one to consider it a drab and boring matter or paper pushing means an absence of appreciation of the real philosophy and function of administration. Intellectual leadership is one of the crying needs of the world of hospitals today. *No amount of technical, including clinical, competency can be applied and utilized with full vigor and force without good, practical administration which such leadership can bring.*

Even casual observation can tell us that the hospital with its departments, services, various professional groups and multiple relationships, is not the unified institution as visualized by some. It is more a collection of cells, each somewhat semi-autonomous, a hierarchy unto themselves (sic), yet all must be so organized, related and directed as to work harmoniously toward a common end. To *activities toward adequate patient care and a satisfactory level of service for the community through bring harmonious action from such groups directed efficient administration is no job for the narrow mind, the limited technician.* It requires basic understanding of principles of administration and skill in application of the administrative processes.[4] (Emphasis added)

178

2. BASIC PRINCIPLES OF ADMINISTRATION

Before getting into the basic or general principles of administration, it is necessary to mention briefly the theory of organization which has evolved over time.

The principles of management practice and theory are based on empirical (trial-and-error approach) evidence of old and past experiences of practice approaches to organization management, which we now call the classical theories. The literature, in this area or subject, first appeared early in the twentieth century in the writings of people like Max Weber, Henri Fayol, and a few other pragmatists of the period. Organizational problems, coupled with the empirical method, forced the jelling of the collective ideas and experiences of both intellectuals and manager into an administrative thought that was based on practice into a theory.[5] Interestingly enough, though, some aspects of the classical approach are still in vogue and use, while reactions to its shortcomings have led adherents to the administrative process or processes of the modern times. Needless to say, the old serves as the base for the new, and the two then become integrally intertwined[6] from the basis that form, serving as foundation for future developments and of improvement in this area of research.

A. THEORIES OF ORGANIZATION

The earliest theory of organization was perhaps first expressed by the apostle Paul and recorded in 1 Corinthians 12[*] in the Bible. And yet no organizational theory, whether classical or neoclassical, has made any reference to it, and I have my doubts that this has been pointed out anywhere in administrative picture or literature.

In this text of 1 Corinthians 12, the apostle Paul propounds the concept of the common good (verse 7) from a religious perspective, which

---

[*]   1 Corinthians 12:7, 12-27: "Now to each one the manifestation of the Spirit is given for common good—The body is a unit, though it is made up of many parts; and though all its parts are many, they form one body-Now the body is made up of one part but many—As it is, there are many parts but one body—If one part suffers, every part suffers with it-and each one of you is a part of it."

has an implied meaning that can benefit every organization, if only it can be applied to its system of operation. He explains this clearly and subsequently in the text by using the body and its parts, stating that a problem in any member or part anywhere in the body spells trouble for the entire body.[5]

1. CLASSICAL THEORY

The management of organizations has evolved over time, dating back to the early years of the last century. I, however, wonder as to what methods were used and what effects did they have on the organizations. We, however, know that at least they were functional administrative methods; for had that not been the case, how else could organization have been run and with some level of success?

Improvements and gains in management practices are, without question, based on theories that were then in effect, which were used with some success to solve organizations' problems that did emerged in the process of or running of organizations of the period. It was the process of organizational management and implementation of policies that the classical theory eventually emerged.

An effective management tool that was also used is bureaucracy, the development of which was ideal for use of classical in the process of running organizations. The main part of this theory or concept rests on the division of labor and chain of command in a hierarchical setting, uniformity of rules and procedures for all employees, bureaucratic rules and procedures in an impersonal manner, and rigidity in the bureaucratic process of hiring and firing employees.

It is noteworthy that modern methodology in the administration of organizations still employs the old device called "bureaucracy" even on a lesser scale. The classical theory is eloquently summarized by Clifton Williams (1978):

> Most organizations are strongly influenced by classical theory. Some of its assumptions are questionable, many of its principles are deficient, its assertions are too sweeping, and its application often led to undesirable results. It is, nevertheless a brilliant

expression of organization theory and a standard of reference which cannot be ignored or considered insignificant by theorists or practicing managers.[6]

In this context, therefore, the ensuing concepts and their definitions are here presented.

a. **Bureaucracy**. The term, in plain language, means "red tape" as a result of grits, perhaps even bug downs and delays in the processing of pushing papers in order to follow organization policies. Max Weber, the one who originated the application of the term to organizational process, according to Peter Bali (1950), describes it as an ideal method in business organizations, even though it does not represent the average business method or process of the period.[9] The characteristics, which include benefits of bureaucratic process, according to Weber (1952), includes the following:

i. *Division of labor*—this establishes and legitimatize official jobs and employees' performance.
ii. *Chain of command*—an official hierarchical arrangement of functions from the top to the bottom.
iii. *Uniformity of job procedures*—the criteria for each job that needs to be performed and to be governed by the same rules in every situation.
iv. *Impersonality*—applying the most impersonal perspective of the bureaucratic procedure in dealing with all employees when hiring or selecting them for new positions.[8]

b. **Classical Principles of Organization:** The major classical principles of organizational management are the following:

i. **Specialization:** The idea of specialization was first proposed by Adam Smith (the economist, not Adam Smith the inventor). Specialization deals with the mastery of one or a few tasks by specializing in a specific area, a sort of a "jack of all trade" mentality that was much pervasive at that time, a significantly different mind-set of the present of specialty orientation. In other words, an eclectic type of knowledge base, proficiency, and efficiency lead to increased production in any given area in the entire organization setup. And goodness gracious, is this idea now in vogue, even to the point of bastardization! Just imagine the hundreds and even thousands of specialties and subspecialties in all areas of disciplines, in almost every profession today, even the podiatry (foot doctoring a subspecialty of medicine has subdivided into manicurist), all in the home of specialization!

ii. **Departmentalization:** This means the grouping of specialized areas together based on function. For instance, in a teaching hospital, the department of surgery assumes responsibility for all surgical issues, including the training of professionals and paraprofessionals in that area. An important aspect of departmentalization is the benefit of a specialized training, which professionals and paraprofessionals get from such an arrangement.

iii. **Span of Control:** This refers to a limited number of levels of subordinates that any supervisory level or management can effectively supervise. There is debate as to the actual number that this should be; but there is also a general agreement, by most theorists, that this number should not exceed eight people at any given level or tier, at the very maximum. Generally speaking, and with all practical considerations, the fewer the number, the better for a supervisor. Interestingly, though, there is a difference between "a span of control" and "a span of responsibility" in the principles of management, which Joseph Massie and John Douglas (1977) argue are essentially different with the latter as bigger in scope than the former.[9]

iv. **Authority and Responsibility:** Authority connotes power—the weight or influence which accompanies a position that allows the subject of an office to perform his or her prescribed duties as defined in job description, as well as defined by policy and procedure of the organization. Responsibility, in this context, denotes to the subject and the power and ability to command and enforce his or her authority. Put differently, it means legitimate authority for a superior to command and to be able to enforce policy decisions on subordinates in their job performance and expect compliance. This classical principle incorporates the idea that implies the existence of equality between the administrative responsibilities and the authority to carry out described duties.

v. **Delegation:** This refers to the assignment of tasks or duties to subordinates by a superior in order to expedite the accomplishment a specific goal, but within the broad frame of the organizational goal and objectives, ultimately. Delegation is especially expedient in complex organizations that are laden with bureaucratic processes. It facilitates freedom and allows the administrator to attend to those matters that require his/her personal attention, that is, matters that cannot be delegated to anyone.

vi. **Unity of Command:** This is a principle of linear relationship, in a scalar setup, where a subordinate takes orders from only one superior and no more.

ISSUES WITH THE CLASSICAL THEORY

The major problems of the classical theory include neglect of the human element in the organization, and it does not factor in the changing nature of environments around organizations or that of the workers. Therefore, bureaucratic organizations have difficult characteristic for these types of setups, as they usually face in the process of running their programs. Furthermore, there is the constant facing of the problems of inaccessibility of top management level by the lower levels of workers. Another aspect is the intransigent formality of procedures. This, in some instances, leads to increased specialization, which frequently leads to confusion and dissonance between certain formalities with organizational goal and objectives, which usually are detrimental to the latter of the two.

B. THE NEOCLASSICAL THEORY

From the 1940s to 1950s, research work was carried out on the basis of the classical theory and its underlying assumptions about the human behavior. This then became the cornerstone, the foundation if you will, of the classical theory. The main premise of the neoclassical theory is the assumption with some level of consideration for employees and how to manage human behavior at the workplace. This is called the X and Y theory, postulated by Douglas M. McGregor[10] and summarized in the following manner:

1. *Theory X.* This holds that there is an inherent aversion to work by the average person, who will avoid it if and when possible. This, therefore, makes it necessary to use control mechanisms, like threats, coercion, or on occasions, force in order to achieve organizational goal—productivity; and that an average individual has an inherent

desire to avoid work and responsibility, has little or no ambitious drive, and so would rather be directed.

2. *Theory Y*. This theory holds that the effort to perform physical and mental work is as natural as play and rest and that people will self-direct as well as control him/herself, with some effort directed toward areas of interests and goals that appeal to them, that the commitment to objectives is associated with reward, that the average individual under normal conditions seeks and will accept responsibility, and finally, that the ability to activate great imagination and creativity in solving organizational problems is high in the general population.

To some degree, both theories apply to the management of organizations as well as to some aspect of employee behavior. In other words, none is completely true and none is absolutely wrong either.

Other neoclassicists like Abraham Maslow's and Frederick Herzberg's work on human behavior will not be covered here but are just as well very important nonetheless. Their work on human behavior, but especially on motivation in organizational settings, will be explored further in the following chapters.

C. MODERN THEORY

The modern theory is not separated from the classical or neoclassical theory and interacts with the two since it is itself in a state of transition. The principal distinguishing features of the modern theory are the following:

1. It focuses more on the organization, as is the case of the general system theory which integrates all parts that are unrelated to work in an interrelated manner as one system. This usually is not the case with either the classical or the neoclassical theory, nor is it even with the modern theory. The maxim that a "system is more than the sum total of its parts, applies here, but particularly in this context, as it is the entire system, the sum total of all functioning parts, that produce or meet organizational goal, not individual parts functioning separately.

2. The structure of an organization depends on its environment and, particularly, all things being equal.[11]

ADMINISTRATION

Literally, the meaning of this word, *administration*, actually means the processes of managing the business of an organization or group of people so charged with developing and ensuring that all processes in the organizational setting working as designed.

The terms *administration* and *management* are usually used interchangeably; and administration is charged with establishing policies for the organization, while the determination, execution, and evaluation of the organizational policies is the domain of management.[12] Peter Drucker, (1994) indicates that

> the manager always has to *administer*. He has to manage and improve what already exists and is already known. Re has to be an *entrepreneur*. Re has to redirect resources from areas of low or diminishing results to areas of high increasing results. Re has to slough off yesterday and to render obsolete what already exists and is already known. Mc has to create tomorrow.

> In the ongoing business markets, technologists, products and services exist. Facilities and equipment are in place. Capital has been invested and has to be serviced. People are employed and are in specific jobs and so on. The administrative job of the manager is to optimize the yield from these resources.[13] (emphasis added)

H. S. Rowland and Beatrice L. Rowland (1984) indicate also that the administrator of an organization generally oversees all the activities that take place within the organization by ensuring that policies are interpreted and implemented by all employees correctly.[14]

Management, according to Peter Drucker, (1974) is useless in and of itself if it is separated from the organization in which it is meant to operate.[15] R. M. Hodgetts and D. M. Cascio, (1993) refer to management as a complex

185

process and an instrument for getting goal-directed work done through other people.[16]

Finally, Levey and Loomba (1984) describe an administrator as someone who guides the implementation of organizational policies, not their formulation, while the manager is concerned with the policy formulation and its appropriate implementation. Peter Drucker (1954) was the first to coin the term *management* by objective.[17]

D. MANAGEMENT BY OBJECTIVES (MBO)

Management by objectives is a control mechanism for operations in the organization meant to ensure that the policies and planned programs are being implemented appropriately. They are a source of motivation for employees as their standard of work measures up to the set goals of organization in each section.

There are three main areas that are central to the administrative process, which are specific to the mission and clearly aimed at the existence of the organization. The mission or main purpose of the organization is production, social responsibility within time constraints. The following discussion will elaborate on these concepts and their function in the administrative process. In management by objective, the employee discusses and defines his own objectives in terms of his supervisor's set goals and objectives, sets standards for reaching set targets and then determines the results.

a. Mission and Purpose

Everything created in life, from the single-cell amoeba to the galaxies has a purpose. Each and everyone was also created equal, has a system with objectives that propel him or her to function toward a set purpose and goal. Purpose and mission are literally one and the same concept that summarizes the goals and future of the organization. The main reason for a mission statement is to give the organization a clear focus and motivation. For instance, a mission statement might read something like this:

> ... The mission of the hospital is to provide health care in
> an ethical, professional and holistic manner for all patients,

inpatients, as well as ambulatory patients. Proficiency by all employees will be maintained through continuous in-service programs and other such efforts. The hospital is of the expressed philosophy for a fair and equal treatment to both patients and employees. This philosophy and other concurrent objectives are clearly stated in the hospital information and employment manuals. Each department or unit will have its own philosophy and objectives that are consonant with the expressed purpose of services therein rendered. All objectives will, on a continuous basis, be evaluated and a written statement of progress is to be sent to the administrators' office by the end of every January.*

Of course, the statement of mission will vary from organization to organization, depending on the nature in which business that the organization is engaged.

b. Productivity
Peter Drucker (1974) argues that the one and only true resource for all human institutions is the human labor, without which no organization can exist or operate. People perform the work that translates into the commodity of production, therefore, so making productivity the central function of all organizations.[18]

c. Social Responsibility
Peter Drucker states that all organizations or businesses are organs of the society:

> ... They do not exist for their own sake, but to fulfill a specific social purpose and to satisfy a specific need of society, community, or individual. They are not ends in themselves, but means. The right question to ask in respect of them is not, what are they? But, "what are they supposed to be doing and what art their tasks?" Management in turn, is the organ of the institution. It has no function itself, indeed, no existence by itself. Management divorced from the institution it serves is not management.[19]

---

* Author of this sample of mission statement is unknown.

The same argument applies to all business and social institutions in the society. Apart from the society, organizations cannot exist, but they may also cease to exist, should they fail in the mission of service to the society within which they operate. Therefore, organizations exist at the behest and benefit of society (the altruistic aspect) at the local, international, or global levels. They thrive only when they service those needs that have been prescribed by society, which necessitate and justify their existence; otherwise, they cease to be of value and so fold up, either gradually or abruptly. It is to this end, therefore, that it behooves organizations to focus on the goals that constitute their responsibility to the society by considering the needs and concerns of the immediate communities in which they are located.

d. Time

Time is an essential element which figures prominently into the administrative process with every required activity based on its own rights. For a better administrative perspective, valuable time is saved when responsibilities that need to be delegated are so done, and those that required the personal attention of the administrator are carried out in such a manner accordingly.

The general principles of administration will be discussed in the following paragraphs. The purpose of these principles is to give the administrator or manager guidance in the effort to stir the proverbial "ship" of the organization in the right direction. As Troyer and Salman (1986) adequately put it, the administrator is responsible for the proper policy implementation and intelligent use of its limited resources every day.[20] The description of hospital administration as they portray it summarizes the role of administration in this manner:

> ... It is the CEO who is responsible for installing and maintaining the controls to ensure that the established standards of patient care and safety are enforced, given the quality of available medical and supporting staff. In a word, the CEO is the manager of the hospital, bearing the heavy responsibility of establishing and maintaining an organizational structure that is both effective and efficient.[21]

F. CHIEF EXECUTIVE OFFICER (CEO)

The CEO is essentially in the same position as the administrative officer, general managing director, or president of the organization,[22] as these terms are all used interchangeably.

The previous concepts and administrative activities or processes have been discussed in the foregoing pages in addition to the basic principles of administration. Since each organization has its own mission statement, goals, and objectives or op-docs,* staffing needs, management styles, public need(s) to service, and a plethora of other variables—all of these impinge administrative duties.

1. Planning
It is the most important part of all administrative functions and responsibilities. It is future oriented and, as such, bears heavily on forecasting in decision-making process. It deals with the whys, the how, the why-not, the what, whereas, and the now ifs, etcetera, in all organization, which pertain to meeting organizational goals. Planning enables the administrator to select and plan appropriate steps for activities for the institution. The planning process is organized by selecting objectives, making appropriate policies for programs, procedures, and the necessary guidelines toward the realization of the overall goals and objectives of the organization.[23]

2. Organization
This refers to the formation and grouping of functions into working systems within the organization. This entity is distinct from all the other structures and their processes, whether internal or external to the organization. It determines administrative responsibilities, designs all levels of work within the circumscribed borders of the organization. It is concerned with hiring staff and filling available positions with skilled

---

* The word *op-docs* stands for "operating documents" for an organization. This term was coined by Dr. Barbara Stephens, chairperson of the Department of Nursing Teachers College, Columbia University, New York City, in I 9~Q. Dr. Stephens is a prolific writer in her area of expertise.

staff. Organization then is the art of putting together separate departments or parts and making them function as a united entity. As it has already been pointed out, policies designs, and others are under the purview of enforcement of the administrative role, which ensures that the goals and objectives of the institution are met in a timely manner. Failure in this respect is usually inimical to the very survival of the organization. This is especially so when the goals of the different departments within the organization are at variance with the overall goals of the institution.

3. Staffing

Making organization work effectively does not end with pulling all the physical mechanisms together, such as buildings and machinery, into one place. It entails more than that, for example, it requires recruiting skilled and qualified personnel to run departments, which are all very important or the organization is doomed.

If, for instance, there are no people to run the departments, units, and programs; but even if robots were to do those duties, someone in the final analysis, a person, would have to at least inspect to assure that processes are running correctly to ensure that the final outcome is the right product. An appropriate technique of personnel administration must also be a factor in the general and overall organizational setup,[24] if the organization will be successful in a world of reality.

4. Budgeting

This is another very important part of the responsibilities of administration. It includes cost analysis and the expenses of equipment, supplies, repairs, and other miscellaneous items atop the capital budget. Good budgets always have provisional funds for contingencies of the unanticipated, such as inflation, increased living expenses, and similar problems.[25]

5. Logistics

Procuring supplies from both dependable as well as irregular sources is another administrative duty that requires diligence, scrutiny, and intelligence, whether this concerns the supply of drugs, detergents, produce, or whatever. Each item may be procured either on a prearranged basis, such as periodic deliveries to a designated area—i.e., an area of need—or to a centrally controlled storage area where these items will be handy and ready to be dispensed to units from central supplies for use.

6. Coordination

The coordination of programs, activities, or projects is another angle through which interdepartmental programs are harnessed and executed effectively.[26] The degree to which the personnel is supervised may differ from unit to unit and individual to individual. This is so because some people require constant surveillance while others may need it sparingly. The policy, procedure, and process of supervision can and do vary from organization to organization, just as the extent and need for these processes vary from person to person. Any of the three styles of leadership—authoritarian, democratic, or laissez-faire[27] can be used as judge appropriate by the upper and middle management levels.

7. Records and Reporting

Some form of records of all procedures is kept by making it possible for report and inspection by regulatory authorities at regular, specified times. These are a form of control to be able to gauge the direction of activities, detect problems, and ensure that some redress or resolution is available. So doing ensures progress toward the organization's mission measurable by its overall goals. Records on policy, procedures, accounts, and fiscal matters are absolutely essential to all organizations regardless of the type of organizations.

8. Consultation

This is akin to supervision except that consultation deals mainly with the technical performance whereas supervision offers both but also ensures, on a regular basis, that a variety of activities are done correctly. Simply put, supervision may offer both technical advice in problem situations and direct behavior toward productivity. Consultation, on the other hand, is strictly a problem-oriented activity, which can be both highly technical and specialized, either for an individual, a group or groups on a regular and/or sporadic basis.

9. Directing

Directing means guiding and/or directing a program and its activities in a particular direction and/or setting. It is closely tied to planning and organizing functions by the administrator. Moreover, it is also associated with the style of leadership (authoritarian, democratic, or laissez-faire)[28] exhibited or exercised by the administrator. Communication, motivation, and delegation are important elements and tools of management.

10. Controlling

The main purpose of control is to ensure that the "goods are delivered" or the product is not only finished, but done so in a timely manner in terms of employee performance. This is compliance with the expressed mission statement of the organization to effectively control the standards and measurement of those set standards.

Control is primarily directed toward people, their behavior at the workplace, in relationship to the machines.[29] It also means the effective manipulation of external forces, like the financial lending institutions in procuring low interest rate for loans and other public resources, i.e., political groups, governmental agencies, etc. Lobbying and negotiation methods, for instance, are ways used for more revenues to the organization. These avenues help to get funds for expansion, benefits, and other hygienic factors to employees in improving their working conditions.[30]

11. Evaluation

This refers to appraisal or assessment of policies, programs, and procedures put into place for the expressed purpose of

    a. Making the system work, and
    b. Achieving the goals and objectives of the organization.[31]

When these are done well, then the organization's mission would have been met. This process is achieved by the following:

i. **Monitoring the System and Its Product.** This serves as a control and feedback mechanism, i.e., a high-quality product means that the system, its policies and all the control mechanisms, are working well and need to be maintained. It also means that the processes of the system do not need radical changes, but gradual steps to make sure that quality is maintained in order not to reduce the quality of the product.

ii. **Continuing Evaluation of Policies and Procedures.** Monitoring constantly requires the awareness of environmental changes; it is a crucial element in the survival of organizations. Economic, social, and other regulatory changes are frequently imprecise and, at times, springing up unawares that infringe on the organization without warning. These changes must be met with quick responses by an administration that is astute and knows how to "roll with the punches."

iii. Understanding the historical, social, economic, and political environments that encamp organizations is a factor in the daily thinking of all astute administrators, who monitor the performance of their organization on a daily basis.

iv. **Records** and **reports** system are factors that make the evaluation process easy and also help stem the tide of abnormalities and irregularities that can prove dangerous to organizations. Any problem in any of these areas should be considered a potential threat to meeting organizational goals that should promptly be addressed.

v. **Supervision** and **consultation** with employees usually lead to early identification of behaviors inimical to the goals of the organization. These enable the management to learn enough time to initiate corrective measures early. When detected, it is dealt with swiftly. All these are methods of evaluation that can, directly or indirectly, be applied to ensure the smooth running of an organization.

12. Contingency Plan

This refers to a plan that can be used in the advent of a major change or emergency. It is a plan that can easily replace the strategic plan that is operation. Rackich, Longest, and Darr, (1992) suggest that it can be used in a specific emergency situation[32, 33] or in an MBO style of management method, according to Norman Metzge, (1981).[34]

13. Managerial Roles

Other administrative responsibilities include leadership qualities such as acting as a leader, a figurehead without the real power accorded the office. The person in this position only act by performing ceremonial duties, which are also roles that the manager plays. Managers act as liaisons within the organization as well as with outside organizations; they monitor and disseminate information in the organization. Furthermore, the manager acts as a departmental spokesperson by playing the role of entrepreneurial decision-maker for the organization by handling disturbances and effecting corrective measures, allocating organizations' resources to its various departments, and conducting negotiations on the behalf of the organization with all outside authorities.[35, 36]

C. THE APPLICATION OF ADMINISTRATIVE PRINCIPLES IN THE HEALTH CARE SETTING

Before discussing the above topic, let us first consider the dynamics of a health system. Components include the historical, political, economic, socio-cultural, developmental, environmental, and organizational policies, programs, and administration.

1. A Historical Perspective

The aphoristic statement implying that "ignorance is bliss" is never tenable or true even today. If this were ever true, then earthquakes would only strike people that are aware. By the same token, nobody should again die from any disease or accidents, simply because most people most of the time are ignorant about these things and when they take place before they even happen. It is, indeed, a wishful thinking on the part of anyone to think that way. This assumption has a stack of empirical evidence that has been repeated time and again and has been proven such beliefs to be unrealistic.

Ignorance is not bliss either; otherwise the lessons of diseases and deaths that have been foisted on humanity, time after time and from time immemorial, need not have been repeated, since only one such a lesson needed to be given to suffice. All the repetitions point not only lack of knowledge, ignorance, if you will, but also the resistance of the human mind to learn from past mistakes. People right now still die of typhoid fever, measles, accidents, and so on, even after knowing how to avoid these killer situations. The experiences of the past have served only as reminders, not as preventers of the hideous past encounters to prevent future repetition of some of the same mistakes. Milton Roemer (1991) aptly echoes such a sentiment this way:

Those who do not know the past are condemned to repeat it.

History is not only a matter of the record of the past but also of the present, and while the gift of prophesy is the domain of prophets, the gift of science and of interpreting events is up to us in the now and present time to benefit by preparing for the future.[37]

2. Policies and Political Impact

Politics play an important role in the determination and self-direction of every social system. Many a times, politics impacts positively the health care system in Nigeria, but at other times, it does so negatively.

The War Against Indiscipline (WAI) of the Buhari-Idiagbonic era, for example, had a positive impact in many social services and, in the economic sphere as well, in Nigeria that the differences witnessed before and afterward were just simply glaring. There were queues everywhere and every social service, including health care services, when people had to wait their turns for needed services. The greatest benefit, however, was observed in the management of health care facilities in the country, as care providers showed up for work punctually and all the time and performed the work that they were employed and paid to do. Equipment, supplies, and other necessities which professionals needed to work with stayed exactly where they were placed; none developed legs to enable them to disappear mysteriously. Pharmacies had drugs inpatient units had the necessary materials to do patient care with, including medications to serve patients.

3. Economic Level

The fundamental that underlies the viability of all social systems, including human governments, is a strong economy. Milton Roemer makes the following summation:

> . . . Most fundamentally, the economic level of a country determines largely, although not entirely, its ability to generate resources for the health care whether it is done by governmental or private educational institutions. In fact, the high cost of modem medical education has made the great majority of medical schools in nearly all countries dependent on government for their support. This is true whether the schools and their parent universities are sponsored entirely by government or sponsored by private bodies and subsidized with public grants.[38]

This and many other examples make it abundantly clear that there is a specific role for economics in the health system setup, as is clearly exemplified by the United States health system with its "better to none" care services arrangement.

However, a salient point raised by Roemer is the cost of health care, which depends on the economy, with government and private enterprises sharing that cost. In Nigeria, not only is the high cost of training medical personnel born by the government alone, but so also is the high cost of running health facilities. It is, therefore, little wonder then that the health needs of the people are not being met since the responsibility of health cost (namely, employees' salaries and the infrastructures, e.g., building, equipment, and drugs, which are always unavailable) is born largely by government.

4. Socio-cultural Development

The socio-cultural aspect of a society influences the health system and the way that services in it are delivered, even more so than the economic impact. Sure, the economy enables and maintains the viability of services, but so are the socio-cultural aspect—namely, values, religion, tradition, customs, environment, politics, etcetera—determines the type of policies by the types of laws that would regulate the system.

And Milton Roemer summarizes the idea in this manner:

> ... The social influences, historical, economic, political, and cultural are obviously intermeshed, constantly changing, and operating in different ways at different times and phases. They combine to shape the character of the health service system one finds in each of the approximately 140 nations of the globe.[39]

5. Organizational Policies and Programs

There must be harmony between the institutional policies and the norms of the society; otherwise, the health facility within that would cease to exist. Furthermore, not only there must be harmony between the two, but the health institution must satisfactorily service the needs so specified by communities within that society.

6. Management

The important role that the management plays in health facilities is indisputably apparent. An effective management results in an effective health organization, which meets the demands of its community. With society's needs satisfied, there is in turn more demand for its services and an increase in services programs.

This cycle, in effect creates more need and becomes a vicious circle, i.e., demand for more services due to an increased in patronage. However, if the management is a flop, then, the reverse of the above description will be the ultimate result, that may eventuate in the demise of the organization.

7. Regulations and Legislation

These are both a part of the political process and so the socio-political aspects of culture. They are also very important as they play significant roles in the society. Laws affect all the social institutions and regulatory systems of the society equally, if not, they should be.

a. Regulations stipulated by law become the responsibility of management in health facilities to ensure conformity to laws of the society by developing organizational policies that would meet the demands laid down by the law.

Regulation concerns surveillance of organizational activities by governmental agencies and authorities with such a responsibility of state-owned health facilities. Regulatory concerns may cover environmental issues, i.e., waste and chemical wastes disposal from hospitals and industries like the pharmaceutical companies, etc.

b. Legislation by state and federal governments, directly or indirectly, affect the health care industry.

8. Administration

It was Oliver Shelton (1930) who aptly describes the interrelationship between the administrative and the institution being managed:

> . . . Management proper is the function in industry concerned in the execution of policy, within the limits set up by administration, and the employment of the organization for the particular objectives set before it. Organization is the process of so combining the work, which individuals or groups have performed with the faculties necessary for its execution that the duties so formed provide the best channels for the efficient, systematic, positive and coordinated application of the available effort. Organization is the: formation of an effective machine, management of an effective direction. Administration determines the organization management uses it. Administration de lines the goal, management strives toward, organization, is the machine of management in its achievement of ends by administration.[40]

Simply put, management is the tool and authority through which administration uses to accomplish organizational goals. The organization of the hospital as an institution remains essentially the same as other enterprising organizations with the following division of labor:

1. Board of Governors/Trustees

This is the general governing organ and the locus of authority, the highest administrative body in the organization with an overall long-term policy formation. Its membership varies but comprises of physicians and prominent people in the community. Usually, the hospital administrator is a member of this body.

2. Administrator/Chief Executive Officer

The administrator or CEO or managing director is the administrator for the hospital who sees to the design and execution of policies of the hospital organization. The board of governors appoints the administrator who is given authority to manage the organization; establish the mission statement, goals, and objectives; plans and directs the execution of policies; coordinates services; and controls all other activities. Of course, the administrator can and should delegate authority to his subordinates to perform some, if not all, of these duties, as it is not at all possible for one person to do it all on his/her own. The board of governors and administration constitute the membership of executive at this level of management.

3. Lower Management and Supervisory Level

The lower managerial and supervisory levels are actually considered commonly known as the middle management.

a. The **department heads**, vice and associate vice presidents of services, fall into this category. It is to them that the administrator delegates duties and the running of day-to-day services that the hospital delivers. This group is responsible to the administrator for enforcing policies, seeing to it that procedures are developed to conform with hospital's policies and the law of the state or land. They are also responsible for formulating departmental policies, hiring people with appropriate skills to staff the various units, budgeting for all departments and staff discipline, etc.

b. **Supervisors**, program **coordinators,** and **unit managers** are the next group down the scale and are responsible for the actual execution of programs in delivering care services. Any one filling any of the positions in this group must have the clinical savvy in that particular area and must also be holding any of the other offices in the higher levels. The hiring and disciplinary action may, as it is usually done, be referred to the superior by his/her superior in that department. In addition to the previous responsibilities are evaluations, promotion, and the determination of the kinds of incentives or remuneration method to be used, but in accordance with institutional policy, for employees and other delegated duties given by the CEO.

4. Staff

Although this term is a misnomer, as its appropriate meaning comes from the organizational structure and relates to authority and relationship with other employees on a horizontal plane. However in this context, it refers to the ordinary employee who is responsible for giving the actual health care may mean a doctor, a nurse, or a laboratory technician, etc.

Line authority is another aspect of the structural relationship within the organization,[46] referring to authority in a vertical or perpendicular plane from the superior to the subordinate. Staff relationship, for instance, in a linear line relationship—the director of nurses delegates authority to the nursing supervisor and the supervisor to the head or charge nurse who in turn directs the staff nurse.

Staff relationship, on the other hand, is something similar to that of the chief of surgery delegating to the unit chief or team leader, who in turn directs the inter-unit operations. The leader directs the residents and medical students rotating in that unit.

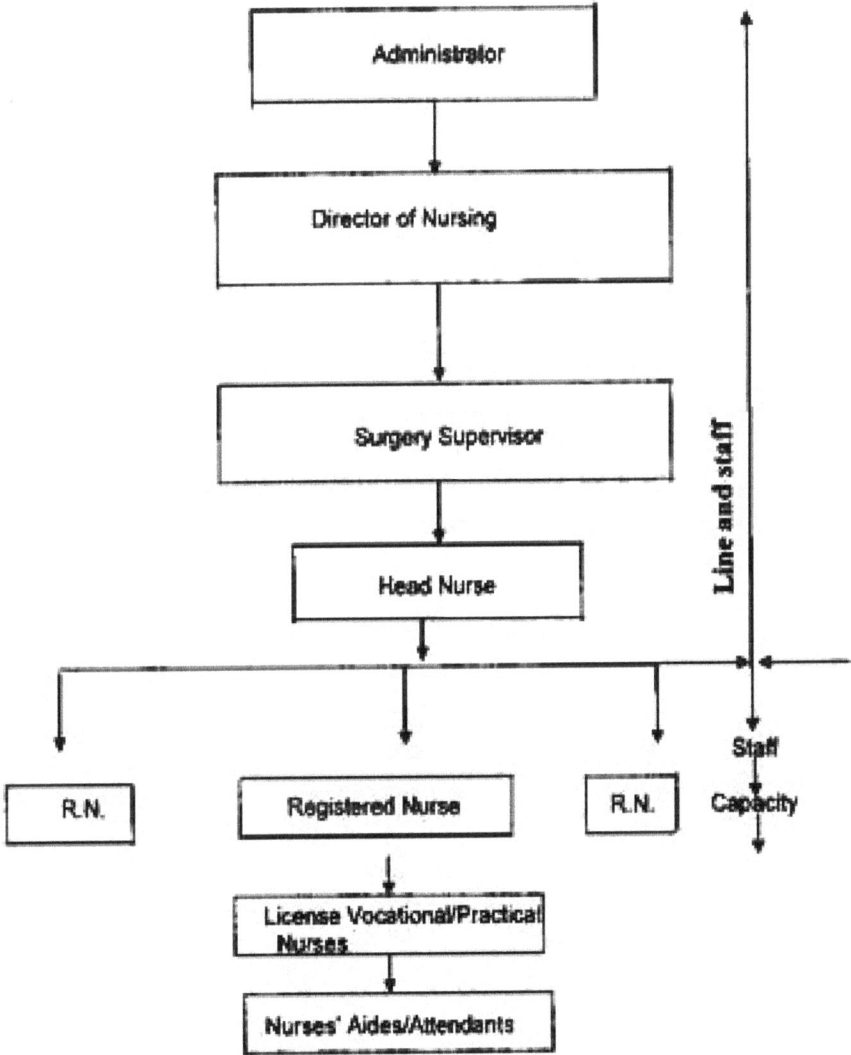

Diagram: Line and staff authority—a nursing service in a hospital organization

An informal structure, on the other hand, refers to the way employees socialize with each other on a horizontal plane at the workplace. This is an informal socialization, which can be a positive or negative force;for instance, an formal activities like going out to bingo or out to lunch by an informal group, whose membership may include a superior mixing with subordinates. Such an association with subordinates can and may enhance full participation in unit or departmental programs by employees members of the group. This is a positive development, one that aids toward organizational goals with enhanced productivity.

On the other hand, the exact opposite can result if certain group activities undermine the goal and objectives of the organization. A good example is taking an extended lunch period by group members that a supervisor is an active member. In this example, the supervisor can lose the ability to control subordinate on the job, due primarily to personal involvement and participation in such a group. The popular saying that "familiarity breeds contempt," is true and has application here, as the organizational goal is clearly undermined.

5. Departmentalization

This refers to the creation of departments or divisions with authority and funding to carry out specific activities. The guiding principle for departmentalization is the same principle that governs work division. The more an organizational structure reflects the internal activities necessary to attain its goals, the more roles are designed to meet such expectations and, according to John Halff, "the more effective and efficient and organization structure will be."[41]

There are advantages and disadvantages in creating departments. The combination of methods in creating departments with effective organizational skills and good programs greatly accentuate institutional goals and objectives, which, as a consequence, leads to a higher demand of services, as earlier indicated. However, creating a department just for the sake of doing so as the organization feels it can is fiscally irresponsible.

REVIEW OF LITERATURE

The general principles of administration serve in a sense as a road map to administrators in every organization, as to how they can effectively manage the affairs of their institutions. They guide managers in their effort to make their particular organization work and do so in a simple way.

However, for a health care facility to achieve its goals and to fulfill its stated mission, it has to both adopt and adapt the principles of administration that fit its particular need. This is why different organizations operate differently, even if their mission statements may be the exact replica of one another. This, in addition, is so because their mission statements, policies, and some other variables may not be the same. In an entrepreneurial atmosphere, there is the need to beat the competition, in the effort to expand services, while maintaining balance at the same time. Organizations that fail to take this advantage may jeopardize their mission and head toward the demise of their organization altogether.

Peter Drucker (1974) indicates that societies have become pluralistically ridden with organizations aspiring to provide every social service to every available group, ranging from the economic aspect to environmental protection servies.[42] He argues by enumerating the various segments of administration, from the management dimension with its different tasks to the top management using business enterprise paradigms and management techniques of Sears, IBM, and Deutsche Bank, as good examples, in the Concept of the Corporation (1964).[43] In *The Frontiers of Management* (1980) and *Managing for Results* (1964), he further delves into the general concepts of corporations as they operate in industrial management settings in the United State.[44, 45]

Edith Penrose (1959) discussed management, performance of firm growth and the theory governing it,[46] while Elton Mayo (1946) describes the problems that people face in industrial work areas.[47] Jay Forrester (1961) discusses the dynamics of industries as they relate to managerial tools and employee skills.[48]

Finally, Ernest Dale (1960) and Henri Fayol, (1949) explain the structural designs of organizations and the general principles of industrial management.[48, 50] Marvin Bower (1966) argues on the virtues of top management in organizational settings,[51] while William Guth (1974) lays out analytically the structure, strategies, and implementation of organizations,[52] as John Dunning (1971) applies the principles of management from a multinational entrepreneurial perspective.[53] And Douglas McGregor (1957) shows the effect and impact of organizational management process on the professional manager.[54]

NOTES

1. Peter Drucker, *Management: Tasks, Responsibilities, Practices* (New York: Harper and Row Pub., 1974) 6.
2. Marshall W. Raffael, *The U.S. Health System: Origins and Functions* (New York: John Wiley and Sons, 1980) 263-264.
3. R. M. Hodgetts and D. M. Cascio, *Modern Health Care Administration*, 2nd ed. (Madison, WI: WCB Brown and Benchmark Pub., 1993) 19-70.
4. John R. McGibony, *Principles of Hospital Administration* (New York: G. P. Putnam & Sons, 1969) 195-196.
5. The New International Version (NIV) Study Bible, Kenneth Barker, ed. (Grand Rapids, MI: Zondervan Publishing House, 1995) 2271-2273.
6. J. C. Williams, *Human Behavior in Organization* (Cincinnati, OH: South Western Pub. Co., 1978) 26.
7. Peter M. Blati, *Bureaucracy in Modern Society* (Chicago: Univ. of Chicago Press, 1950) 34.
8. R. K. Merton et al., eds., *A Reader in Bureaucracy* (Glance, IL: The Free Press, 1952) 18-27.
9. J. L. Massie and J. Douglas, *Managing: A Contemporary Introduction*, 2nd ed., (Englewood Cliffs, NJ: Prentice-Hall Inc., 1977) 143.
10. Douglas McGregor, *The Human Side of Enterprise* (New York: McGraw-Hill Book Co., 1960) 33-34, 47-48.
11. Beaufort B. Longest, *Management: Practices for the Health Professional*, 3rd ed. (Reston, VA: Reston Pub. Co Inc., 1984) 111.
12. Peter Drucker, *Management: Tasks, Responsibilities, Practices* (New York: Harper and Row Pub., 1994) 45.
13. Ibid.
14. H. S. Rowland and B. L. Rowland, *Hospitals Administration Handbook* (Rockville, MD: Aspen Pub., 1984) 3.
15. P. Drucker, *Management: Tasks, Responsibilities, Practices* (New York: Harper and Row Pub., 1974) 39.
16. R. M. Hodgetts and D. M. Cascio, *Modern Health Care Administration*, 2nd ed. (Madison, WI: WCB Brown and Benchmark Pub., 1995) 16.
17. S. Levey and N. P. Loomba, *Health Care Administration: A Managerial Perspective* (Philadelphia: J. B. Lippincott Co., 1984) 49.

18. Samuel Levey and Thomas McCarthy, eds., *Health Management for Tomorrow*, (Philadelphia: J. P. Lippincott Co., 1960) 28.

19. P. Drucker, *Management: Tasks, Responsibilities, Practices* (New York: Harper and Row Pub., 1974).41.

20. Glenn T. Troyer and Steven L. Salman, eds., *Handbook of Health Care Risk Management* (Rockville, MD: Aspen Pub., 1986) 75.

21. Ibid.

22. Melon I. Roemer, *National Health Systems of the World*, vol. 1 (New York: Oxford Univ. Press, 1991) 68.

23. Howard S. Rowland and Beatrice L. Rowland, *Hospital Administration Handbook* (Rockville, MD: Aspen Pub., 1984) 7.

24. M. I. Roemer, *National Health System of the World*, vol. 1 (New York: Oxford Univ. Press, 1991) 68.

25. Ibid., 9.

26. Theo Heimann: *Supervisory Management for Health Care International* (St. Louis, Missouri: The Catholic Hospital Association, 1993) 230.

27. H. S. Rowland and B. L. Rowland: *Hospital Administration Handbook* (Rockville, MD: Aspen Pub., 1984) 11-23.

28. Ibid., 9.

29. Harold E. Smalley: *Hospital Management Engineering: A Guide to the Improvement of Management System* (Englewood Cliffs, NJ: Prentice-Hall Inc., 1982) 18.

30. Ibid., 16.

31. Ibid.

32. J. S. Rakich, B. B. Longest, and J. D. Kurt Darr: *Managing Health Service Organization*, 3rd ed. (Baltimore, MD: Health Profession Press, 1992) 538.

33. Norman Metzge, ed., *Handbook of Health Care for Human Resource Management* (Rockville, MD: Aspen Publication, 1981) 759.

34. Ibid., 305.

35. Samuel Levey and N. Paul Loomba: *Health Care Administration: A Managerial Perspective* (Philadelphia: J. B. Lippincott Co., 1984) 60-61.

36. Howard S. Rowland and Beatrice L. Rowland: *Hospital Administration Handbook* (Rockville, MD: Aspen Pub., 1989) 978.

37. Milton J. Roemer: *Comparative National Policies on Health Care* (New York: Maral Dekkar, Inc., 1977) 2.

38. Ibid., 35.

39. M. I. Roemer, *National Health System of the World*, vol. 1 (New York: Oxford Univ. Press, 1991) 68.

40. Oliver Sheldon, *The Philology of Management* (London: Sir Isaac Pitman and Sons Ltd., 1930) 32.

41. John Malff: *Management: A Studying Guide to A/C Company Koonts, O'Donnell and Weibrich* (New York: McGraw-Hill Book Co., 1989) 77.

42. P. Drucker: *Management: Tasks, Responsibilities, Practices* (New York: Harper and Row Pub., 1974) ix.

43. P. Drucker: *Concept of the Corporation* (New York: New Amer. Library, 1964).

44. P. Drucker: *The Frontiers of Management: Where Tomorrow's Decisions Are Being Shaped Today* (New Year: Truman Talley Books, 1986).

45. P. Drucker: *Managing for Results: Economic Tasks and Risk-Taking Decisions* (New York: Harper and Row, 1964).

46. Shigeru Kobayashi: *Creative Management* (New York: American Management Assoc., 1971).

47. Edith T. Penrose: *The Theory of the Growth of the Firm* (London: Oxford Univ. Press, 1959).

48. Elton Mayo: *The Human Problems of an Industrial Civilization* (Boston: Harvard Business School, 1946).

49. Jay W. Forester: *Industrial Dynamics* (Cambridge, MA: MIT Pres, 1961).

50. Ernest Dale: *The Great Organizers* (New York: McGraw-Hill Inc., 1960).

51. Henri Fayol: *General Industrial Management* (New York: Pitman, 1942).

52. Morviz Bower: *The Hill to Manage* (New York: McGraw-Hill Inc., 1966).

53. William Guth: *Organizational Strategy: Analysis, Commitment Implementation* (Homewood, IL: Irwin: 1964).

54. John W. Gardner: *Self-Renewal: The Individual and the Innovative Society* (New York: Harper and Row, 1964).

CHAPTER EIGHT

OATHS OF PROFESSION AND ETHICS IN PRACTICE

INTRODUCTION

No book can discuss a subject in its full scope and include all that there is to know about the subject. Similarly, this book is in no way complete, nor is it capable of containing all there is to be discussed on any particular subject including the subject at hand. I am not, neither can I, to be expected to cover the full scope of all the ethical issues in the health field and health care facilities in Nigeria in this book. An attempt will, however, be made to discuss at some limited degree pertinent ethical matters of the issues at hand.

I will first attempt to define certain words, like *ethos*, *ethics*, and similar others. This will enable me to establish some perspective on this elaborate topic. *Ethos* in a Greek word, according to Williams Grahams Summer, refers to the sum total of all ideas, codes, and usages that characterize and also differentiate a particular group of people from all the other groups. Ethos of a particular society, therefore, sets it apart from all others, by some particular set of "guiding beliefs," which provide the people within that society "a distinguishable makeup"[1] that separates it from all others.

Ethical issues begin with personal moral values, as already discussed— which, inevitably, are manifested in practice—and certain ethical values do already exist in the nature of codes of conduct for both personal and professional practices in most professions. Ethics, however, is a subject that deals with the moral duty of man to his fellow man; this primarily means action, which is either good or bad toward another person.[2] It is a set of moral principles, discipline, if you will, that deals with good or bad conduct or actions in every situation that are in the realm of moral obligations of one person to another. It also means the code of conduct that governs professional behavior that pertains to some complex ideals, beliefs, or standards that are characteristically pervasive in the conduct of groups of people in a society.

The philosophical, sociological, medical, administrative, and other approaches to ethical issues are as varied, indeed, as the different fields of professional practice. To the physician, it means compliance with the professional standards as well as meeting the expectations of society by acting in a certain manner toward patients. To the health administrator or manager with special responsibilities to the profession, there is a deep sense of responsibilities to the profession, the organization, and ultimately to the society that health care services are provided properly, in a timely manner, and in compliance with policy and letter of the law.

The social worker's view of ethics focuses particularly on the cultural aspect and mores of a people, while the philosopher may view it as a formal approach to the subject of mortality.

However, ethics is a topic that includes all of the above and perhaps more. It is more than just the observance of the law, as it is meant to help facilitate better interaction, professional practice, and relationships among all groups in the society. The basis for this stems from the biblical injunction of the golden rule: "Do unto others what you would want them do unto you."*

In essence, therefore, ethics is an essential part of morality—a code of conduct found in every civilized society that has an established system of acceptable, as well as unacceptable, behaviors with commensurate punishment for violators. In professional practice, however, ethics is a

---

*   Matthew 7.21: "Therefore, all things whatsoever you would that me should do to you, do ye even so to them, for this is the law and the prophets."

code of conduct for all the health professions with the underpinning that reflects a sense of right and wrong within the society.[2] Henry Hazlitt (1988) says that this ethical or moral principle applies to each and every human being since everyone of us practice them in our daily lives. He thus states,

> ... Each of us has grown up in a world in which moral judgments already exist. Those judgments are passed every day by everyone on the conduct of everyone else. Each of us not only finds himself (sic) approving or disapproving how other people act, but approving or disapproving certain actions, and even certain rules or principles of action, wholly apart form his feeling about those who perform a follow them. So deep does this go that most of us even apply these judgments to our won conduct, and approve or disapprove of our won conduct in so far as we judge it to have conformed to the principles or standards b which we habitually apply to others, we feel guilty; our conscience bothers us.[3]

A. C. Edwin (1953) agrees with this premise and suggests that we already have some idea of the concepts of good and bad, right and wrong, which are precisely ethical concepts of good and bad as he argues that

> ... ethics is concerned with two main, kinds of questions, first, with deciding the general principle on which ethical terms. i.e.: good, bad, duty, etc., are to be applied to anything, and secondly with deciding precisely what these terms mean.[4]

These ethical principles exist or are learned from our childhood, as they enable each of us to judge the actions of other people as we compare them to ours. Variations, on the other hand, do exist between individuals, cultures, and societies, past from present.

In the health system, the role that ethics plays concerns the harm or benefit that may accrue to the patients, who are the beneficiaries of such actions, by the action of the practitioner. The mere fact that someone stands to gain or to get hurt by any procedure becomes an ethical issue, to say the least. Erich Loewy (1989) makes the following point:

> . . . Our ethical concerns are prompted by the benefit, or harm that can, directly or indirectly, result from our actions to another. Primary moral worth attaches to an object which in itself is capable of being self-knowingly benefited or harmed, which, at the very least, has the capacity to suffer. The capacity to suffer the necessary condition of primary worth may be actual or potential (sic).[5]

The professional obligation for a health care professional in a health care setting covers three main areas of concern, namely, decision-making in the giving or termination of care, deciding not to give care in certain conditions, and setting up the criteria for initiating any decision to either treat or not treat. Jonsen, Siegler, and Winslade (1986) make the following observation:

> . . . The ethical principle underlying much of this chapter is the principle of "beneficence," the duty of assisting others in need and avoiding harm. This principle is expressed in the history of medicine by the Hippocratic maxim: Be of benefit and do no harm. This duty of beneficence, incumbent upon all persons, is particularly weighty for physicians who have by profession, undertaken to care for the welfare of patients. The ethical duty of physicians and the ethical importance of the contract between physician and patient are directed to fulfilling the goals of medicine (sic).[6]

Ethical issues in health care generally are front and center of any legal and/or psychological problems, ability to choose or inform consent and patients' rights issues. It is not only a given as it is routine that in health care facilities, practitioners often face ethical issues which appear in a variety of ways. Some as very dramatic, while others not so obvious, even subtle at times. Issues of ethical import range from the permission for simple treatment of a common cold to the most complex, like brain surgery or a variety of surgical procedures. The basic premise of ethics in health care is based on the biblical principle of "Thou shall not kill,"[*] a general moral code which the Hippocratic Oath enunciates so clearly

---

[*] Exodus 20:13, one of the Ten Commandments that God gave to the children of Israel through Moses on Mount Sinai.

and as summarized (Thomas A. Mappes and Jane S. Zembaty, 1986) in the medical maxim for all physicians:

> ... I will apply dietetic measures fir the benefit of the sick according to my ability and judgment; I will keep them from harm and injustice. I will neither give a deadly drug to anybody if asked for it, nor will make a suggestion to this effect.[7]

ETHICS IN HEALTH CARE

The very root of ethics, besides the moral code used by society, is the principle mentioned above and the Hippocratic injunction that is binding to all practitioners. This oath was written not by Hippocrates, but by Pythagoreans, some of his disciples in the fourth century BC. This is the oath,

> ... I swear by Apollo Physician and Asclepiads and Hygieia and Panacea and all the gods and goddesses, making them my witness, that I will fulfill according to my ability and judgment this oath and this covenant. To hold him who has taught me this act as equal to my parents and to live my life in partnership with him and if he is in need for money to give him a share of mine, and to regard his offspring as equal to my brothers in male lineage and to teach them this act if they desire to learn it without fee and covenant; to give share of precepts and oral instruction and all the other learning to my sons and to the sons of him who had instructed me and to pupils who have signed the covenant and have taken oath according to the medical law, but to no one else. I will apply dietetic measures for the benefit of the sick according to my ability and judgment; I will keep them from harm and injustice.
>
> I will neither give a deadly drug to anybody if they asked for it, nor will I make a suggestion to this effect.[8]

Ethics is a collection of moral values of people. Its application for medical, dietary, and other uses are based on the ability and judgment of practitioners to apply to practice in the effort to prevent harm or injury and injustice or refusal to administer or apply any substance or advice based on request that would cause harm or death.

The core of any and all ethical decisions, in clinical settings, is the four broad generalizations under which the rest fall: the need or indication for care, the desire or preferences of patients, the quality of life after intervention, and the surrounding circumstances of the particular situations.

These constraints require the health practitioner to exercise good judgment by employing ethical and moral principles in the delivery of care.[9]

The need for care generally presents the first ethical challenge to the professional health provider, be that a doctor, nurse, or just about anyone providing the care (in the event of an accident). This is because anyone—in an emergency situation such as accident, heart attack, and myriad of other life-threatening situations—can make a life-saving decision. At the scene, usually the first determination is whether or not care is indicated. Paramedics are also involved in this role in many instances and can be referred to as the "professional triage," since it involves a professional decision to determine the need for intervention—where, when, and how soon it is provided.

However, once the patient is in the confines of a health care facility, a hospital preferably, nurses and physicians usually take over and make such determination. Patients' preferences in emergency situations become secondary ethical, even non-ethical issues, but under ordinary circumstances, they do matter.

In an emergency, the focus is on preserving the life of the patient while comfort, patient's desires and idiosyncrasies become secondary concerns. However, under normal conditions, the patient's personal choices and desires come into play during treatment. For instance, should a patient object to any procedure, after a thorough explanation to him or her with a reasonable understanding as to the implications of their action, the procedure may not or should not be done or it becomes an unethical practice. This, of course, is so only if the patient is conscious and emotionally sound with the choice not interfering with life. If it should interfere with a life process, it becomes injurious to life and, therefore, a non-ethical issue.

The ethical obligation of the health care provider in such a situation would then be to ensure that the patient understands the pros and cons of action choices. The health professional would then proffer acceptable method of care of safe standard of practice, as opposed to the one advocated by patient's choice, and the differences in results between the chosen method and the one being rejected as well. However, in the event that the situation turns out otherwise due to impaired mental status of the patient for any reason, professional decision should then outweigh the patient's desire and legal sanction for treatment is then sought.

Equality of life is also another ethical aspect that is not a central issue in a life-threatening situation, but becomes one after the emergency situation is over. The surrounding circumstances of external forces and factor and availability of equipment, affordability, etcetera.

PRINCIPLES OF ETHICS IN HEALTH CARE

The aim of professional code of ethics, like the medical code of ethics, is to establish and provide a standard of care for practice, which will serve as a guide to health professional practitioners, their relationship with patients, colleagues, and to the rest of the society.[10] The health professions, like other organized groups, exist purposely to service the needs prescribed by the society. In the words of Peter Drucker,

> ... Business enterprises—and public service institutions as well—are organs of society. They do not exist for their own sake, but to fulfill a specific social purpose and to satisfy a specific need of society, community or individual. They are not ends in themselves, but means.[11]

The American Medical Association, in complete agreement with this premise, makes the following declaration as indicated in the preamble of the Principles of Medical Ethics:

> ... The medical profession has long subscribed to a body
> of ethical statements, developed primarily for the benefit of

214

the patient. As a member of this profession, a physician must recognize responsibility not only to patient, but also to society, to other health professionals and to self. Principles adopted by the American Medical Association are not laws, but standards of conduct which define the essentials of honorable behavior for the physicians.[12]

Most health care activities take place mainly in health facilities and primarily in hospitals, clinics, and to a lesser degree, in some other forms or settings. The obligation of the health care provider begins with the patients and extends to the community or the society, as the case may be. Professional obligations furthermore include patient's right to good professional care, the right to confidentiality, the right to courtesy and courteous treatment, the right to refuse care or treatment, and soon.

The Society
The well-being of the family and the general welfare of everyone else remain the bedrock of community and of the society. Remove that indispensable part and the society is reduced to nothing, as it disintegrates in no time. Show me a nation whose citizenry suffers from poor health and sicknesses, and I will show you a weak nation.

The Profession
Professional allegiance is the cornerstone of a profession—any profession that is without an ethical standard is hardly a profession. Similarly, a profession whose members do not adhere or observe its tenets and, worse, if the profession does not discipline members for infractions when its ethical and principles rules are flaunted at will enjoys little, if any, public respect; nor should the public support such a profession, as it only deserves to be proscribed.

The Professional
Strong and influential professions, like the medical and legal ones, have ascended or descended, as the case may be, to those levels and command influence in most societies today because their memberships hold their profession in high regard or disregard. This is not to suggest that all doctors and lawyers behave ethically and professionally, as a majority of them do, while some within their ranks do not. These professions discipline their members who flaunt professional ethics.

The Organization

Allegiance to the organization, as far as professional practice in health care is concerned, is beneficial to the profession and the organization. By maintaining professional conduct and standards, the organization enjoys a good repute with the locals and expansion with other positive things that are natural outcome of such a good relationship.

Failure of an organization, on the other hand, can be attributed to the failure of professionals who are responsible for the daily running of the affairs of the organization.

The general ethical principles in health care include, but are not limited to, the following:

   a. Dedication, competence, compassion, and respect for human dignity in delivering health services.
   b. Honesty in dealing with the people whom they serve, and as well as with colleagues. This means discussing the conditions of patients honestly with them, the cost of care and other matters, and the exposure of illicit activities of colleagues who are incompetent and deficient knowledge or skills.
   c. Respect for the law of the land and its application in the various aspect of practice.
   d. Respect for the rights of patients and other health professionals within the constraints of the law.
   e. Freedom of choice as to who should render health care except in emergency situations.

A PERSPECTIVE ON NIGERIAN HEALTH CARE ETHICS

Nigerian-trained physicians take the same Hippocratic Oath after their training to become doctors and practice in the Nigeria in a similar manner, just like doctors in other societies. It is fair to assume that these health professionals also share similar ethical principles with their counterparts in other societies. Whether this assumption is true or not, we will see later on, but for now, detailing just the clinical and ethical issues will suffice.

Ethical considerations, in the context of Nigerian health system, need not be discussed in their entirety to appreciate the degree of its problems and so only a few examples of some of these problems should serve the purpose at hand.

Let us start with patient's rights in health care facilities in Nigeria, i.e., the right to good or appropriate care, at the very least, for patients who are already inside the confines of a health care facility. Most patients in these health care facilities, private or public, do not have the luxuries of medical care or treatment, but only after their relatives have paid the levied amount that has been stipulated and purchased the needed medications prescribed for treatment from drugstores outside these facilities and brought back to the care facility before treatment can commence, including in emergency situations.

This is not the way that health care facilities are run in most Western societies. The availability of essential equipments for treatment are other areas lacking in ethical consideration in health care settings in Nigeria, which health care professionals do not seem to mind to exploit for money, which is a direct contravention of the Hippocratic Oath, now rendered meaningless by such awful behaviors.

REVIEW OF LITERATURE

There is an avalanche of topics in literature which deals with ethical and moral conduct in health care situations, and as it has already been pointed out earlier, ethics and morality deal with the values of people in societies. In reviewing these values and their application in the context of the Nigerian health care facilities, as professionals perform these essential health services in Nigeria, it is clear that most of the health care practitioners have not lived up to their commitments.

Henry Hazlitt (1988) shows the presence of moral judgment in rational human beings in all human societies. Moral judgment, he maintains, is a learned cultural behavior, which also varies from society to society and group to group. He maintains by implication, however, that this basic instinct to preserve life vis-à-vis adversity and danger that pervades the entire animal kingdom.

Adherence to established codes due accrued empirical experiences, he continues, leads to social cooperation in societies and that moral rules are by no means static, but dynamic, constantly changing as they undergo refinement. Furthermore, he explains, ethics and economics influence both human actions and choices and that ethical values are not only framed for the individual but are also meant for his good ultimately. He also indicates that all moral rules are universally impartial and that their violations occur mainly at the individual level—that the main purpose of moral rule is to prevent conflict and collision between individuals. He continues by stating that mutualism is the results when self-interest and concern for others fuse into each other as one within the society, with asceticism as an aberration and immoral and, that ethical rules are prescriptive, not descriptive.

Ethical judgment, according to this reasoning, therefore, is always cognizant of facts, while morals enjoy autonomy that is often reinforced by religious values. In conclusion, he makes this following stern, and yet prescription concerning corruption and immoral society:

> . . . Immoral action is nearly always a short sighted action. If it occasionally helps an individual to achieve some immediate particular end that he might not have achieved without it, it is usually at the cost, even to Iii m of some more important or enduring end. *And immorality can achieve even these minor success only to the extent that it is rare and exceptional and confined to a tiny minority. A corrupt or immoral society is ultimately an unhappy or dying society.*[13] (sic) (emphasis added)

Jonathan Daney (1993) discusses the various moral concepts and refutes contrary arguments to his stated position, by strengthening earlier positions, on moral reasoning, taken by moral philosophers of the caliber of Humes, Negel, Sturgeon, Boyd, Cornel, Brink, Hare, Wolf, and others. Victor Grassian (1981), on the other hand, provides a thorough and critical abstract on moral questions and their practical effect on everyday situations that affect peoples' lives.

Eliseo Vivas (1963) discusses their solutions, values, and functions in human settings individually or in an organizational setting in *The Moral Life and The Ethical Life*, while Aurel Kolnai (1978) presents a synthesis on various topics on moral values, complexities, and their ethical influences on society. Anthony Cartese (1990), in *Ethics*, presents ethical analysis on key moral issues with critical implications that affect aspect of moral cognition on culture, ethnicity, and language, concepts with problems linked to justice, interethnic tensions, and the methodology in approaching moral judgments.

And George Snell (1988), on the other hand, analyses the moral role of science for humanity and the pragmatic principles that shape individual behavior, which may lead to satisfaction. He sees no use for the return to traditional and religious values or the need for sacrifices, and yet he emphasizes the importance and role of knowledge in human biology, an argument that, to me, does not make any sense. If religion has no role in human societies, then neither is biology or any of the social sciences, since all of these are, ultimately, for the benefit of "man." He concludes his argument by suggesting that the binding fabric of the society (a clear contradiction of his argument) is that, indeed, ethics is progressively being downplayed by almost all professional practices in recent years. This part makes sense. He warns,

> . . . Indeed, rational ethics and true democracy are dedicated to the same end—the general welfare and the two are totally inter-dependent. In the long run, only the moral can be free. This is no moral concept. It was voiced by Samuel Adams more than 200 years ago when he wrote . . . We may look up to armies for our defense, *but virtue is our best security. It is not possible that a state should long remain free, where virtue is not supremely honored.*[14] (emphasis added)

He concludes by adding that:

> Ethical Theory is meaningless unless it is put to work.[15]

Moral issues or the principles of ethics as applied to health and medical situations are summarized well by the statement of Torn Beauchamp (1989):

> . . . The objective of this book is to provide a moral framework for determining our obligations in the wave of these developments.

We do not ignore the history of moral reflection in health care, indeed, we assume its relevance. But we emphasize the development of a theory and set of principles for the treatment of problems. That even the most elevated and ancient forms of medical ethics are ill equipped to handle.[16, 17]

Moral reasoning in medical ethics, he continues,

. . . may be theoretical—such as whether physicians or nurses may ever legitimately hasten the death of patients or the practice of killing—such as whether or not a particular patients should die. In either form, our perplexity about these matters and our desire for resolution drive us to moral reasoning.[18]

Finally, he concludes,

. . . Systematic work in biomedical ethics is a recent phenomenon, despite decades and, in some cases centuries of discussion by philosophers and theologians. Within the health care profession the most influential reflection on these problems has evolved through formal codes of medical and nursing ethics, codes of medical ethics and reports by government-sponsored commissions. These writings include specific rules that apply to persons in the relevant professional roles in the practice of medicine and nursing, in health care institutions, and in research. We should distinguish between these particular moral codes, which govern such groups as physicians, psychologists, and nurses, and general moral codes, which government whole societies and apply to everyone alike. A general moral code consists of the society's cherished moral principles and rules. The word *morality* often refers to this general code and the practices it spawns. An example of a single rule in a general moral code is whenever you have promised to do something then you have an obligation to do it. By contrast, a special or professional code specifies action-guide for a particular group, such as physicians or nurses. These action-guides should be justified by reference to more general principles and rules, which may not be explicitly identified in the codes themselves.[19] (emphasis mine)

Jack Dowie and Arthur Eistein (1988) provide some analysis on moral and ethical judgments and decision-making process in professional practice. Robert Veatch (1989) points out key ethical principles of normal ethics as it applies within a health care setting, a guide to medical students, physicians, or the public at large.[20]

Richard Wright (1988) presents a philosophical perspective on ethical issues that are pervasive in the health care system by portraying the moral and philosophical basis, an ethical decision-making process in the general framework of organizations,[21] and Managle and Thomasma, (1988) describe changes that occur in the health care system that result in its constant state of flux with other changes that affect health professionals.[22] In *Health Care Ethics of Critical Issues* (1994), emphasis is placed on the handling of bioethical and other contemporary issues.[23]

Freedman and McDonnel, (1987) portray an empirical application of moral values in decision-making during practice in ethical situations in a paradigm,[24] while Frederick Herter et al., ed., (1986) give explicit examples of the effects of ethical values and their implications for all categories of health care professionals in long-term settings. They warn that illustrations are no answers for clinical situations, as each case differs on presentation, approach, and management.[25] Finally, Jonsen, Siegler, and Winslade (1982) identify common situations in which ethical problems do present and the way of solving, since they are rarely taught in medical schools.[26]

NOTES

1. William Graham Summer: *Folkways* (New York: The New America Library Inc., 1960) 48.
2. Kurt Darr: *Ethics in Health Services Management* (New York: Praeger,1987), xxxxiii.
3. Henry Hazlitt: *The Foundations of Morality* (Lanham, MD: Univ. Press of America, 1989), 7.
4. A. C. Ewing, *Ethics* (New York: The Free Press, 1953) 9.
5. Erich H. Loewy: *Textbook of Medical Ethics* (New York: Plenum Pub. Corp., 1989) 29.
6. A. R. Jonsen, M. Siegler, and William J. Winslade: *Clinical Ethics: A Practical Approach to Ethical Decisions in Clinical Medicine*, 2nd ed. (New York: MacMillan Pubs. Co., 1986), 11-12.
7. Thomas A. Mappes and Jane S. Zembaty: *Biomedical Ethics*, 2nd ed. (New York: McGraw-Hill Book Co., 1986), 54.
8. A. R. Jonsen, M. Siegler, and William J. Winslade: *Clinical Ethics: A Practical Approach to Ethical Decisions in Clinical Medicine*, 2nd ed. (New York: MacMillan Pubs. Co., 1986), 5-6.
9. Thomas A. Mappes and Jane S. Zembaty: *Biomedical Ethics*, 2nd ed. (New York: McGraw-Hill Book Co., 1986) 59.
10. Ibid., 55.
11. Peter F. Drucker: *Management: Tasks, Responsibilities, Practices* (New York: Harper and Row Pub., 1973).
12. Henry Hazlitt: *The Foundation of Morality* (Lanham, MD: University Press of America, 1983).
13. Ibid., 357.
14. George D. Snell: *Search for a Rational Ethics* (New York: Springer Verlag New York Inc., 1988).
15. Ibid., 260.
16. Ibid., 264.
17. Ibid.
18. L. Beauchamp: *Principles of Biomedical Ethics*, 3rd editor:, New York: Oxford Univ. Press, 1989).
19. Ibid., 10-11.
20. Jonathan Dowie and Arthur Eistein: *Professional Judgement: A Reader in Clinical Decision-Making* (New York: Univ. of Cambridge Press, 1988).

21. Richard A. Wright: *Human Values in Health Care: The Practice of Ethics* (New York: McGraw-Hill Book Co., 1989).
22. John F. Managle and David C. Thomasma: *Medical Ethics: A Guide for Health Professional* (Rockville, MD: Aspen Pub Inc., 1988).
23. John F. Mangle and David C. Thomasma: *Health Care Ethics: Critical Issues* (Rockville, MD: Aspen Pub. Inc., 1994).
24. John M. Freeman and Kevin McDonnel: *Tough Decisions: A Casebook in Medical Ethics* (New York: Oxford Univ. Press, 1987).
25. Fredrick P. Herter et al., editor: *Human and Ethical Issues in Surgical Care of Patient with Life-Threatening Diseases* (Springfield, IL: Charles C. Thomas Pub., 1986).
26. Albert R. Jonsen, Mark Siegler, and William J. Winslade: *Clinical Ethics: A Practical Approach to Ethical Decisions in Clinical Medicine* (New York: MacMillan Publishing Co. Inc., 1982).

CHAPTER NINE

COMMENTS AND INFORMATION ANALYSIS

INTRODUCTION

... We have need of history in its entirety, not to fall back into it, but to see if we can escape from it. (José Ortega Y. Gasset)[1]

... I have but one lamp by which my feet are guided, and that is the lamp of experience. I know of no other way of judging of the future but by the past. (Patrick Henry).[2]

... To be ignorant of what occurred before you were born is to remain always a child. (Cicero)[3]

... From the least to the greater, all are greedy for gain; Prophets and priests, police, all practice deceit. They dress the wound of my people as though it were not serious: Peace, peace they say, when there is no peace. Are they ashamed of their loathsome conduct? No, they have no shame at all, they do not even know how to blush . . . Hear, Oh earth. I am bringing disaster on these peoples the fruit of their schemes. Because: they have not listened to my words and have rejected my law. (sic) (Prophet Jeremiah)[4]

Who was the prophet Jeremiah* Jeremiah 6:13-15 & 19. Who was the prophet Jeremiah speaking of in the context of this quoted passage? Was he talking about Nigeria or some other nation? No the Prophet was speaking to Israel and its citizens, because Nigeria was not even in existence then, as the nation or country known as Nigeria is a creation of the 18th and 19th centuries dreamt up by the colonizing British empire. Having said this, then let me say that the fact that the British economic gluttony does not in any way manner or shape, limit God's foreknowledge and plans for the nation of Nigeria and its citizens, simply because the prophet makes no mention of Nigeria in this prophesy. I dare say that in spite and despite of the behavior of Nigerians, God in His divine grace and mercies have been abundant to the country of Nigeria and its people; even during its short tenure (from 1900 to the present) of merely just over a century.

To analyze is to examine primarily the different components that form an entity. Such examination assumes any number of ways including:

1. Deduction—looking at the total whole of an entity by breaking it down into its component parts.
2. Induction—looking at parts of the total whole separately and then weave them back into a whole again.

Analysis, then, is defined in the dictionary as "to break up" or "loosen" up to something; "the separation of whole into its component parts for an examination of the complex, its elements, and their relations"; or "an examination of a thing to determine its component parts," a deductive analysis. But when the whole is examined from the perspective of its different parts that then is inductive analysis. The key issue in analysis is the relationship of component parts, i.e., the influence of each part on the others. Thus, analysis here, on a critical examination of the health system in Nigeria and issues arising from it, is the main purpose of his presentation.

Furthermore, another purpose is to analyze available and scientifically collected data as well as that which is empirical—not so totally and scientifically collected, both subjective and objective that is duplicatable. This is because not all information or data collected here was totally and flawlessly collected by the scientific method. No such claim is being made here, either directly or indirectly, implied or otherwise. However, it is not only the intention but also the aspiration in this presentation to look at all the information or data presented in the first seven chapters critically to objectively analyze that information and let the chips—and that is the opinion of you the reader,—fall where they may. The governing concern here is not so much the information or data and how it has been collected, but what obtains currently in the Nigerian health care facilities. Should the interest and understanding of the reader be held to the end of the entire presentation, with the arguments fully comprehended, then the purpose and the objective for this book would have been met. And that is all I ask of you my audience—understanding and rapt attention if possible. Let's face it, every Nigerian reading this book has observed, heard, or experienced some aspect of this disaster or catastrophe called medical care in the country. This madness has now become the expected rather than the unexpected events or happenings in our health care facilities in Nigeria. Should that be the case, then no amount of write-up can explain any better than your personal experience and/or observation. That is it—empiricism at its very best!

As it has been indicated elsewhere in this discourse, the white man, according to some, is responsible for all our ills' past, present, and future! The white colonialists did this, that, and a million other things that "pull us down" even when we now know that the white man relinquished power to us some forty-five years ago. The residues of the white man's method of governance did not go away with the white man when he left after he relinquished power, but have lingered on, I dare say, all these forty-plus years. The "divide" rule and principle has continued to be the bedrock of all governmental policies ever since this nation obtained its independence in 1960. Nigeria's republic civilian administrations and the dictators of the army regimes alike have all seen it fit to change nothing.

However, being the hypocrites that some Nigerians are, as well as also being known to be undisputed copycats, most administrations—present and/or past—have seen it fit to conveniently suspend credulity and want to have us believe that changing the constitutions of the country, purposely to accommodate despicable acts of government officials or their administration, somehow makes such a misdemeanor okay. To them, and in this instance the head in the sand principle (where there's no light but total darkness), the silence of the poor populace equates ignorance and/or acceptance of such a criminality. Nigerians have remained inseparably wedded to the British influence and their legacy and principles of governance, but at the same time failed to learn from the British that corruption, nepotism, cronyism, and despotism are all detrimental to the functional governance and, thus, the survival of any and all nations, because these corrupt values are archenemies of the "public good."

On this account, I do not excuse anyone as everyone in the Nigerian society has played a contributory role, which has led to this tailspin. The people of Nigeria (who are, for all intent and purpose, the bedrock of every government administration that has ever come to power in the country) could have demanded change and be ready to make necessary sacrifice in defense of such a stance, if they wished, but Nigerians have chosen volitionally, I might add, not to not only not change these wrapped value system but accept the policy of status quo from their government and that of every administration that comes along. For instance, black leaders or politicians in Africa constantly, as it's always the case, gang up on any white person or country with obstreperous and boisterous condemnation of any and all misdeeds of other racial groups in the present-day global community. Except, of course, for act that they themselves or any of their own have committed, then the silence is deafening as they have all of the sudden found that there is virtue in being numb and dumb. When apartheid was the official policy of the defunct South African white government from its inception through the 1980s, the unison of the African leadership in its condemnation of the apartheid regimes was very clear and unmistakable. Yet these self-same-sanctimonious hypocrites practice apartheid in their own countries right this very minute under the nose of the world, and no one dares to say a word or point it out for fear of being branded a "racist." The heinous acts of the Idi Amin of Uganda, Mugabe of Zimbabwe, Sergeant Doe and Charles Taylor of Liberia, Babangida and Sani Abacha of Nigeria, and many more—all in Africa—and Baby face Duvall of Haiti did not and have not generated any level of interest close to the drumbeat of opposition that greeted the South African situation, especially when Nelson Mandela was still in prison.

However, and amazingly enough, we continue to blame the white man. At any rate, we also all know deep down our labile minds that the white man was not all that despite all the noise to the contrary. In fact, the white saved us from ourselves (or none of us could have been left on this continent called Africa had the white man left us to devour one another. We would have all been sold to white people all over the world by our greedy brothers, knowing what we all know now). Otherwise, how come that the white man's ideas of governance has remained the model for government in running this country since we complain so much that the white man is evil? This and other pertinent questions concerning the attitude and behavior of the ruling groups in Nigeria will continue to be asked at least here anyway, if not in the consciences of our government officials, who are mostly from the dominant groups of this country!

PUTTING HISTORY INTO PERSPECTIVE

> . . . Those who do not remember the past are condemned to relive it. (George Santana)[7]

> . . . We have to do with the past as we make it useful to the present and the future. (Frederick Douglas)[8]

Systems, after they have diagnosed a problem that seems to be disrupting normal functions or operation, do their level best to try to prevent or minimize loss or suffering that might ensue. The next step is to find support system for the part that is weak and causing the problem. This is to improve the general situation and to make the functional aspect of the entire system less strenuous.

Finally, the system or organization takes steps to effect a permanent solution that eliminates the problem entirely, if that is possible. In so doing, the system is then capable and prepared to deal with similar situations in the future. This, essentially, is what constitutes self-preservation that is based on experience. However, the failure to commit such experience into memory leaves a system open to similar happenings or situations reoccurring in the future. Thus the words of George Santana,[10] "Those who do not remember the past are condemned to relieve it," ring very true. But George Orwell's[11] observation that "he controls the past, controls the future" as well appears on the surface as an oxymoron, and yet a paradox and an axiom, because past experiences serve as education sources, if used properly and sensibly.

ANALYSIS

The history of health issues in the health system and health care facilities in Nigeria need some analysis that is necessary, and a relevant matter requires some comparison with the attitude of some of the ancients. People of ancient civilization—like the Minoans, Egyptians, Greeks, and Romans—valued the importance of good health for their citizens and did all that they could do, certainly more than the governments of modern Nigeria have been doing to ensure the health of the citizens of Nigeria of today, ever since the first military coup d'état in 1966.

While it is true that no new nation has ever gone through its early beginnings without experiencing social problems, similarly, Nigeria has gone through all experiences without benefiting from them. Most other nations grow to be better nations than they were from the very start, except for Nigeria. It is also amazing to observe a nation like Nigeria, in the modern era, which places a premium on all other aspects of national development, except for health and comfort of its citizens.

The Roman Empire realized the importance of good drinking water and so provided it, building aqueducts that carried this precious commodity to all areas for its citizens throughout the empire. However, I believe that had electricity been available then, nothing would have stopped the Romans from providing that too to every household in the empire. A similar assumption also goes for the Greeks, Egyptians, Jews, and even Arabs, but not Nigeria.[9] As far as some Nigerians are concerned, some of these basics are both too good, and would cost too much, for some ordinary citizens in Nigeria.

Another area is the disease transmissibility. Ancients knew that certain diseases were transmissible, and they took preventive steps and actions to forestall their acquisition. People in the Middle Ages were aware of this concept of contagion (as mentioned or as discussed earlier), a theory that was espoused by Girolamo Fracastorius in 1546.[*12*]

However, in Nigeria, there remains a hefty majority, and this cuts across all segments of the society, which still runs around in a sort of dead stupor, still believing in witchcraft. These people call on God's name daily during prayer and recital in their religious rituals, but who don't show any evidence that God has power over their lives. Witchcraft is believed to have the power to kill if and when anyone dies, when this is hardly the case as there is no evidence to support such claims. They are totally enslaved by these pagan or animist thoughts and beliefs, which are not helpful, but actually harmful. So, when, not if, a debilitating disease strikes, they run around from one witch doctor to another searching for cure. They utter the name of God more times in one breathe than anyone can count, which is usually very superficial because it is not from the heart. They truly believe witchcraft, or *boka*, nonsense and its attendant balderdash, yet they are the very ones to engage in all kinds of dubious activities that are anything but religious! This word *Allah* means absolutely nothing to them. Every word that comes out of their mouths is "Allah, Wallahi, Tallahi"—Allah this and Allah that! When you hear a Muslim in Nigeria swear "Allah Wallahi," you know that what comes after that is nothing but concentrated, calculated, and purified lies!

Education is definitely a change agent, which no sane person can deny. To some, that change may be a positive one, and yet to others, it can be a negative force as we have also witnessed in the Nigerian situation. The West has used education to improve the living conditions of its general citizens, and in the course of time, it has also used others in geographic locations of the globe. Even during periods of hostilities, the West has shown not only maturity in restraint but also caution in its application of kind acts as displayed in its past dealings with defunct Soviet Union and even with Germany, Japan, and China today after the World War II animosities. Yet even during the periods of hostilities, there were and still are educational cooperation, shared knowledge, and to some degree, even economic cooperation between these old and bitter enemies.

The point here is this, the white man knows when to put away feelings of hostility during a period of human suffering and intense need. At the same time, he always keeps hostile feelings in check during moments of emergencies. Dominant tribes in Nigeria and especially the Hausa/Fulani groups, on the other hand, are always insensitive to such needs, while claiming at the same time to be pious. A piety and religion that teach and demand of its adherents to hate others and neighborhoods alike as perpetual enemies, because they are not only of the same time, but also have a different religious beliefs.

Governmental policies have been based on religion to such a point that the Nigerian government now appears to be synonymous with Islam, since it sanctions Islamic fanaticism. This excludes all other Nigerians, who are not Muslims. Based on the level of hatred and rank barbarism that one witnesses from some of these groups, one cannot help but wonder that if Nigeria were a nation with a civilization during the ancient times with the Hausa/Fulani as the dominant group, would there be any archeological finds by archeologists of the remains of other ethnic groups in that country? I wonder!

The mere fact is that the society comprises roughly over four hundred different ethnic groups (with an intense repugnance toward one another), according to the Federal Research 1992,[14] which alone was a major concern during the colonial years that made the "divide and rule" very attractive to the colonial masters.

However, some of these social institutions—like family values, education, political parties, etc.—are only in name, as they do not serve their purposes as their counterparts do in other societies. Their idea of equality of every individual has, for long, been swept under the rug. In its place, Nigerians have institutionalized the ideals of pride and materialism with corruption as the means of achieving those ends. These ideals are blatantly observed in the so-called economic development which, Olu Ajakaiye and Bayo Akinbinu (2000) claim, imply an increase in human production as they opine in the following statement:

> . . . By development then, we refer to an increase in human productivity that is sustainable and that enhances, rather than degrades the quality of both human and ecosystems.[13]

But according to a proclamation made by UNESCO in 1968, which I am sure Nigeria was also a signatory,

> . . . if man is the origin of development, if he is the agent and beneficiary therefore, he should, above all, be considered as the justification and finality of development.[14]

Well, let us analyze some of the figures in the economic spectrum put out in the *Economic Development* (2000) by Ajakaiye and Akinbinu and see where Nigeria fits in in this so-called agent and beneficiary . . . justification and finality of development.

As of August 2000, the per capital income, an economic indicator, showed South Korea with $76,600 per year; Japan with $31,490; United State of America with $24,740; South Africa with $2,980; and Nigeria with $300. When these figures are converted to Nigerian currency, the naira (N), at the rate of US$1 for N100, it would amount to N7,660,00 for South Korea; N3,149,000 for Japan; N2,474,00.00 for United States; N298,000 for South Africa; and only N30,000 for Nigeria!

For practical purposes, a big schism exists and separates Nigeria from most of the others of the international community in terms of economic development! Enough with this constant drumbeat of economic development of this so-called giant in Africa! Nigeria pats itself on the back as it cranes its neck like an ostrich that has swallowed a tennis ball, but being laughed at by the whole world!

This idea of development implies not just economic increase in human productivity but also the enhancement of human quality of life. It then only stands to reason for one to surmise that all the governments in Nigeria that have come and gone, from the colonial period up to this point, have all failed, except for the colonial governments. The colonial government had some success because the health system functioned and serviced the needs of most Nigerians in their era of administrations. There were areas in the nation that had health care facilities, there were drugs for treatment and equipment to work with, there were pipe-borne water that was always available—and even electricity was constantly available—because mischievous NEPA was not yet born. And so could not be an obstacle.

President Olusegun Obasanjo, in August 2001, announced that Nigeria was to launch a satellite into the space for some technological advancement purposes. This was to enable the so-called Nigerian scientists to better forecast the weather. The weather is not the problem, the problem is corruption, the police, the NEPA, the legal system, the health system, the Water Board and all the services, the military—all and every social institution in the country stinks, they all stink! Even the major hauling system (a necessary part of every industrialized nation) in the country does not work because it has been undermined so badly and now proscribed. Just take a hard look at the dismal performance by all these services! Yet launching a satellite is the worry—how is it going to be launched, with electricity or hush lamps, and what is the purpose?

It is commendable that in August 2001, the new Obansanjo's administration was making plans to provide up to 23,000 drilled wells in the rural areas as announced during the same broadcast. That effort was a noble one and whose aim was in the right direction, yet more is not always better. It would be interesting to know how many of the intended new wells were actually drilled in. Even better, how many of the actually dug wells in the targeted and all the social service institutions in the country have run amok? Not some nebulous pie in the sky project by nature of a satellite program that could easily be manipulated by a government already filled to the brim with corrupt politicians, who could, just as they are, be ever ready to convert this lucrative opportunity into another scheme of self-enrichment.

Just imagine how the standard of living could change and how may lives would be saved by these simple measures that palpably benefit people's lives! Furthermore, just imagine how many of the listed services can be provided to improve the lives of Nigerians with just half of the amount to be wasted in launching a satellite to forecast weather, which, in the first place, will not work, and that is, if it is finished and not abandoned before it is completed. But if it is finished, it will not work or be damaged because of the irresponsible and willful acts of NEPA who will make sure that it cooperates as it will give the perennial excuse of the need for a new "transformer." Now, President Olusegun Obasanjo has come and gone, yet he installed Mr. Walking Sedative, who is putting the nation to sleep. Because he is so slow, no one seems to know what he is going to do as we are passed by half of his first term, and he still do not know what he intends to do. No, Mr. President, get things done right, right here on earth in Nigeria, and forget about the skies, the space, for now!

But then again, Nigerians are well known for their violent allergic reaction to laws, their own laws, even God's laws—also rules, regulations, and common sense; then is it any wonder that they have also ignored sociologists' prescription of UNESCO, an arm of WHO, which Nigeria is also a member?

The Nigerian cultural background, nevertheless, guarantees the employ of common sense as a part of practicing it. The declaration on culture as adopted by UNESCO World Conference on Cultural Policies in 1982 in Mexico City—which Nigeria, I am again sure, was a signatory—states this:

> . . . Culture may now be said to be he whole complex of distinctive spiritual, material, intellectual and emotional features I hat characterize a society or social group. It includes not only arts and letters, but also modes of life, the fundamental rights of the human being, value systems, traditions, and beliefs.[15]

We are here again faced with the dilemma of human beings, but in the Nigerian context. In Nigeria, Muslims can say anything they want against anyone or any religion, and even question the fundamental tenets of other religions anytime, anywhere, with no fear, retaliation, or ramification of any sort. But no one dares say a word against Islam, whether expressed or implied, or hell and its ugly agents break loose, in their attempt to devour the non-Muslim infidels, even if it is they, the so-called holy agent of Allah, are the ones who started it in the first place!

It is not enough that this group of people has pillaged the country, but to them, it is not enough that they dominate every one and everything. They still continue to want to entertain the dominated with depraved and wanton acts of barbarism and ask a total allegiance in return. They cry foul even when they know they are wrong, knowing full well that their leaders will, without investigation, jump to the defense of these inhuman acts. They break every law, regulation, ordinance, or rule no matter how simple, yet no one dares to say a word about such uncivilized conducts. Any such criticism is considered anti—or un-Islamic and punishable with death. For instance, just consider the cockamamie sentence that Ayatolla Khomenei of Iran passed on Rushdie in the 1980s for his writings that were considered to against Islam.

Is it not silly to think that flaunting God's laws here on earth can gain one entrance into God's heavenly abode? It stands to reason that if you can't obey laws and regulations stipulated by people, or God, here on earth with people that you can see and interact with, how is it possible that they would admit into his heavenly abode for you to contaminate it? God is not biased and has never been and will never break His own laws in favor of Muslims or anyone for that matter. He is not, nor is He going to admit not only unconfessed, and yet willing murderers into a sinless pristine heaven. Nor will He, for that matter, take that chance of affording such people another opportunity—mind you, an opportunity that that they have rejected here on earth to mess things up in heaven (tongue in check, of course!). If you have no respect for people whom you see, it is virtually impossible for you to claim that you respect the divine Almighty God who is altogether invisible to the human eye!

ECOLOGY

The ecological boundaries of the country and its ambiance have been shifting, over the last three to four decades, in favor of physical development. There is no doubt today that there are a lot more roads that are just slightly better than just a few decades or so ago, and equally true, the big towns and cities have expanded and continued to expand, with forests, arable land even marshlands continuing to recede, by giving way to uncontrollable urban sprawls. These sprawls have now become the symbol of modernism in the eyes of material-minded Nigerians, at least, so it seems.

In truth, though, these are mere façades, a so-called signs of superfluity and displays of affluence, because this is a sign of superfluity, of grand-looking buildings on the outside and empty on the inside, nicely developed areas and great to behold during the day, but without lights at night—thanks to NEPA as an unknown cartoonist once said, "In the beginning, God created the heavens and the earth, and the darkness he called NEPA," a body in charge of producing electricity for the nation, but closes operations any time there is a storm or even no signs of it but the sound of a passing train or a jumbo jet. There is no comparison between the defunct Electrical Corporation of Nigeria, which did a splendid job as it provided electricity regularly compared to the current demon and prince of darkness called NEPA, none whatsoever! Believe it or not, NEPA switched off the lights in Kaduna, even as President Olusegun Obansajo was delivering the independence message in his address to the nation on October 1, 2001, and assuring Nigerians that the electrical services problems in the country were a "myth" that had been concocted by the active imaginations of his critics, as electricity supply in the country had, indeed, stabilized.

POLITICS

Most of the problems that Nigeria faces today owe their beginning, at least in part, to this nebulous social institution called politics. Politics has become, practically, the sole domain of the Hausa/Fulani group. Ajakaiye and Akinbinu (2000) indicate that customs and traditions are part of culture and traditions—I add religion to the mix. It is the position of the dominant groups in the North that belonging to any of the two major group automatically earns one the support of the whole of the group, but only so long as that person remains a Muslim. An individual has no right except as a group member, and of the Islamic faith, they can then behave or misbehave anyhow in the society and not be persecuted either by the group or society.

Members of these same ethnic groups also have the right to any office in any of the governments of the land, elective and/or appointive. It is such type of belief that prompted a politician, Shehu Shagari in the election cycle of 1979-83, an attempt to incite Islamic crowds during one of his campaign tours in the North, urging his supporters not to vote for a *karfiri* (a heathen or an infidel), referring to the candidate and chief opponent, Chief Abafemi Awolowo. Later on, he was to be surpassed by retired General Buhari, former head of state and a Muslim who had himself toppled another, Shehu Shagari—viciously and vituperously made and debasing pronouncements in the 2000/2001 election cycle about other non-Muslims—who was himself toppled in 1985 by yet another Muslim, all brothers in the faith of Islam, the now retired general Ibrahim Badamosi Babangida (IBB) in 1983.

Above all else, politics has been the main vehicle, to my mind, that's mostly responsible for subverting and corrupting influence on the morals of Nigerians, which Islam has not only been used as a vehicle, but has sanctioned, so long these adherents donate portions of stolen public fund toward building of mosques all over the place. The moral character of some Muslims in Nigeria is not grounded in the fear of God or in any moral principle, but in material acquisition. That is why some of these adherents easily fall prey to such practices as murder, thievery, etc., as the basic tenets of the religion condones atrocities committed in its defense by people who only profess God by mouth.

Chapter 2 has dealt with some definition of terms and health concepts, leaving very little to analyze or comment on. However, it is pertinent here to point out the fact that not all of the terms and concepts defined in chapter 2 comport with accepted definitions or meanings of these terms.

The definition of *health* should be the same in Egypt, Norway, Cuba, Taiwan, New Zealand, or New Guinea, even if the understanding of that concept may vary in all these different societies. Similarly, the concept of hygiene is equally universal, although the application of this concept may vary from one individual to the next. Sanitation, environmental health, and other health risks have the same application and management. On the other hand, the definition of *health risk* in a society like Nigeria may clearly be understood and accepted on face value, but its implementation is not acceptable and must be rejected because of the gross negligence and failure, with regard to it, in this country.

Health risks mean virtually nothing since practically nothing is done to discourage lack of compliance with the blatant disregard of environmentally hazardous, poor or lack of sanitation, as human waste products and disease harboring material anywhere to overflowing in all areas of human habitation. Open gutters in every community are replete with sewage brewing with imaginable disease carrying insects, rodents, and many other nasty little creatures—you name it—as they wallow in open human waste products. Environmental health and sanitation definitely do not include any part of this, and definitely, the uncontrollable urban sprawl does not deal with this particular aspect, because food ready for human consumption is being sold in these infection-infested environments and has never or will it not ever be considered for any type of regulation.

Health education and promotion, disease control, or any other effort for that purpose is an absolute sham and waste of resources. Above all, the concepts of treatment and rehabilitation in government hospitals are the worst aspects of health and/or health care that could be visited on people of only society. Most of the so-called hospitals are empty. There are no equipment to work with, and just as well, because the attitude of some health care providers stinks to high heavens. Moreover, the trouble that patients go through in search of genuine drugs just to bring back to these so-called health care facilities, so that a sick relative could be treated, is simply despicable and unacceptable and should not be happening anywhere in any modern society. Patients or their relatives should not have to have written prescriptions filled outside and, particularly offensive to any civilized mind, at a drugstore or pharmacy that is owned by the same professionals who are the primary care provider of the patient, outside the confines of the hospital, as this brand of professional misconduct defies every description!

Last but not the least, poor patients, in some of these inhuman amphitheaters, dare not object, ask for simple questions or explanation related to their sickness or they draw the ire of the professional and so be denied treatment for "questioning professional judgment." No wonder the mass exodus and flight of the corrupt politicians to developed countries to have for better care, for themselves and members, but the same care that they so readily to their fellow countrymen and women!

In chapter 4, the dietary aspect of Nigerians has also been discussed, even if it was discussed in a rather superficial level.

For one, most people eat what they eat, usually because they have grown accustomed of doing so; yet in many other instances, people from different cultures all across the globe eat and enjoy everywhere these days. The Nigerian society is certainly a part of this global scene, including some selected locations in towns and cities in the country today, like Lagos, Abuja, Kaduna Jos, Enugu, Port Harcourt, where foreign restaurants serving foreign dishes can be seen. Equally true, there are restaurants that serve African dishes, including ebba/teba, jollof-rice, moi-moi, and others in places like London, Los Angeles, New York, Houston, Dallas, etc.

In chapter 5, health professions, their training programs and their induction into the health care practice, are laid out. It points out, in the introduction, how the health system, in so far as it is meant to service human needs, cannot service those health needs adequately, without the professionals with appropriate professional conduct.

Furthermore, human resources is an absolutely necessary part of every organization which, according to Charles Taff, (1984), exists so for the purpose of meeting the needs of people by rendering necessary health services to the society. If that goal is to be met, health professionals must be employed for that purpose.

In this chapter, it is also pointed out how a society can play an effective role in meeting the health needs of all its citizens, by first defining what those health needs are, their scope, and then going about in meeting those needs. Ranking health issues in the order of priority, but especially among other national issues, indicates the level of priority given to the issues of health and of what importance does the government considers health issue. One of the definitions was one advanced by Kostrzekski*, a paraphrased version is particularly interesting as it defines health as that state that represents the absence of disease while the individual goes about performing all normal activities. It also points out that an individual may perform his role and duties as prescribed by the society and yet be very far from being a healthy individual.

In chapter 6, the distribution pattern of health facilities is discussed. The approach and criteria for such a determination is still not based on need, as indicated by the spread of the population or of the number of people in an area, but based purely on ethno-religious centralism. Put simply, this means that certain groups and their religion or religious affiliations continue to define the criteria such that need, which reminds us of the fictitious characterization of a political ideology of Marxism as symbolized by the communist party of the defunct Union of Socialist Soviet Russia that George Orwell portrays in *Animal Farm*.

The defeated Marxist system preached equality of all the comrades, not just some comrades. Yet the pigs in the fiction were "more equal" than the rest of the animals. This meant that the ruling class in the Soviet political system was "above" the proletariat or the laboring class as it has already been pointed, even though it preached egalitarianism. The faint similarity between the Nigerian and the Soviet Communist governing class resides in this wisdom: with the majority of the population of the country residing in the rural areas, more health care facilities should, as a matter of common sense, be allocated to those areas, but that is not the case. The

---

*   Information about this article and its author is not available for similar circumstances that transpired before the publication of the first edition in Nigeria that were far beyond my control as earlier expressed.

dominant Hausa/Fulani residential areas of every town, city, or section of the country have everything given to them, to the disadvantage of those rural areas, that have had nothing, almost, in comparison. It should be obvious to the reader as to what the similarity with communist politburo of the defunct communist party, whose religion was atheism, has with the Hausa/Fulani majority domination in present Nigeria.

Chapter 7 addresses the general principles of administration and the various theories of organization. As indicated in the introductory section, the success of administrators is generally couched in honesty, abiding by the laws of the nation, proper use of authority or responsibility, and accountability with good a management style. This claim is especially true in organizations, whose administrators have these attributes with irresponsibility and accountability.

The concept of bureaucracy, on the other hand, would warrant further comment here, as all other administrative concepts are pretty easy as they, at some length, address various aspects dealing with the process of bureaucracy. While the term *bureaucracy* means "red tape" or "delays" employed in the process to ensure control, accountability with accuracy in dealing with any given issue, it has become a means of embezzling public funds in Nigeria that even the bureaucratic protocol is no match for the corrupt mind of some Nigerians who are so bent on making money anyhow and at all cost. The unabashed use of bureaucracy as a vice to an end, for the bureaucrats to enrich themselves, is a vice no longer hidden!

From the clerk who types up the voucher and the cashier who pays out salaries, to the department head, all demand and receive graft for services they were employed to perform in the first place. It is only in Nigeria that people are doubly, even triply, paid—that is, paid and repaid for the work that one should do. It does not really matter whether you are in a government office corporation premises, telephone or electrical office, or department store, the story is the same, and that, too, can only happen in Nigeria! The police, for example, play both ends against the center in matters of public safety, as they demand payment from both the complainant as well as from the defendant. This is not the role of the police, i.e., dabble in the adjudication of civil or criminal matters; its role is to make arrests and present evidence in the court of law, and that is it.

But what they should not do is precisely what is being done in Nigeria, as these extortionists do not discriminate because, to them, there is no difference between the guilty and the innocent!

Another example is the telephone service. When this government parastasal had no competition, it will not only give you bellyache for applying for phone services, but will give it to you doubled dose when you get your phone installed. Telephone workers will use your line, without authorization, to make illegal calls all over the globe and then charge it to your account without any records to prove that you actually made such calls. Yet you the customer cannot even protest, let alone contest the unlawful charges—again, only in Nigeria that this can happen! These workers get paid for what they do as government workers and get paid again, illegally, by the citizen whom they are supposed to serve or help when they come for such help or services.

Chapter 8 deals, primarily, with the ethical issues in the health professions. It is in this section that the word *ethos*, a Greek derivative that means the sum total of characteristics that differentiates any group of people from all others is discussed. This then leads us to the definition of *ethics* and/or ethical issues. Ethics specifically deals with the morality of man's responsibility and his actions to other people, which is either good or bad. This is a moral code that is present in every human being by nature of conscience, as reflected in our daily conduct within our social settings.

Generally, therefore, the ethical code in health practice centers around the legal and psychological problems faced in the health system. Similarly, just as the ethical values of people are reflected at the societal level and vice versa, it can also be postulated that the ethical values of practitioners of the health professions reflect the ethical values of the professionals and of the society within which they practice.

The importance of individual health in Nigeria has been supplanted by the corrupt desire for money by many in the health care professions. The way that patients are spoken to by doctors and nurses, in some of these health care institutions, does not inspire confidence or leave any room to give these corrupt professionals any benefit of the doubt. Patients' relatives are treated and spoken to in insolent and uncouth manner that there is no room for any explanation as such callous attitudes are never warranted, no matter the cause. Relatives are expected to do everything for their sick relatives, except performing surgical procedures. Some of these doctors, nurses, and assistants fold their arms as spectators of the struggle between sick patients and relatives as though it is some funny game.

For example, my uncle was admitted to a university hospital here in Kaduna in August 2001 for a leg infection, but what I witnessed in that so-called teaching institution or teaching hospital during the period of my uncle's hospitalization was gut-wrenching. It left me with no option but to think that some of the nurses were anything but nurses. Some of them spoke to patients as if the poor patients deserved what had happened to them.

Besides the fact that a teaching hospital is supposed to be clean, which this very hospital was an exact opposite of, the place hooked and smelled like a camp of shepherds. It had no good wheelchairs or stretchers to convey sick patients unable to walk; the only one available was broken and squeaked in gross protest when moved with or without a patient on it. The stretcher was not any better. It emitted noisy screeches, the thrills of which sent birds in nearby trees to flight. To crown it all, I had to dash outside the hospital premises to purchase drugs from local drugstores for nurses to administer to my sick uncle.

One could say that this serves us well, as this was the kind of self-governance for which politicians—the like of late Sardauna of Sokoto, Sir Abubakar Tafawa Balewa, Awolowo, Nnamdi Azikiwe, etc.—had clamored. But again, as good as the colonial rule was, it was bound to end, at some point in time. It had to. As for teaching hospital mentioned earlier, to my mind, that institution does not qualify for a university teaching hospital, regardless, because it is a super disgrace!

Since this is the condition in our so-called teaching hospitals, just imagine the conditions in government nonteaching hospitals, health centers, and private clinics! Allow your imagination to run wild! No wonder that they are referred to as robbing, instead of hospitals! Most of the health care professionals do not give a hoot about anyone or anything, not even about their very profession, and much less, the suffering of poor people under their care. All they care about is themselves and that they are employed, that they will collect a salary at the end of the month, period!

There is no accountability or any modicum of professional ethics in caring for the sick—none, *nada*, *zilch*! This is simply the case because it seems that these professionals, as products of a deprived society, have no ethical or moral values in their personal lives. The result this is the lack of accountability, as no sanctions is required from professionals or the public at large, since human life has little or is of no value in the Nigerian society of today. It is little wonder, therefore, that the society's problem of corruption is so widespread and has become insolvable, when coupled with the crazy notion of ethno-centralism and religious (or irreligious) bigotry, as the situation has become hopeless.

Any profession that is devoid of ethics in its daily practice is not worth its salt or much. However, when a health system with a list of professions and professionals has abandoned its ethical values in its daily professional conduct of services to the society, then that society is no longer just immoral but amoral.

NOTES

1. George Orwell: *Animal Farm* (New York: The New American Library, 1970) 418.
2. Rhonda T. Tripp: *The International Thesaurus of Quotations* (New York: Harper and Row Publishers, 1970).
3. Ibid., 319.
4. __The New International Version Large-Print Study Bible (Grand Rapids, Michigan: Zondervan Pub. House, 1995) 1469-1470.
5. Ibid., 417.
6. Fredrick C. Mish, *Webster's Ninth New Collegiate Dictionary* (Springfield, Massachusetts: Merriam Webster Inc. Pub., 1991) 82.
7. Fitzhenry, editor: *The Harper Book of Questions*, 3rd edition, (1993) 204.
8. Ibid.
9. Rhonda T. Tripp: *The International Thesaurus of Quotations* (New York Harper and Row Pub., 1970) 670.
10. Ibid., 699.
11. M. J. Cohen: *The Penguin Thesaurus of Quotations* (New York, NY: Penguin Putnam Inc., 1998) 386.
12. Lloyd E. Burton, Hugh H. Smith, and Andrew W. Nicholas: *Public Health and Community Medicine*, 3rd edition, (Baltimore: Williams & Wilkins, 1980).
13. Roy, Porter: *The Greatest Benefit to Mankind: American History of Humanity* (New York: W. W. North & Co., 1997) 428-429.
14. __Federal Research, Division Library of Congress, (1992).
15. *Dorland's Pocket Medical Dictionary*, 24th ed. (Philadelphia: W. B. Saunders Co., 1982) 142.
16. Melvin L. Defleur, Wm. V. D. Antonio, and Lois B. Deflueur: *Sociology: Human Society* (Glenview, IL: Scoff, Foresman & Co., 1973) 95-96.
17. Olu Ajakaiye and Bayo Akinbinu, editors:, Strategic Issues in Nigeria Development in Globalizing and Liberalizing World, 2000.
18. Ibid., 212.
19. Kunle Adeniji: "Transport Challenges in Nigeria in the Next Two Decades" (Keynote Address, August 2000) 220 & 221.
20. Charles Taftt: *Management of Physical Distribution*, 7th ed., (Homewood, Illinois: Richard D. Irwin Inc., 1984).61.

21. M. A. Raffael and N. K. Raffael: *The U.S. Health System Origins and Functions*, 3rd ed., (Albany, NY: Delmar Pub. Inc., 1949)11.

22. Ruth M. French: *Dynamics of Health Care*, 3rd ed. (New York: McGraw-Hill Book Co., 1979) 21.

24. George Orwell: *Animal Farm* (New York: American Library, 1996) 116-118 & 133.

25. Peter Drucker: *Management: Tasks, Responsibilities, Practices* (New York: Harper and Row Pub., 1974) 6.

26. Wm. Graham Summer: *Fallways* (New York: The New American Library Inc., 1960) 48.

27. Kurt Darr: *Ethics in Health Services Management* (New York: Praeger, 1987).

28. Henry Hazlitt: *The Foundations of Morality* (Landam, MD: University Press of American, 1989).

CHAPTER TEN

CONCLUSION

The use of force alone is but temporary. It may subdue for a moment but it does not remove the necessity of subduing again; and a nation is not governed, which is perpetually to he conquered. (Edmund Burke, speech on Conciliation with America, March 22, 1775)[1]

The supernatural virtue of justice consists of behaving exactly as though there were equality when one is the stronger in an unequal relationship. (Samuel Well)[2]

I have a dream that one day this nation will rise up and live out the true meaning of its creed. We hold these truths to be self-evident that all men are created equal . . . I have a dream that one day every valley shall be exalted and every hill and every mountain shall be made low, the rough places will be made plain and the crooked places will be made straight and the glory of the Lord shall be revealed and all flesh shall see it together . . . Let freedom ring from from every hill and mole hill of Mississippi and every mountainside. And when we let it ring from every tenement and every helmet, from every state and every city, we will be able to speed up that day when all God's children, black men and whitemen, Jews and Gentiles, Protestants and Catholics, will be able to join hands and sing in the words of the old spiritual, "Free at last. Thank God

Algmihty we are free at last." (Dr. Martin Luther King, Jr., August 23, 1963)*

It is the Roman Empire they referred to in Latin as "divide et impera", literally translated as divide and rule, or an "indirect rule." In 190 BC, the Romans, according to H. A. Clement,

> . . . defeated the King of Syria at the Battle of Magnesia(sic). As in the case of Macedonia, the country was not made a Roman province at once. Instead, the Romans used their power to place on the throne Kings who would favorite (sic) them, and to split the country up into smaller Kingdoms that would be too weak to resist any demands. This was a favorite Roman way of ruling a country, and is often called a policy of divine et impera, or divide and rule.[3]

Although the Romans in ancient times subjugated a lot of people in their vast empire of conquest and used the "divide and rule" concepts, they did so only as a means to an end, which was to extract total obedience in compliance with Roman laws. In all fairness, I should not compare the defunct Roman Empire with any modem nation because the Romans lived in ancient times, ruled the worlds with violence and rank barbarism, which was the order of the period.

Moreover then, there were no League of Nations for the entire world. The League of Nations came into existence in the twentieth century, over fourteen hundred years after the fall of the Roman Empire, when some Western nations came together to form the League of Nations, now known as the United Nations. At any rate, with these two goals accomplished and besides the violence, the Romans treated their subjects really well by making all the provisions available to all peoples in conquered territories, similar to what the Romans themselves enjoyed. Clement further makes the following point:

> Rome also founded many garrisons or colonies among her conquered peoples. These colonies were composed of Roman

---

* The text of Dr. Martin Luther King Jr's I Have A Dream Speech, August 28, 1963 (from the Internet).

citizens, many of them soldiers, Their task was not merely to put down disorders, but to settle down to the arts of peace and to mix with the people around them. By this means, Roman customs would be introduced and the people would be "Romanize." These Roman colonies, you will observe, were far different from the old Greek colonies. Whether "Roman lived in Rome itself or in a colony hundreds of miles away, he always remembered that he was a citizen of Rome and that his duty laid first and foremost to the Roman state . . . In order to join up these colonies and make the movements of armies easier in case they were needed, many roads were built. The roads were like the veins and arteries of the Roman state, and the city of Rome was like the heart at the center. So well were they made that many of them in Italy, and elsewhere still remain as the foundation of modern roads (sic).[4]

The Romans had the political sense, will and power that is backed up by a very powerful military might, which led to the conquer and then, the rule of vast areas of different people with divergent ethnic and religious backgrounds. They ruled their subjects through surrogate rulers chosen from among the conquered people. Except for the use of force to ensure allegiance and compliance with Roman laws, the Romans did not force their own religion down the throats of their subjects, even when they could have. Neither did they deliberately ignore certain ethnic groups and refuse them amenities enjoyed by either the real Romans or the other ethnic groups in the empire because of ethnicity, religious views, or anything else, even when they differed significantly from that of the ethnic Romans in power. They knew, as did Edmund Burke, that no "nation is governed, which is perpetually to be conquered."

This was precisely because they believed in the virtue of justice, which Samuel Well agrees with, as the virtue of governance and tacitly behaved "exactly as though there was equality" between them and their subjects when actually, "one is the stronger in an unequal relationship." In the context of today's world, ancients have for long been viewed as brutes, and yet we find ancient Romans acting more humanely toward their subjects than today's dominant groups of modem Nigeria.

It is abundantly clear that the ancient Romans had better common sense and better political judgment even then than some leaders in today's

Nigeria. In almost every situation, instead Nigerian leaders, from the dominant groups, do not view each situation objectively, as they almost always view situations through the tinted lens and prism of religion. They have made Islam synonymous with life itself so that everything must he interpreted in the light of Islam whether one is a Muslim or not. Everything must conform to their understanding of Islam and always, whether or not people under such an arrangement agree. This also goes for every world situation involving or affecting Muslims.

The white man is blamed for everything wrong in the world, including slavery. This type of accusation is so senseless, baseless, and tasteless that if it were not so serious, it would be laughable, yet Muslims that level such accusations against the West are very serious, dead serious. When it comes to the serious questions of all the terrible things of repressive regimes of the likes of Saddam Hussein, the Mommar Ghadaffi, and the Hafad Assad of the Arab world, who have done more egregious deeds in their countries and to their own people, the silence is deafening. Hardly a whimper is heard from the lips of these false and self-appointed "apostles of peace" who constantly parade themselves as goodwill ambassadors and merchants of love, but at the same time, they wish the white man dead.

As a good example, as recently as in 2005, "slavery was and perhaps is still taking place, perpetrated on black Sudanese by their white Arab Muslims in southern part of Sudan. There is not even a whimper uttered by Muslim in Nigeria. In fact, Muslims should be very unhappy for what their Muslim" brothers are doing to the Kafir Christians in Sudan, but nothing, except dead silence. The most frightening thing about these people and their line of thinking is that they do not tolerate any kind of criticism whatsoever, as any criticism is misconstrued to a personal attack. In the first book, I recounted word for word an intense discussion that took place between me and one Musa Kallam, a Muslim who was working at the Nigerian consulate at the time in New York in 1985. Mr. Kallam was one of those who did not like the white man, but was living in a white man's country, used the white man's language in his entire school life and communicated in it. Yet Mr. Kallam railed against white people and did not like anyone pointing some inconsistencies on the position he had taken against white folks. Mr. Kallam and his ilk, because of their hate of the white man, would prefer we all spoke Arabic, then everything, according to them, would be okay. The only problem with that position is that, these people are hypocrites, as they peak English, a white man's language, to communicate their ideas to us because that is the only way can get large audience since nobody almost speak or even care about Arabic, period!

Also, how can anyone forget the memories of the sight of the jubilating Muslims that erupted in Islamic communities all over Nigeria after the 9/11 incident in New York, which remains very fresh in the memory of all people of goodwill in every nation.

> . . . We all know the old saying: "beggars have no choice," yet black leaders here in Africa, or in the United States, make all kinds of demands, on white people after poking their proverbial "fingers" in white peoples' eyes and still get what they want. Beggars do not make demands, they "make-do" with whoever is given them or leave it. Yet time and time again black people will say all kinds of foolish things about white people, then turn around right-away, forgetting what they have just said or done, and ask for financial assistance. These so-called black leaders do not want to forgive or forget the past but at the same time claim to be Christians and disciples or ministers of Christ. They are like some Moslems, who do not want and will not accept any culture that is not Islamic. Otherwise how do you explain the demand on white organizations like Nascar, Coca Cola and others, who are coerced to make financial contributions every year to Jackson's Rainbow coalition out of fear that Jesse Jackson would sabotage them and not call them racist organizations? Well, after all that, he still calls them racists after collecting their money anyway!

> Or say, for instance, the Mugabe phenomenon in Zimbabwe against white farmers, and then be embraced by France and other white countries? I know that white people have a soft spot for people who are suffering, and so the concern of white Christian in U.S.A. over the plight of black Sudanese. So why is Jesse Jackson silent about Sudanese black massacre could it he that he has been bought by the Arabs? Some white Christian organizations constantly raise funds to purchase the freedom of black slaves in Sudan from white Arabs and speak

out against the Moslem treacheries Christians in Nigeria. The black leadership is, on the other hand, missing and quiet on these current black situations, but continue to appear as carrying a "collective" chip on its shoulders.

Like the Moslems and some Christians in Nigeria, they constantly worry over what the world can do for them instead of what they can contribute to calm the turbulent interracial relations n the world. In the subsequent paragraphs and pages, an attempt will be made to present a classic case or paradigm to illustrate a game of blame-the-white-man from the West by some fundamentalist Moslems. This was a heated exchange of views between a Hausa-man Moslem who claimed to he a postgraduate or a one time "Ph. D" student in one of the universities in the state of New York in 1985 and this writer. This graduate student gave me a copy of one of his write-ups and solicited my frank appraisal. Here we go:

Take a broad look at the universe we live in. You probably will find out that citizens of great nations like China, Japan, Germany, Russia, France, Italy, Greece, Portugal and Spain to mention a few are supposed to he "cousins" of England in terms of genetics or biological looks compared to we in Nigeria (sic). But yet (sic) each of these Western countries including those nations from Asia (with the exception of England and America) have (sic) rejected the use of English language as its official language. As a result, each of the above mentioned nations speak (sic) indigenous language rather than a foreign language i.e. English. The French speak French, the German speak (sic) German, the Italian speak (sic) Italian, the Russian speak (sic) Russian, the Greeks speak Creek, Portugal speaks Portuguese and Spanish is the official language of Spain. Why then is Nigeria subjected to English which even fellow white people oppose to using (sic). We should not he indifferent with other Europeans who saw the use of foreign language as social ill and pride less (sic). Just like English language is to us as social ill, so the other principles are to Nigerians (sic). Needless to talk of the social conflict those religions are playing in our society (sic).

WHAT IS THE MEANING OF ALL THIS?

SERVICES IN GENERAL

Culture of Greed: The culture of greed, self-centeredness, religion, and tribalism has taken over in Nigeria. The employ of reason and rationality in dealing with the natural consequences of actions taken in the country in view of the above debates or dialogues is no more tenable. Nigeria is a pariah nation and deservedly so, not only because corruption reigns supreme with materialism and the mismanagement of public funds are all done only for the sake of money. In the event that you have not been following the arguments, all government services in Nigeria are for sale and to the highest bidder. NEPA does not provide electric light up to two hours a day, but charges consumers for twenty-four hours a day every month. The disruption in electrical services are never preceded without any notice or warning to customers. The spurts and surges of electricity return results in enormous damages to electronics and other electrical equipment and at great expenses to customers. Shutting electricity off by NEPA is real easy: a passing locomotive or a low-flying jumbo jet (747) and just about anything (including a dark sky) are reasons for electricity to be shut off in this nation, the giant of Africa. But this does not bother NEPA or the government. Visiting any office or business, customers are expected to call everyone in sight "sir," "madam," or "ranka shi dade", to every Dick and Harry or be denied the service they came to seek.

CORRUPTION

Corrupt behavior and practice can only happen in Nigeria with official sanction by both the executive arm of the government and the judicial system. I say this because inaction is a tacit approval of all that is happening with regard to the corrupt behavior of Nigerians. Water Board in the country charges a full amount for only a fraction of service that is supposed to be provided, but no one has done anything about it. Yet the customers did not question the Water Board because they will not listen, yet water bill hikes are constant without the commensurate improvement of service.

The telecommunication industry behaves as though it is a special gift from God to the fraction of humanity that lives in Nigeria. You have to spend a lot of money both officially and by bribe to have services connected or be reconnected, but when that service is installed, you are given bills for phantom phone calls that you never made. These are only a few examples, but in general, virtually every service area of the government, state or federal, participates in this mess. The government cannot invoke ignorance about the state of affairs in every social institution, but especially that of the health facilities in the country.

Anyone visiting the hospital, clinic, or some other health care facility must be prepared to bring everything that will be needed during the period of hospitalization. People visit such places because they are sick, yet these facilities are so empty to the point that food, medication, bed sheets, etcetera must be carted to the health care facility, on top of the high charges one must be prepared to pay, as no one will provide anything for you. Some of these points have already been made, so I will not beat this horse to death here again. On this account, all professionals in all areas of the health field are implicated, no one exempted, as a result of unprofessional conduct, and it must be reiterated that the unsavory conduct of government officials at all levels sanctions this shoddy and unsavory situation.

Official corruption is now so high that in 2004, Nigeria gained the undesirable title of the most corrupt society in the entire globe; this evil practice is anywhere and everywhere of all aspect of the society! This is true because the reference is always referred to in business deals, bureaucracy of government offices: "This is Nigeria," "We are Nigerians," and/or "Don't forget the Nigerian factor"—all of which refer to bribery, graft, and other unsavory corrupt practices. Nigerian politicians have the "honorable" title before their names, but most of them behave in less than honorable ways as a result of corruption.

THE HEALTH PROFESSIONS AND HEALTH CARE FACILITIES

Corrupt and unethical practices should not have any pail in the health care facilities in a civilized society because peoples' lives are involved and depended on it too. But as we have seen, that is exactly what is being perpetrated on patients by professionals who are supposed to be custodians of their health care services. It seems that no segment of the Nigerian society is exempted from this unholy bug or virus of corruption. If one should take a good look at the social institutions that used to be venerable (for instance the military, the police, the clergy, the judicial system, customs, schools and educational institutions of higher learning) this debased culture or "tradition of corruption" has affected or contaminated each and every single one—I should say, all of them—to the point that one is forced to admit that all these past glories are no longer the same.

THE MILITARY AND ALLIED FORCES

An institution which fails in its bid to service the needs of society, including ethical matters, is similar to organization that fails in its mission. That institution is no longer useful to the society which needs to altogether be proscribed. The military is a clear example of a social institution that has not measured up to the ethical mandate of its calling. Among others, the military has, for the most part in the past few decades, allowed selfish interests to make it dive into or dabble with politics, instead of strictly sticking with the business of national defense issues that are supposed to be its focus and only concern. In fact, in so doing, it has relegated the safety of the nation to a secondary concern. Furthermore, the military has allowed itself to be used by a segment "of the country with an ulterior motive" to the disadvantage and detriment of others who are equally important and part of the total whole of the nation. In so doing, it seems that the military and other men in uniform also continued to hack or subscribe to the notion of superiority by dominant groups. The protection of our borders is of paramount importance, but even more so is internal peace and unity within our so-called secured borders, without which there could be no Nigeria.

THE POLICE

The decadence in the police force witnessed today started over three decades ago. The police are now so corrupt that they openly demand graft from innocent citizens for no reason and sometimes crimes committed only in the active mind of imaginations of the police—a corrupt system. To the police, every one of us is fair game and defenseless victual. At one time in the distant past, people used to believe that the police were underpaid, and thus their inclination to corrupt practices. This belief is no longer tenable as members of the police force are among the well-paid and salaried employees of the federal government. On the other hand, the police brasses at the very top, who are charged to see as to the smooth running of law and order, have very little concern for those very vital areas or arc their subordinates. This is because it does not bother them at all that their subordinates have no materials to work with, no paper to write on, or even no pens to do the writing with. Just think of it, no pen or paper for a police to take reported complaint of crime committed. It is this group of people or what I call "thugs in uniform" that have the charge and the unequivocal support of the government to enforce the laws of the land. To me, this is worse than knowingly appoint a wolf to keep an eye or hang around an unlocked chicken's pen. This is worse than even that; it is actually locking the wolf inside the pen with the chicken!

It is when someone with concerns comes to make a complaint that the police would ask the complainant to furnish them with these essentials with which to do their work. On top of that, the complainant is asked to provide transport to and fro for the police. And God forbid that based on your complaint, the respondent would have to be detained, in which case the police would ask you the complainant to pay for the feeding expenses of the detainee. This then puts the complainant into a catch-22, meaning of situation or double jeopardy—damned if you do, and damned if you don't. It is now common knowledge and a joke that police's word is no longer worth anything, not even the paper it's written on. As far as police writing is concerned, there's no such thing as indelible ink because whatever is written can be erased, pencil ink—indelible or not. All that matters is money—cash, that is—which when brought can put broad smiles on the face of every police person on duty and erase anything in the police report books (*rubutun yan sanda ke nan*), the implied meaning is, everything that the police write in their report can be erased with just the right amount of money. We do understand that the police need to protect us from armed robbers quite all right; they also need to eliminate or stamp out armed robbers too, as there is the need for it. However, we need more protection from members of this very group hired, provided with armory to be employed in our protection, the police, but who have turned every single one of us into victim and prey on a daily basis.

I am speaking from a firsthand experience as this happened to me in 1997. I had brought a complaint against a suspect to the Kachia Police Motor Traffic Division (MTD). First, I was asked to either take the police to the village where the crime was committed or give them some money for traveling expenses. I offered to drive the police to the village where the crime took place and back to Kachia to investigate and take evidence. After a few days, the suspect was apprehended and brought to the police office in Kachia. The Kachia police then demand money to buy "foolscap" or the paper to write with and a *biro*, the pen to write with. This is after I had given them money for traveling expenses in addition to trips made to the crime scene. After all that, I was asked to give some money for the feeding of the suspect, but to this additional demand, I refused to comply and left. I had a feeling that they were in cahoots with criminals in the area and do not think or believe that anyone can blame me for feeling the way I do, or do you?

CLERGY

The clergy has left itself open to daily criticism due to the proclivity of some of its members to high living. They seek earthly glory and honor and demand money from both their church treasuries and parishioners alike for selfish reasons and to the detriment of evangelism and other biblical mandates. Granted, certain churches and some denominations do help and assist the needy, but a lot of these "men of the cloth" who have lent themselves to seeking the comfort of material things and do not really care about their calling or the spiritual well-being of their parishioners. Some of these clergymen care more about worldly glory, honor, and money than all else and have forgotten that we have been warned to be in the world, but not be of it. They prefer or demand that they be called "our father" (*babanmu*). This is contrary to the injunction given by Jesus, not to call anyone father, because there is only one father who is in heaven,[15] yet if they are not addressed this way, they simmer in anger and disgust, not caring for what the Bible has to say and, worse, do not believe in the biblical admonition not to lay for ourselves treasures here on earth but in heaven. They want to be salt to the world and ride the best cars now, today, and have a tantrum if they should be denied these by their churches. A pastor's wife once questioned a parishioner who was seeking admission to study theology abroad if he were truly called to be a minister! This kind of behavior is indicative of jealousy and anger toward competitors or competition! So far, as I know, this is not the lot of any Christian—pastor or otherwise—as taught in the Bible.

CHRISTIANS IN GENERAL

> ... These people come near to me with their mouth and honor me with their lips, but their hearts are far from me. (Isaiah 29:13).

A lot of Christians in Nigeria are worshipping God with their mouths and only on Sundays, but from Monday through Saturday, they are nominal Christians pursuing money and material wealth. The pursuit of money and other worldly materials has turned these Christians to ungodly misbehavior in their homes and places of work, but very much to the delight of non-Christians and some Muslims. They demand graft just like these groups do and sometimes worse. Most of the other Christian sects, on the other hand, whether in the private sector, have conveniently become emulators or what I call "Muslim-lite" or come across like a Muslim in behavior and conduct. Worse, some copy exactly what Muslims do without becoming Muslims through baptism or *wanka* or *bow* in the sallah ritual. Instead of following Christ and be His ambassadors—i.e., light in a dark world, salt to a tasteless society as we are clearly enjoined by Holy Scriptures—they do exactly as the Muslims do without the sallah, a sign and practice characteristic of Muslims. They themselves do not worship the Muslim's Allah, or so they claim. Some Muslims behave in a "holier than thou" manner while some Christians have followed suit. That is wrong both morally and as well as on a religious account!

This is what I also call the "reverse" (R-driving) Christian. By puffing your car in an R-gear, you will be going backward instead of forward as the D-drive is the only mode setup for that. They have actualized the freedom that Christianity affords them by taking bribe money in their offices (public or private) and practice the other misdeeds, characteristic of non-Christian and some Muslims with their "motif operandi" to economically cripple the nation. At any rate, it does not matter how this behavior is practiced or who practices it, duplicity remains as it has always been and will forever remain, a vice and true Christians need to know this and avoid it! Yet being good is and always will forever be a sign of strength and not of weakness!

MUSLIMS

Islam is a religion that is said to mean submission to Allah, with some of its adherents possessing a strange, and perhaps a rancid, sense of proportions. The premise that this religion is a religion of peace, or peace loving, runs counter to as it is diametrically in opposition to everything that is peaceful and of peace. It frowns or has no love or tolerance to all other religions or religious beliefs (meaning, non-Muslims = *arna da kafirai*), people with different faiths. It is very disdainful of others' ways of life (cultures); it detests with absolute repugnance any proselytizing efforts by any and all the religious faiths outside of it, but it believes in its own absolute divine right to conduct activities of proselytization using all means from all the other religions who then are fair game to Moslems. Its adherents can criticize anyone—religion, system, or belief—but this same right, or any other rights, is not reciprocated or reciprocal to any outside the Islamic faith. Some of its adherents' hideous and heinous atrocities—as they visit mayhem those who either refuse or reject this religion and threaten mass death through decapitation on people who are not Muslims with cultures not governed by the sharia law, but dare to reject it—are wrapped up in religious activities which are propelled by hatred that can only be based on the inability to forgive others and racism. So then, Islam is religion that seems to have a form of godliness but in practice and in actuality, minus God, as these acts of evil practices have nothing, absolutely nothing, to do with a kind and merciful Almighty God!

However, some of these same people think—no, they go about thinking or believing that they own the whole world because they are the only ones who follow "Allah." That God created other people not as co-inhabitants with them but subjugates on earth. They also forget that their religion was founded in the sixth century, five-good-plus centuries after Christianity and two-plus millennia after Judaism. They carry out all kinds of atrocities and damages to property without feeling the slightest compunction. They fill every nook and cranny of available space with mosques, and yet they are not satisfied with that because, according to them, everyone has to believe as they do or else. All these activities done in the name of religion without a commensurate change of heart means nothing at best, at worst are useless, not withstanding, even prayer five, ten, or a million times a day!

JUDICIARY

The judiciary is no different from all the other social institutions of this society. Bribery is rampant and has perverted justice in many societies, but the Nigerian situation is really and totally in a class of its own. While the police can change evidence in favor of the guilty after they have stuffed their pockets with graft money, sending the innocent to disappear, similarly the judges who are supposed to know better are easily influenced by bribe and let the guilty go free, making judgment in their favor. And lawyers, a group so good at its profession, can actually bend, twist, and turn iron in every which direction without the benefit of heat of fire. They can change the truth to become a lie, prima facie (in face of evidence) and vice versa, all the while knowing that they are defending the indefensible. Simply put, they call black white, but to them that is too easy to grasp, so they have to try the impossible by calling black red or any other color of their choice. Even more despicable is the idea that someone could be exonerated of a crime they have committed by the simple reason that they belong to a particular tribe or a member of a certain religion.

Some of the Muslim judges are notorious for this type of behavior, letting crooks off the hook often with the concocted cockamamie claim that the Muslim brother was in the first place, falsely accused (without a shred of evidence to back the claim. Remember that this is what some Muslim do all the time, what psychologists call projection) and only because he is a Muslim. Yet they go out and around doing as they please, claiming that Muslim live holier lives than non-Muslims and are in the majority. They are so cruel, and yet the first to cry foul is being persecuted even as they prosecute the non-Muslims and resent Western influence, but then try to ram Islamic traditions, influences, and other cultural practices down non-Muslims noses and throats, whether or not they like it.

CUSTOM AND OTHERS

Our customs officials are a downright disgrace. Recently, I traveled from the United States to Nigeria, and prior to my transit, I had some packages that I had shipped by air cargo to Kano. The six pieces of luggage were checked and cleared with all payment made, and I was directed to go and collect my bags when I arrive Nigeria in Kano. Upon arrival, I proceeded to Kano, and for two good weeks, the Nigerian customs in Kano dribbled me around as if I had committed the worst of crimes. On the third week, I went to see the custom overall boss, a Yoruba man, in Kano. He told me my papers indicated I had done all that in the United States, but not in Nigeria. Those papers were not sufficient to have my luggage released to me in Nigeria, and then he ran by me some new Nigerian rules and regulations that govern luggage claims in Nigeria. I told him that neither I nor the officials in the United States were aware of the new regulations, that we did not know of any problems since the regulation were new anyway. He then cockily said that "ignorance of the law is no excuse." I was so amazed that I wondered aloud by asking him which was worse, ignorance of the law and breaking it or knowing the law and breaking it? What he said next shocked me! He told me to leave his office; that as far as he was concerned, my case had never come across his desk! I was asked to go back to the airport, and if his "boys" released the luggage to me, well and fine, but if not, he would not take kindly if I should return to his office again.

Well, your guess is as good as mine! I spent that whole week again in Kano shuttling from one custom office to another every single, solitary working day with everyone in those offices, and from the clerk to assistant controller, they were soliciting money that I had to pay before my bags were finally released. The most galling and despicable area was the narcotic section, whose staff sniffed, handled, and re-handled my luggage over and over after opening each of them, piece by piece. They finally told me that while they found nothing, they were not prepared to affix their seal of approval on the final document that would clear my luggage for release unless and until I had given them N500. I left Kaduna with N30,000 (naira), but ended up having to borrow N20,000 more in Kano, thus making the sum total of N50,000. I had to spend to claim my personal luggage that I had properly and legally paid and shipped to Nigeria. The money spent for luggage I could hardly afford, but even if I could afford it, it was wrong to spend that amount of money, which I did not want to spend in the first place, to callous custom officials.

SCHOOLS AND UNIVERSITIES

As earlier indicated, the virus of corruption has afflicted all Nigeria's social institutions, and its educational system is not exempt. This particular section's involvement has culminated in lowered educational standards and at all levels of the education endeavor. This is very much to the chagrin and dismay of parents who have no other recourse to educate their children, but then, who cares or bothers? Before the advent of this debacle of education, schools were owned either by governments (local or state governments) or parochial interests—private, church, and/ or missionary entities. Under that type of arrangement, the standard of education was not only high but excellent, and school buildings were symbols of pride for students and parents alike. However, with state government taking over ownership of schools following a decree by the federal government for universal primary education in 1976, which, tacitly was aimed at promoting Islam, the standard of education in the entire nation started dipping. There are those who would argue that the UPE program was not meant to promote Islam but to meet the educational needs of the times to these skeptics. I say take a look at the issue again and not just view it at face value. Certainly, behind this diabolical scheme, a foolish proposal at best was the aim and goal to Islamize the country. If not then, at least the seeds were planted; but had these goals and objectives been clear then, they would have been opposed vehemently.

The standard of education has never been the same since that change. Our universities graduate thousand of graduates every year, but these know perhaps only one-half of the subject matter in which they majored after completing their education at some of these institutions of higher learning. This is because during their study careers, they spend over 75 percent of the time at home due to strikes, time they needed to have spent in school studying. If the students are not agitating for strikes, their lecturers and professors are. This has now turned into a vicious cycle of one strike after another all the time, while Nigerians and their politicians "play the proverbial ostrich head in the sand" game. By doing so, they indicate that what you do not see has not happened or will not happen simply because their collective "head" is under the sand. It is dark in there since they can see nothing. The fact that it is dark where the head is buried in the sand does not stop the sun doing its preordained job, and doing it very well, to the enjoyment of the rest of God's creation. Well, it is not all that well in Nigeria, and it is foolhardy to think that way because the rest of the world knows and sees what is happening in Nigeria whether or not we realize it.

NIGERIANS ABROAD

The behavior of Nigerians at home and abroad has placed a collective tag of stigma on all Nigerians, who are looked upon as "social rejects" outside the borders of this nation. Things are so bad that Nigerians are neither able to live in Nigeria, nor are we comfortable outside it; therefore, we are or have been marginalized! Because many of us left our country of Nigeria for a variety of reasons, but since we grew up there before leaving, we were infected by that awful virus of moral decay, leading to corrupt behavior that has now become the mainstay of every activity back home. Some of us transported some of these unholy characters and behaviors into our new abodes and environments. Some even carry their criminal conducts to extremes by getting involved in criminal activities such as robberies, distribution of drugs and/ or narcotics—all in the effort to get rich quickly. In so doing, some of these fools think out ways in hopes of outsmarting the white man in his country of birth; but then their worlds almost always crumble in on them as many of these "smart Nigerian thugs" have been languishing in foreign prisons.

Just a few years back, a Nigerian and his wife schemed to defraud an insurance company based in the United States. They both came home to Nigeria, but only for the husband to return to the United States and declare that his spouse had deceased, while he presented a fake certificate of death which he had obtained in Ghana to the insurance company. He collected the first payment and was about to collect the last part of payment, when his supposed late or decease wife returned to America. They were both hauled to jail and are sitting in prison. Another Nigerian is also serving a jail sentence for fraud and crimes that involved stocks exchange business acts in Wall Street, New York. All these corrupt behaviors do not help, but only enhance the turbid reputation that Nigerians have so very well earned as result of misdeeds outside the confines of Nigeria. Hopefully, children born to these people outside Nigeria will turn out to be good citizens in their respective countries, and not be like their parents, that they will learn to live within their means and not thinking that they are entitled to can have everything material in this void.

OTHER AREAS OF CORRUPTION
AND THE IMPLICATION

Our institutions of higher learning are phenomena onto themselves, in addition to the incessant strikes by lecturers, students, workers, and administrative staff. The university libraries are empty shelves with no books. Nothing seems to work as designed as when the white man was in charge and running things. The most sobering aspect of the corruption madness is the temerity that lecturers, who refuse to teach, but are always asking for salary increases. Bribery is everywhere, from admission to graduation. These lecturers are what I call "dons with an attitude." If they are not striking, they are planning for one or are on a sabbatical or vacation. If they are not on vacation, you can be sure that since teaching is only a side issue to them, they are scheming methods to extort money from their poor students. Let me be blunt but spare you the gory details. Some of these lecturers do not only ask for money from students as payment for lecture notes, but demand sexual favors from poor female students. Some female students cannot even graduate without succumbing to gratify immoral sexual desires of some of these creeps on twos.

What does all this mean, you ask? Well, for a start, black people—whether in Nigeria, Africa, or elsewhere in the world—are in a very bad shape. Slavery officially ended with the emaciation of slaves in the 1862 when President Abraham Lincoln signed an edict that proclaimed slaves to be freed.[15] After this great humanitarian act of emancipation, it was only a matter of time that freedom of all blacks everywhere would follow. Slaves in America were freed and allowed to return and settle in Liberia. Freed slaves in Britain likewise were repatriated and settled in Sierra Leone. Following these examples, colonial power in colonized Africa started succumbing to both internal (civil unrests) and external pressures (by the international community of nations) by relinquishing colonial rule and occupations of countries in Africa over to Africans. In a nutshell, without circumlocution and its attendant verbiage, this particular act of emancipation implicated as it affected all black people everywhere, who are both free and responsible for their own state of affairs.

ALL BLACK PEOPLE

Slavery is over and has been over a long, long time ago. In the first place, white people did not invade Africa, hunted the Africans down, and took them captives as slaves. The truth of the matter is, Africans themselves sold their fellow Africans—their brothers and sisters—to the white man and then blamed the white man. It is therefore not only unfair, but a sinister misrepresentation of facts to blame only white people for a deplorable inhuman behavior that the black people themselves have been architects of—hook and sinker! Goods in the marketplace are for sale, therefore, what you do not wish to part with, if you get my drift, is not put on display in the marketplace with a price tag with an On Sale sign on!

Furthermore, after the emancipation proclamation and freeing of every slave, all freed slaves were then not only freed—yes, totally freed—to leave and return to Africa. Some did, but a lot more chose to stay behind. Today, their descendants—the likes of Jesse Jackson and other black leaders, a group that has specialized in complaints and misrepresentation of facts and only about white people from Western countries—are asking or demanding for reparation. Sure, I am for reparation, but only after the Jews have been compensated for their slavery in Africa. After all, they were enslaved by the African Arabs for over four hundred years in Egypt. It is guilt by extension or affiliation that the black leaders in America are leveling against the white people in general. No white American alive today owns any slaves, not their fathers, not even their grandfathers owned one, but they are connected to slavery through guilt by extension. Fine then, let us also examine the African record and our responsibility toward the Jews. Black people everywhere in the world, including the ones in American, also owe the Jews reparation because living in Africa connects all of us to the sordid past of the Jews slavery in Egypt, Africa, by extension.

The argument that the Jewish slavery took place in Egypt does hold because Egyptians then and now were and are Africans, and so are we. Moreover, because slavery took place several centuries after the Jews had finished their own slavery in Egypt, it is all the more reason why we are connected to it. Our forebears were involved in that human tragedy, and so are we by implication, because this is exactly what some blacks are accusing whites of doing! It is only after the Africans have compensated the Jews for their slavery in Egypt, where untold millions of them died. Look at the facelift they gave the African nation of Egypt by building the pyramids—now a famous tourist attraction. Any talk about reparation for black can only begin after a Jewish compensation! The Jews were wronged through forced labor first, and this was well over two millennia before slave trade that brought slaves from the African continent to the Americas even began (perhaps early to mid-second millennium after Christ).

It is a fact, whether we understanding it or not, that the white man relinquished power and handed it over to the black people in Nigeria several decades, if not a half century, ago. In so doing, he handed the ugly chains of slavery to black people in general, and African in particular. After the episode of this ugly situation of bondage, white people left the scene. The natural course of action that should have followed was to throw those ugly chains of slavery to sink them in the depth of the deepest ocean and then forget them there! However, this is not what these black leaders have done; they have instead hidden them as secret treasures and have used the same factors that the white people used as they enslaved blacks in Europe, the Americas, and elsewhere here in Africa. There are constant haranguing and preachments about the evils of slavery, racism, and unfairness by the white man from these same so-called black leaders, who actually seem to be allergic to peace and harmony and go about sowing seeds of discord anywhere and everywhere that they are given audience.

Talk about the inability to forgive! Many black people are what I call the "blancophobics," (people who hate anyone with "white" people or anyone with a white skin, just as there are some white folks who are "negrophobics." It is amazing to observe how some black leaders are quick to react with accusatory fingers after any incident between a white person and a black person without knowing or examining all the facts as the case may be, with the black person at the receiving end. Yet by the same token, these same black leaders remain quiet with a convenient or selective amnesia, when a similar incident occurs that involves a white person and a black individual and the white person is at the receiving end!

This group of people do not want to forgive, nor do they want to forget anything or any wrong done in the past, except when it comes their own misdeeds and wrongs they have themselves visited on others, which they do not want revealed or mentioned, for doing so is definitely based on "racist motives." Neither do they wish to speak out on issues like the current slavery situation in Sudan, which, to my mind, has the dollar sign attached to it, as the dollar does not pass them by for any reason whatsoever. I believe that bribery is involved here; they must have been bribed by some of the Arab states to be quite about it; otherwise, how is the deafening silence on this outrageous issue so palpable? The so-called mother ship brings messages to Minister Farrakhan to announce to the entire world—perhaps these evil deeds are perpetrated only by white people and not by blacks!

Moreover, these missionaries of bitterness and confusion prefer to hate, but also at the same time, preach togetherness and pretend to see no contradiction in their messages. They use similar factors to cause bitterness and disunity among the races, while at the same time enrich themselves all during the same process. Call it what you wish, I choose to call it what it really is—inane and capricious stupidity. No one group can or should claim a higher ground in race relations, as far as I am concerned, until it has totally and completely disavowed racism, with all racist motives, nor any traces of racism been seen in any of its actions; and this applies equally both to the white and to the black people alike, or for that matter, whatever other color available to the human race or races there may be!

Another clear example is the mistreatment of other immigrant blacks by some of the American-born blacks that defies description. The descendants of African American slaves—the American "black graftees" or "African rejects"—were sold to white people by black Africans themselves, as white people had nothing to do with hunting down the slaves from their villages in their homeland in Africa, although the role of the white people was a minor one, that of purchasing the goods or wares (the slaves) and transporting those goods to mainland or continental America, but one which was, all the same, wrong for engaging in human-ware trafficking at any rate. To my mind, while the buyer may be at fault, the greater culprit is the hunter and hawker of the human goods that he had captured. Call me naïve, but that is the truth that no black person would want to admit.

These black Americans are among the most racist group of people that stand erect on twos. The attitude of a good lot of black people not only reeks of racism, it is racism proper, through and through. As the adage goes, "If it looks racist, smells racist, and acts like a racist, it is a racist!" Consider the recently held presidential election of November 2008 when well over 95 percent of black people in the United States voted for Barack Obama, simply because of his skin color, as Barack Obama was, as he still is, "black," and against John McCain—because he is "white." Yet this is the same group of people, black people, who would instantly accuse white folks of racism, but would defend the most ridiculous, even defenseless behavior or conduct of any of their own, no matter how racist the behavior! A good number of white people made it possible for Barack Obama to become the president of the United States of America in the last presidential election cycle; this is because a huge number of white people voted for him, and not for John McCain. If white people in America were anything close to being racists, nothing in the world could have made them vote for Mr. Obama, yet today, these same white group are being branded as racists, and swastikas-carrying mob on the grounds that they dare to oppose Obama's tax and spend super liberal views and policies on a number of issues, but especially on health care.

Furthermore, bashing white people draws applause at gatherings, but especially and particularly in black audiences all across the United States in which black people cannot help but indulge at every available opportunity. Yet these same groups are offended at the slightest hint of any poked at any other race, but especially about people, in any public speech, regardless of the setting for which the speech is delivered.

In 1980, my house on 301 North Day street Orange, New Jersey, was set ablaze by a female American Negro who collected more benefits from the state Welfare Department by claiming she lost all her belongings in a fire, but this was not the case. My crime was that I, an immigrant black from Africa, tried to help her with her illegitimate child after her parents threw her out from their house! She could not deal with her parents, but displaced her anger on me and my family by trying to burn our house. You see, according to the thinking of some of these graftees, "foreigners" should not be so successful through hard work. The fact that we are, it is a potent testament against their indolence and culture of dependence of the white man whom they love to hate and fitfully condemn every chance they get. However, this is a totally different subject, which probably, on its own has a life of its own, and it is best to just leave it alone for now. In short, "black leaders" the world over, especially those in the United States, are not interested in racial harmony, but rather in disharmony of the races. These leaders are constantly on crusade and expedition of finding or perhaps inventing reasons for radial restiveness and disunity.

AFRICANS AND NIGERIANS IN PARTICULAR

As earlier indicated, the white man has been gone from the colonial and political scene in Africa for several decades now. Still, the African leader, but especially Nigerian leaders from the dominant groups, the Hausa/Fulani/Muslim triumvirate, like some black leaders in America, continue to find it necessary to apportion blame due to action or conducts of their own that is also volitional and blame it on the white man. Doing that does not make us any better, or different, from the white man—it certainly does excuse us, nor does it grant us black people the right to be or act racists ourselves? This is because, two wrongs do not a right make! A racist is a racist regardless of the color of skin he or she wears! End of the story!

These African leaders were bequeathed or inherited not only the reigns of government from the white man, but also his fanaticism for exploitation. In some instances, they have far exceeded the evil deeds of the white man, some of which are beyond imagination. They are unable to use any of their languages that are native to Nigerians other than that of the white man, whom, as they want us to believe, they hate so much. It is the same white man's language that Nigerians use as a lingua franca in conducting official government business in Nigeria, in case anyone has not yet noticed! We saw the use of the "gun power" as mentioned in the preface, but the "machete" or "adda" power that was unleashed on blacks by their black brothers in Nigeria defies description. It takes satanic possession to hack another person to death without any human feeling, just because they are from another tribe or they practice a different religion.

Let me show you just how racism is deep-seated and cherished in Africa by using Nigeria as a clear example. In Nigerian, this subhuman behavior, racism, has its own off springs—tribalism and religious bigotry—that are potent tools used in the domination of other Nigerians, or Africans, as the case may be. Because they hate each other so much, they cannot even use any of the native or local languages as a lingua franca, but would rather use English, a foreign language—one that they claim to hate very much. Racism, as expressed in tribalism, is a gem that these dominant groups of the ilk of Hausa/Fulani Muslim dyad or triad and/or the Yoruba/Igbo groups or whatever so much cherish. Because the Hausa/Fulani, the most dominant of the dominant groups, are predominantly Muslim, they detest all other groups that happen to be non-Hausa/Fulani and who also happen to be predominantly non-Muslims, or the Kafirs, under their domination. However, that is not the end of the story. The Hausa/Fulani Muslim group considers itself superior to any other Muslim (except for the Saudis) whose members will not be converted, or be *tubabbus*, to Islam. They consider themselves born into Islam as the real Muslims while the proselytes or *tubabbus* are not as real, genuine, or assiduous in the practice of Islam. In short, and to sum it all up, according to them, there is a reason, an ulterior motive, behind anyone's conversion because he/she was not born into the Islamic religion, rather than on purely personal conviction of becoming a Muslim. This is, however, a totally different and larger subject beyond the scope of this book, so a token mention of it has to suffice here.

People's health in every human society is very important. It is not, on the other hand, nearly as important as the moral fiber and values of a society. A person can give money, valuable materials, or something else in exchange or quest for physical health. However, a person—indeed, a society—can give nothing in exchange of his or its moral or soul. The Lord Jesus Christ captures this truth so succinctly when he said,

> For what shall it profit a man if he should gain the whole world and loose his soul, or what will a man give in exchange for his soul?[7]

If the past world empires like the Roman—and before it the Greek, before which was the Babylonia and all the other empires that followed and could not stand because of moral decay, an internal rut that always characterizes corrupt societies—it will take a colossal miracle to see Nigeria survive this state of decadence it has attained and still remains a nation. I, for one, will not be surprised if this country easily falls into the hands of a weak enemy, or breaks into a few countries from its current entity in not too distant future. I may be preaching doom and gloom as some may say, but the degree of corruption has now passed that palliative stage for a mere therapy to do any good. What is needed and must happen to salvage the situation is either shock therapy or radical surgery. If any cancer has metastasized, as this moral disease called corruption has done in Nigeria, a mere palliative tinkering approach will not do. A radical approach must be considered, for it will take a humongous calamity to shake this nation back to its natural senses, and that is radical surgery, period! But again, surgery is not the panacea in conditions; chemical and radiation therapies usually do accompany cancerous surgical excisions, as powerful treatment adjuncts. So I want to see what will happen to Nigeria!

Let us again return to the write-up of Mallam Kallam and analyze a few things that he said. Note in paragraph 10 of his write-up, while Mallam Kallam blames the white man in every imaginable way possible, he uses

English, the white man's language, as the medium of communicating his ideas. Since he is a Muslim, he could have used Arabic, but then few and perhaps no one would read his garbage. Consequently, the circulation of such a crazy material would be severely limited, as it would certainly be restricted as it should, only to the Arab world, which I am sure would applaud him. At any rate, it is in English that he studied and "earned" his baccalaureate and master's degrees in business administration and finance in economics, respectively, and not in Hausa, Fulfulde, or the Arabic language. He is still using English in his PhD program and all other educational pursuits, which he derisively calls the "wrong type of education," including a myriad of other endeavors and some such silly accusations. In paragraph 13, he chides Nigerians for accepting "foreign doctrines without" thought. As a Muslim, which I believe he is, he is supposed to be fluent in Arabic—I doubt he even knows Arabic, much less write it, in order to accuse any of the Arab states about anything, even if he were willing to do so! If Mallam Kallam, an educated Muslim, can express this level of stupendous ignorance, just imagine the degree of such ignorance and the herd mentality that is often characteristic of this bunch. Without knowing the facts and not to talk of thinking for themselves, they are always against everything for no reason. They often abduct the innocent and the unwary into believing this kind of garbage in the name and cause of their religion! And guess what, they are always accepted and believed without equivocation. These people just won't tell the truth, instead they use propaganda to obfuscate it, and that is only a part of the problems facing this country.

FREEDOM OF EXPRESSION

This brings us to the question of freedom of expression, religion, and all other freedoms. For a start, during civilian administrations, there is usually press freedom. However, under dictatorial reigns—i.e., when the military commander takes over power—that freedom is always reduced to zero, as it cannot stand any criticism and does not tolerate it at all. They start the suppression of all human rights by suspending the constitution and then go from there. Second, religious freedom is a myth in Nigeria. If the freedom to believe as you please exists, then it is only superficially and in the minds of those who think it exists.

Christians are allowed to believe and practice their religion in certain areas, whereas Muslims can believe and practice anyhow and anywhere they please. They discuss and insult other religions and their belief without the fear of any retribution. Recently, an article captioned "A Study in Tribalism" accused ex-head of state General Buhari of ethnocentric behavior. He is said to have pursued or fostered sectional or tribalistic goals during his tenure as the executive chairman of the now-defunct Petroleum Trust Fund (PTF). Besides concentrating his PTF efforts for road construction in area of his states of origins, Kano and Kaduna, I also hasten to add that it was also the observation of many people in Kaduna State that General Buhari (Rtd.) concentrated the PTF road construction efforts in Kaduna town in predominantly Hausa and Muslim areas like Tudun Wada, Ungwar Sarki, Kawo, and Badarawa, providing them with good tarred roads. However, in places like Television, Kakuri, Ungwar Sunday, and their surrounding areas, just forget it. Since only very few Hausas-Fulanis and Muslims live in these parts, they were neglected. As recently as the year 2001, General Buhari made statements of profound interest to all peace-loving Nigerians, when the former head of state of this country uttered statements that only illiterates, the likes of Mallam Musa Kallam and other fanatic religious zealots, are capable of making. He is said to have intoned that no Muslim should vote for a Christian in the 2003 elections. If General Buhari, who has been a leader in Nigeria, can display such a reckless level of carelessness in both deed and word, then it all goes to show that no solutions can be available to solve the country's problems. But should it be wrong, so be it, but I at least believe in finding lasting solution. I also believe we can reach some solution, provided they start treating us people and objects. A good star will be for them to stop ramming their religion down our throats. By the way, why does this religion demand defense in a violent manner from its adherents?

What this all means is that some people talk peace with their mouth when their heat is not in it. Others, people like Buhari, believe that they and their dominant groups have a divine mandate to rule this country. They have been endowed by Almighty God to lead this country at any and all costs. Furthermore, they are accountable to no one, including the very God they claim put them in charge. The claim is this, they are in the majority, and because of that, they have to concentrate governmental services in the areas that their dominant groups reside in the country. Health facilities, you name it, including health care personnel, are drawn from all other areas to the neglect of other groups without the feeling of any compunction at all. Worst, it is their belief that there is nothing anyone can do about it for all the above and more reasons.

14. ORDINARY NIGERIANS

Ordinary Citizen

Having dealt with other segments of the society, I cannot be remiss by failing to mention the part played by the ordinary citizen in all this. Nigerians are to blame for what corruption has done to the nation. Dishonesty and corrupt practices pervade the entire society. Our leaders and politicians are not Martians or creatures from some other extraterrestrial bodies. They are born and raise or bred in the Nigerian society, at least the majority of them are anyway. The love of money and material things have so damaged our moral character so much so that one is hard-pressed to find anyone with moral integrity in the country. From the hawkers and market women who sell provisions in the open market to our commerce department in the federal government, none is immune from the above charge. As it has already been pointed elsewhere in this book, Nigerians are allergic to all laws, including laws made by God and their politicians. There is a culture that is countercurrent to law and order. As far as they are concerned, laws are for "my neighbor, not for me. I am too big for that."

I can list every occupational category and their corrupt practices here, but that is not necessary as I believe you get the point. It's no use beating a dead horse to death, it is already dead! I, however, will use only a few other examples.

Think of it, spare parts are not only fake but sold at exorbitant prices. Stop at just any store that sells auto parts in Kaduna, Jos, Maiduguri, Lagos, etc., and ask if the part you are looking for is available. The immediate answer is yes, it is available, knowing full well that the store either does not stock it or is out of it. You will finally arrive at an agreeable price and the dealer of the part then sends someone to "their other store" to bring it. The part is brought, and you remit payment, collect the part, and leave.

Well, what has just transpired is not exactly the true picture. This arrangement is a constant occurrence between mechanics and their customers. What has happened is this: the store owner, for start, did not have another store even though that was the impression he wanted you to have. Second, the agreed price that you paid was a certain percentage over the actual price of the item, which he quickly removes and then sends the actual cost to the store that he got the item from. You see, there is a tacit understanding and agreement among these auto parts sellers who are governed by dishonesty to defraud customers. This behavior violates the moral mores and ethical practices of any occupation or profession. However, this is a detestable behavior, but in Nigeria, it is viewed as being "smart" or fiscally savvy. Also lawyers all over the world have a bad reputation precisely because of the circumvention and/or suspension of personal ethics in certain business practices. In Nigeria, a very close second to the legal profession is this auto part dealership, an occupation with a very turbid reputation, as everyone who owns a car should know by experience what I am talking about.

In order not to belabor the point, one more example should drive this very point—the endemic nature of corruption in Nigeria, home for the reader. Builders are another group among a slew of many others, and not just professionals, with everyday misbehavior. If, God should forbid that, something happens to a place you are currently developing, a house for example, the estimates from the land survey to the architect would only be part of a greater headache that awaits you. The mason, after you have all agreed on the cost price for puffing up the building, would demand for down payment for mobilization from 25 to 50 percent. After you have paid him, he then absconds and becomes a fugitive. But if you are lucky, he might lay the foundation and start building, following which, he would then bolt. Some builders may have several other building contracts for which they divide their time and attention. So a building contract that you expected and anticipated a quick execution may last months, if not years!

In the meantime, prices continue to rocket sky high while you sit, wait, and seethe with anger. If and when the building is completed, well, then, only half of your problems have gone. The carpenter and his crew of helpers is about to unleash his own demands, which all follow a similar pattern as that of the builder and those before him. Call this cynicism or being overly critical or what else you may choose to call it, but to my mind, it displays both unethical and immoral behavior—all of which stems from the tree of corruption and greed and results to an unbelievable level of materialism. There are churches and mosques everywhere, indicating that Nigerians are very religious, but all that is only an outward display of religiosity, which does not really translate into deeds.

Lastly, and by no means the least, I am suggesting that the list of groups or individuals that have contributed to the decadent situation which our society finds itself in today has been exhausted. The list, it is fair to say, is inexhaustible as most, if not every, Nigerians over the age of twenty is either directly or indirectly involved in corrupt practices. Nobody, if you get my drill, is exempt; and if they are, they are certainly not exculpable, or they do not live in Nigeria. The corrupt practices of Nigerians was and continues to be neither contained nor limited to the country's physical and natural borders but has been exported to wherever and whatever societies Nigerians are found in. We drive discarded cars from other nations as if they are flying new jets with a high rate of accidents and mortality in the country. Besides, at home, they are rudely uncouth to each other and park their used cars anyhow, anywhere, and anytime.

Take for example the scholarships awarded to Nigerian students in foreign countries by either the federal government or the state entities in years past. I cannot, as I am not, speak about all embassies or consular offices overseas. However, if what was going on in our consular office—then located at 575 Lexington Avenue, New North, New York—was even remotely similar in London, other parts of Europe, Australia, and Canada, then the suffering of Nigerian students was not only uncalled for but criminal. I can, however, speak with authority about our consular staff in New York. Those of us who were fortunate to have won the privilege and selected for scholarship suffered unnecessarily. True to the saying, we were suffering and enduring absolutely "in the middle of plenty." Every year, the federal government would send tuition, fees, and other forms of payments, but these monies would not be paid out on time for several months, purposely to enable the lump sum sent to yield interest or to so-called collect dust. This so-called dust was the interest on the lump sent before students were paid their tuition and other allowances. This was and is filthy lucre and decried by most religion that I know of.

The implications of the mess in the present state of our health system are simply glaring not to be noticed. For starters, it is already discussed in portions of the previous chapters that the health of individuals, and ultimately that of the society at large, is very important in every human society during one's lifetime. Governments of most societies have health concerns at the very top, among other priorities. In Nigeria, however, this is not the case, whatever available resources apportioned to the health sector are a leftover by corrupted officials who usually take the lion's share. What is left goes to the dominant areas of the majority groups first. Whatever else, a precious title that is a leftover from that is what is then used to address issue emanating from the areas or communities of non-Muslim groups. The downside of all this is that the health care, even facilities in the areas of the dominant groups are not optimum and health care is poor for all the reasons already mentioned. This is due primarily to the lack of equipment and the nonchalant attitude of health care workers followed by the non-caring attitudes of leaders. As far as these corrupt government officials are concerned, the provision of any basic amenities to other Nigerians is tantamount to setting up a well-furnished table of food before rodents. Similarly, but equally offensive to them, is the idea of the provision of adequate health facilities and care to non-Muslims, as tantamount to turning over Buckingham Palace to pigs or swines. Just conjure up any detestable imagery that your mind can dredge up, and replace it with the foregoing examples. This is the attitude of dominant Hausa/Fulani groups, who happen to be Muslims. This kind of a mind-set does not auger well for either peace or peaceful coexistence among neighbors within a nation.

It is high time that Nigerians come to terms with the fact that it is pointless chasing the winds of materialism and hunt for what we cannot catch. Anyone that goes hunting or fishing must carry with him the necessary tools, without which they might themselves become the hunted! In seeking for material gains, we cannot abandon the principles of morality, values, fair play, and justice, but instead hope to succeed using corrupt practices.

COMPARISON OF HEALTH FACILITIES AND CARE IN THE VARIOUS STAGES OF THE NATION'S DEVELOPMENT

Let us compare the state of our health care facilities equipment, services provided, and the availability of drugs in pharmacies in these government health care facilities during the colonial rule, the first civilian administrations, and the subsequent military regimes.

Let us start first with the colonial administration and its efforts about the health system. At the very beginning, health facilities were very few that health care concentrated mainly in large cities and towns with huge populations, places like Lagos, Ibadan, Kano, Zaria, Enugu, Port Harcourt, Calabar, Benin, Ilorin, Bauchi, Jos, Gombe, Yola, Onitsha, Sokoto, Minna, Makurdi, Katsina, Kafanchan, Malunfashi, and a few other places. At that time, the available hospitals, dispensaries health centers, and pharmacies were replete with drugs and other medicinal necessities. The laboratories were functioning very well with proper laboratory equipment and every imaginable reagent; x-ray machines were functioning properly and had spare parts in the event of any breakdown. Operating theaters had functioning autoclaves, and other sterilization equipments were also available. Medical and surgical inpatient units had bandages, instruments, and other implements for dressings as well as thermometers, sphygmomanometers, stethoscopes, etc. Bedpans and urinals were also available for the proper and effective care of patients. Morgues or mortuaries had functioning refrigerators to house dead bodies, cadavers, and so on. Most of all, health care workers employed in these facilities did their work as described and prescribed in their work policies, manual, or schedules; and doctors, pharmacists, nurses, and other administrative personnel came to work on time and stayed at their respective working areas as there was discipline. In short, patient care was smooth and patients received the best of care that the health system could offer even at that time of low education when the educational requirement for training professionals and occupations was very low.

By comparison to today's entry levels for these same professions, the entry levels were really very low, yet after graduation and taking a job in any of these health facilities, health care workers who took their work seriously.

During the first civilian administration of 1960 to 1966,[8] the condition of the health system, its facilities and workers, were not all that different from the preceding colonial administration. In fact, one can say that the conditions in those eras were similar in many respects, but I am not implying that things were rosy good as this was not so, even during the colonial times. This much, too, can also be said to be the situation during the first and second military regimes of both General Aguiyi-Irosi and Yakubu Gowon from 1966-1975.[9] While the general welfare of the average Nigerian in those years was fair, yet because of inflation brought about by the civil war of 1967-1970,[10] with remarkable increase in population, the health of the average citizen did not experience any marked change. Although the society had a lot more health facilities with increases in population, the number of doctors, and generally in all health professionals, increased somewhat. This was due in part to the increased number of secondary schools, technical and tertiary institutions of learning, like polytechnics and universities that were turning out graduates in record numbers. However, it was during these first two military regimes that the seed of corruption began to germinate and rear its ugly head. By the end of the third and fourth military regimes of the Murtala and Obasanjo,[11] due to the oil boom and inflation, corruption took hold in the economic scene. Contracts were inflated to cover the 10 percent or even 25 percent of the graft money that went to those awarding the contracts. The military men, after the second civilian administrations, even forgot that they wore uniforms, even though before induction into the army they had taken oaths of allegiance to the military, a profession charged with the safety of the nation.

The fifth military regime of Buhari-Idiagbon in 1983 ushered in an era of discipline dubbed war against indiscipline, or WAI. This particular effort sought to put on leash or restraint on the ungovernable conduct of Nigerians at every sphere of activity: The Buhari-Idiagbonic military administration also endeavored to correct all the serious missteps of its previous military predecessors. However, before these corrective steps took hold, the self-born Babangida era came into existence through another military coup that dislodged Buhari and Idiagbon in 1985. This latest military regime of Ibrahim Babangida proved to be the worst, not only because it was a corrupt military regime but because it was the most corrupt administration that the country had ever witnessed in its very brief history of less than forty years after independence as a nation.

Following this diabolic regime was the short-lived Shonekan civilian administration which, by all accounts, intent, and purposes, was just another military phased-in regime installed by Babangida, purported to serve him as a puppet or stooge when, not if, he decided to stage a comeback. However, General Sani Abacha thwarted that effort and came to power by default. He ceased on the Shonekan civilian weakness, an opportunity that was ripe and was presented to him on a silver platter! He just walked over the timid civilian leader, who should appropriately be described as the "storekeeper," into the chambers of government and took control with no resistance whatsoever from Baba Shonekan, proving that he, Abacha, after all, was not as dumb as he was made out to be by some. Remember that Ibrahim Babangida had left Abacha in the military, as insurance in the event that the civilian Shonekan nursed any funny ideas by getting comfortable in his storekeeping position and thus did not attempt to pull any pranks before Babangida's messianic return.

So after securing and consolidating power, Abacha then put the country through another squeezer by squeezing any life left by the Babangida administration that was that the brutal regime was not aware existed, but was untapped, nonetheless. He nearly smothered out the little and the remaining life that Babangida left in the Nigerian economy, his careless spending escapades. However, the truth is, Abacha, though shred, was not very bright as he was an absent leader, since it was his lieutenants that ran the show, and very ruthlessly, for that matter. They did so by fiats and edicts. The lust for power that usually accompanies powerful leaders or rulers in Africa, but especially military rulers and their illegitimate regimes that enjoy exercising in Nigeria, is best left epithets of word of description, but not for sight by the human eye. The military (or militiamen in military uniforms, if you will) cannot win elections in any democratic society without the use of force; after which, if the elections are held, they steal them by rigging the results. Whatever methods is used to ascend to power, they would then ransack the treasury of the country silly of whatever precious little that was left from the previous military ruler and his administration.

The country got some sort of a reprieve from Abacha when he kicked the bucket (died) in office. Then came to power another military regime, the short-lived Abdul-Salami Abubakar administration that seemed to have been a much-needed relieve of the combined long, but equally dark years of Babangiad/Shonekan/Abacha (evil triumvirate) administration. But even the benign-looking Abdul-Salami regime was not, after all, immunized to corruption, as we were later to come to learn. Just remember that "not all that glitters is gold." Similarly, the steady decline of health care facilities that started in previous years dipped even further reaching its lowest ebb at this time. As a matter of fact, this phenomenon—poor quality of services—was, and still is, not only peculiar to the health sector alone, but pervades all the social institutions of the country.

Ordinary Nigerians have been neglected for too long—this trend began during the second civilian administration—but by the same token, the nation was relegated to and has remained a beggar nation status despite its vast oil and mineral resources. The perchance for crime—the disregard for rules, laws, and regulations—has pushed us to become the world third-class citizen's status instead of world's second-class, the class to which most third world underdeveloped nations belong. Because the standard of living of some Nigerians, in some instances, is prehistoric—that is, if there ever were such a people. While a few people can afford a car, those that can afford to buy a car can only buy used automobiles from European countries and the Americas. For sure Nigeria assembles Peugeots cars all right, but it does not make a single knot of that car—everything is imported and the prices of the assembled car is so outrageously unaffordable even to the very rich! All this, unequivocally, is as a result of corruption brought upon the innocent people who have had nothing to do with the upheavals in the country by corrupt political leaders, some of whom they did not elect. These corrupt practices make Nigeria a pariah nation with citizens as third-class world citizens. So, Mr. President, it is within your aegis to save us from these corrupt practices, but especially the police force. Please help all Nigerians from these officially sanctioned thugs.

Shortages from oil and oil products made from the very petroleum oil, which Nigeria exports in copious amounts to other countries, to drinking water became daily occurrences. Long queues were formed at every petrol or gas stations which dot every street in every city in the country and were a commonplace while touts in areas like Kano, Plateau, Sokoto, Kaduna, etc., had plenty of supplies of the same scarce petrol, which they use to extort money from motorists in towns and other far-removed areas of the country. They sell it in the back market at exorbitant price, these fraudulent charges yield filthy lucre for them.

We Nigerians suffer from collective amnesia or what I refer to as the Sauna syndrome. Sauna is a fictional character who overdosed on numbskullity, behavior that is progressively and expressively idiotic and foolish in almost every situation that required the employ of common sense. For instance, Sauna saw a white man in the marketplace wearing nice shiny shoes; Sauna approached the white fellow and asked him, "Please give me your shoes." The white man declined the request stating, "I need them myself." Sauna would not be deterred, so he followed the white man everywhere he went, studying the shoes carefully! Satisfied with his observation, Sauna then dashed home, got some money he had saved, returned to the market, bought some leather and rubber materials, then went to work. Before long, Sauna had a pair of shoes which he started wearing right away with his best clothes. Of course, the shoes were not anywhere close to what the white man wore than his skin is any closer to the color of the white man's skin!

THE FUTURE OF HEALTH CARE IN NIGERIA

The future of the health system in Nigeria rests squarely on the shoulders of Nigerians, but the future is not too bright, nor are the portends, as all that good either. In fact, the future is bleak, and that is putting it mildly if there should be no change in conduct and attitude toward money. Abraham Lincoln is credited as having once pointed out by his reply to a riddle "How many legs does a dog have if you count the tail?" His answer to the riddle offers a profound insight as he stated, "Four." He said, "Because counting the tail as a leg doesn't make it one." Could it be Abraham Lincoln had been describing Nigeria? I doubt it because the nation that we call Nigeria today was not in existence in Lincoln's day, and Mr. Lincoln was no prophet. The fact that Nigeria dubs itself "the giant of Africa" does not make Nigeria a giant any more than the story in President Lincoln's riddle. No one commands respects except through deeds of respectable acts. Nigeria would indeed be a giant at least for Nigerians if its government earning that kudos by making the necessary provisions and situations at home palatable. That means by providing not piped, but good water and electricity to every nook and corner of the country, given its vast natural resources. But where and when these services are even found, they are erratic at best. Our health facilities are in shambles, schools look so dilapidated that make one wonder if they are schools at all. Children have no place to sit, nor do their teachers, with everything looking either torn or broken down. The above description is not at all the symbolism of a giant but that of a weakling.

There are no drugs in our government hospitals and health care facilities where the concept of "socialized medicine" is supposedly being practiced. No compassion or courtesy on the attitude of the health care professionals in health care facilities toward sick patients, who are often treated as inanimate objects, is devoid of any human feelings through no fault of theirs. This is clearly portrayed in a few examples of government hospitals, including the teaching hospital in Kaduna. These health care facilities are filthy, and most of the time, they look as if they were the habitation of pigs and not places where human beings receive care. Some of the equipment, like wheelchairs make horrendous noise when patients are being conveyed to and from emergency room of a teaching hospital Kaduna that birds in nearby trees take to flight.

There is, however, a glimmer of hope that the health system situation might change. With the second coming of President Olusegun Obasanjo (first as General Obasanjo, but now a popularly elected politician) and with some governors of his ruling party in office in some of the states, one can hope for change, or should one be hopeful? It seems that some of the health care facilities are getting some facelift only outwardly—that is, structural changes—but no new equipment acquired for workers to work with. If this should be the case, then this new effort and other similar initiatives will inevitably end up in the same way that past efforts ended up. They would be mere cosmetic designs dressed up purposely for aesthetics and, therefore, shallow. But with the procurement of instruments for the health professionals to work with; good working equipment and proper maintenance for all department to function properly; the constant awareness, orientation, and reorientation toward a maintenance of culture of medical equipment by all workers; a real change of attitude of health workers toward their work and care of patients—these and other changes affected would lift the health system from the rotten state it had fallen into to new levels. Finally, these changes must be monitored by competent administrators and managers who are not only responsible but accountable for what happens in their health care facilities under strict supervision by government officials who, in turn, should be held responsible and accountable by the voters. In addition to these, the law enforcement and the courts must unite to make the law work as it should work. In short, it is Nigerians that must change and demand change. They must demand the best in services and attitude in those who provide the services. We can collectively avoid the Sauna syndrome by using our collective intelligence wisely and for the betterment of all.

CONCLUSION

No system, including the human body, is designed to last forever with or without any problems. Similarly, no system, no matter how well-built, can last for long times without the benefit of maintenance and constant vigilance. A system, according to Gordon W. Allport (1960),

> ... is defined merely as a complex of elements in mutual interaction. Bridgman, as might be expected of an operationist includes a hint of method in his definition. He writes that a system is an isolated enclosure in which all measurements that can be made of what goes on in the system are in some way correlated[14] (sic).

The very first statement of Allport's definition makes two claims: complexity of elements and mutual interaction. For the sake of our discussion, "complex of elements" in this context refers or is synonymous with different parts or different functions of a system. Members of a system must perform their individual functions and at the same time cohesively as a member of the group that forms the system, then and only then can harmony result; otherwise, there is disharmony, and the whole system falters. The Nigerian society itself is a system made up of different parts, which include all the social institutions among which the health system is an interval part. Similarly, the health system comprises of components; the facilities equipment, personnel and their various professions, and practitioners are all a part of it. The neglect of any part can wreck havoc for the whole as the Nigeria case has demonstrated. No right-thinking Nigerian, no matter how patriotic, would deny the fact that our health system is, at least, broken.

The second aspect of the definition is mutual interaction. This means mutual or commonality of interest set in specific direction toward specific goal and for a specific mission. This element has been lacking in the health system in Nigerian people who run it and are pulled in different directions. It is precisely this missing element that has resulted or caused the lack of equipment and the lack of repair for broken equipment and the failure by staff to be considerate to patients and so on. Without mutuality of interest and concert of efforts, a system might produce a product, but the quality of such a product would be a disappointing one, to say the least.

Another aspect of this very element is that interaction can and should be mutual. However, if interacting parts have, each with a different aim and also hidden agenda, then the net result will be a disaster. The overall end result will be total confusion at the very best. Parts of a system are designed each for a specific purpose in the overall scheme of the things within that system; well-built systems may endure abuse and mismanagement, but they can do so only for some time, but will eventually succumb to both external and internal pressures, with ultimate cessation of function. Equally true, Nigeria's health system has suffered mismanagement and neglect for a very long time, thus the deplorable state of its facilities and services, which sooner or later must account for the long neglect it had come to. The process of its decline can, as I would like to believe, be in the process of being arrested with all the new developments instituted by the Obansanjo administration if he should carry through. However, as previously indicated in other chapters and parts of this one, outward change must be more than mere cosmetic alterations. The change has to be a real one that would bring health care from its present fallen state back to its former glory, mission, and noble state. For instance, the government has a role to play in all this and so does every single solitary citizen. Self-help initiatives at individual and other levels are equally very important. No government can do everything for everybody, so citizen should not just wait and look to the government for everything all the time!

Furthermore, changes cannot just be made randomly at any level, but they must be made at every level, from the CEO down the hierarchical ladder of each health facility, government, and all other concerns. There is an old English adage that states, "A bird in hand is worth two in the bush." Personally, I believe that a bird in hand is worth two, three, ten, or even a million in the wild. It is very clear that President Obasanjo was doing his best to stave off corruption in the Nigerian government during his first term. These changes, hopefully, would filter down to the rest of the society, and that is our only hope. However, now no one is sure if he will stick to his guns or not. If he should continue, then we can say he has done a very good job and is a noble leader. Nigeria is lucky to have him as its leader at this trying period.

However, the problem of Nigeria is not more programs, but making the ones already in the books work. Recently, in 2001, the president in a televised interview indicated that he was planning to launch a program that would send a satellite into the space. Why throw more money into programs that don't work? Consolidate the ones that are already here on earth that don't work. Giving politicians and heartless people working in our deplorable social institutions that more money to grab or steal is like dressing a monkey in a cute designer's suit and then releasing it into a marsh area with mud. It's a waste of money that should not be contemplated or entertained. This is simply because you are fighting corruption and in Nigeria, for that matter, for heaven's sake. More government money for corrupt bureaucrats can only mean more opportunity to be corrupt.

Hopefully, all my railings—directed at all Nigerians, the nation, its social institutions, politicians and every form of corrupt behavior—would lead readers to serious thinking and then to some action. If that should be the case, then the monologue in this book, with its scathing criticism, should lead to the direction of that desired change. In that instance then, I should be glad, very glad! This is because it would have accomplished its objective no matter what my critics may say—all I would then say is tough! However, if the criticism is not viewed for what it is, but worse, if it does not lead to change, then no matter what degree of criticism leveled against me would not matter as I would have failed and all this talk would simply be an exercise in futility. But that is for you, the reader and all Nigerians, to decide—you can and should be the judge!

NOTES

1. M. J. E. Cohen, *The Penguin Thesaurus of Quotations* (London: Penguin Books Ltd., 1999) 183.
2. Ibid., 271.
3. H. A. Clement, *The Story of the Ancient World: From the Earliest Times to the Fall of Rome* (Toronto, Canada: George Harrap & Co. Ltd., 1971) 198.
4. Ibid., 489.
5. *The Post Express*, August 7, 1999, 5.*
6. Ibid.
7. *Matthew 16:26,* The New Testament of Our Lord and Savior, Jesus Christ with Psalms and Proverbs (The Gideon's International, 1985).
8. David Williams, *President and Power in Nigeria: The Life of Shehu Shagari* (London: Frank Cass & Co. Ltd., 1982) 9.
9. James O. Ojiako, *Thirteen Years of Military Rule* (Lagos: Daily Times of Nigeria Ltd., 1992) 3-73.
10. Ibid., 45.
11. Ibid., 77-159.
12. *The Post Express*, August 7, 1999.
13. Buhari Brouhaha, "African Market News," *Worldwide Free African Newspaper* vol. 7, no. 8 (August 1999): 6.
14. Gordon W. Allport, *Personality and Social Encounter* (Boston: Beacon Press, 1960) 42.2.
15. The NIV Study Bible, 10th Anniversary Edition (Grand Rapids, MI: The Zondervan Corporation, 1995), 1912.

BIBLIOGRAPHY

Abbeggle, James. *The Japanese Factory.* Glencoe, IL: Free Press, 1958.

Abernethy, David. *The Political Dilemma of Popular Education: An African Case.* Standard Univ. Press, 1969.

Abu-Saad, H. *Nursing: A World View.* St. Louis: The C. V. Mosby Co., 1979.

Adeniji, Kunle. *Transport Challenges in Nigeria in the Next Two Decades: Key Note Address.* August, 2000.

Ajakaiye, Olu, and Bayo Akinbinu, editors: *Strategic Issues in Nigerian Development in Globalizing and Liberalizing World.* Ibadan, Nigeria: Institute of Social and Economic Research, 2000.

Allport, Gordon W.: *Personality and Social Encounter.* Boston: Beacon Press, 1960.

* Anderson, C. L. and C. V. Langton. *Health Principles and Practice,* 3rd ed. St Louis: The C. V. Mosby, 1989.*

* Anderson, C. L. and C. V. Langton. *Health Principle and Practice,* 3rd ed. St. Louis: The C. V. Mosby Co., 1967.*

* Anderson, C. L., and C. V. Langton. *Health Principles and Practice,* 3rd ed. St. Louis: The C. V. Mosby, 1961.*

Anderson, R. E., and L. E. Carter: *Human Behavior in the Social Environment.* Chicago: Aldine Pub. Co.,1974.

Annual Abstract of Statistics, Federal Office of Statistics, Lagos, Nigeria, 1982.

Argyris, Christopher: *Organization and Innovation.* Homewood, IL: Richard D. Irwin, 1965.

Arrison, F. M: *An Introduction to the History of Medicine,* 4th ed. Philadelphia: W. B. Saunders, Co., 1929.

Austin, Charles. *Information System for Health Services Administration*, 3rd ed. Ann Arbor, MI: William J. Harvey, 1988.

Awolowo, Obafemi: *The People's Republic*. Ibadan: Oxford University Press, 1968.

"Back to Genesis." No. 93 of the January Issue of ICR (Institute for Creation Research): Acts and Facts, Vol. 24 No. 1., 1994.*

Bailar, J. C. III et al: *Assessing Risks to Health Methodological Approaches*. Westport, CT: Auburn House, 1997.

Bainton, Roland H. *The Reformation of the Sixteenth Century*. Boston: Beacon Press, 1956.

Barefoot, P. and P. J. Cunningham. *Community Services: The Health Worker's A to Z*. London: Faber & Farber, 1977.

Barron, Jerome A., and C. Charles Dienes: *Constitutional Law*. St. Paul: MN: West Pub., Co., 1991.

Bassett, Lawrence C. *Achieving Excellence: A Prescription for Health Care Manager*. Rockville, MD: Aspen Pub., 1986.

Beauchamp, R. L. *Principle of Biomedical Ethics*, 3rd ed., New York: Oxford Univ. Press, 1989.

Benenson, Abraham S., ed. *Control of Communicable Diseases in Man*, 15th ed. Washington, D.C.: American Public Health Association, 1990.

Bennis, W. G. *Changing Organization*. New York: McGraw-Hill, 1966.

Biehl, Bobb, and Ted Engstrom: *The Effective Board Member*. Nashville, Tennessee: Broadman & Holman Publishers, 1998.

Birnbaum, R. W. *Health Maintenance Organizations: A Guide to Planning and Development*. New York: Spectrum Pub., June 1976.

Blum, H. L. *Expanding Health Care Horizon: From a General System Concepts of Health to a National Health Policy*, 2nd ed. Oakland, CA: Third Party Pub. Co., 1983.

Blau, Peter M. *Bureaucracy in Modern Society*. Chicago: Univ. of Chicago Press, 1950.

Boissoneau, Robert: *Health Care Organization and Development*. Rockville, MD: Aspen System Corp., 1986.

Boris, Emet, and John C. Jeneth. *Catalogues and Computer: A Mystery of Sears*. Chicago: Univ. of Chicago Press, 1950.

Bowditch, H. I. "Address on Hygienic and Preventive Medicine." Transaction of International Medical Congress, Philadelphia, 1986.

Bower, Morviz: *The How to Manage*. New York: McGraw-Hill, 1966.

Brown, M., and H. L. Lewis: *Hospital Management System Multiunit Organizations and Delivery of Health Care.* Germantown, MD: Aspen System Corp., 1976.

Bryant J.: *Health and the Developing World.* Ithaca, NY: Corneal Univ. Press, 1969.

Buhari Brouhaha: "African Market News." *Worldwide Free African Newspaper,* Vol. 7.

no. 8, August, 1999.

Bullough, B., and V. Bullough, editors: *Issues in Nursing.* New York: Springer Pub. Co. Inc., 1966.

Burnett, G. W. and H. W. Scherp: *Oral Microbiology and Infectious Disease*, 3rd ed. Baltimore: Williams and Wilkins, 1968.

*Burns, Sir Alan. *History of Nigeria.* Old Working Survey: Wilkins, 1968.

Burns, Alan: *History of Nigeria.* Old Working Survey: Union Brothers Ltd., 1972.*

Burton, Lloyd E., Smith, Hugh H. and Andrew W. Nicholas: *Public Health Community Medicine*, 3rd ed. Baltimore: Williams and Wilkins, 1980.

Carter, L. Marshal, and David Person: *Dynamics of Health and Disease.* New York: Appleton-Century-Crofts: Educational Division, Meredith Corporation, 1974.

Cavins, H. M. "The National Quarantine and Sanitary Conventions of 1857-1860 and the Beginning of the American Public Health Association," *Bulletin Mist Med.*, December 1944.

Chadwich, H. D. "The Diseases of Inhabitants of the Common Wealth." *New England Journal of Medicine* 216:8, June 10, 1973.

Charns, Martin P. *Collaborative Management in Health Care: Implementing the Integrated Organization.* San Francisco: Jersey Bass, 1993.

Chemnichosvskv, D.: *The Economic Theory of the Hospital and Impact Measurement of Related Health Programs.* Washington, D.C.: World Bank, 1978.

Clement, N. N. *The Story of the Ancient World: From the Earliest Times to the Fall of Rome.* Toronto, Canada: George G. Harrap, Co., Ltd., 1971.

Cohen, M. J.: *The Penguin Thesaurus of Quotations.* New York: Penguin Putnam, June 1998.

Cole, George F. *Criminal Justice Law & Politics*, 4th ed. Monterey, CA: Brooks/Cole Pub., Co., 19 Russell C. Coile Jr: *The New Medicine: Reshaping Practice and Health Care Management.* Rockville, MD: Aspen Pub., Inc., 1990.

Conley, V. : *Curriculum and Instruction in Nursing.* Boston: Little Brown & Co., 1973.

Conrad, L., and E. B. Collagher, eds. *Health and Health Care in Developing Countries: Sociological Perspective.* Philadelphia: Temple Univ. Press, 1993.

Cortese, Anthony. *Ethics: The Restructuring of Moral Theory.* Albany, NY: State Univ. of NY Press, 1990.

Covello, V. T. et al. *Effective Risk Communication: The Role and Responsibility of Government and Non-Government Organizations.* New York: Plenum Press, 1989.

Covey, Lawrence et. al. *Medicine in a Changing Society*, 2nd ed. London: MacMillan Pub., Co., 1977.

Dale, Earliest: *The Great Organizers.* New York: Pitman, 1942.

Daney, Jonathan. *Moral Reasons.* Oxford, UK: Blackwell Pub., 1993.

Darr, Kurt: *Ethics in Health Services Management.* New York: Praeger, 1987.

Davies, J. B. *Community Health: Preventive Medicine and Social Services.* London: Balliere III, Tindall, 1979.

De Fleur, M. L., William, V. D. Antonio, and L. B. DeFleur: *Sociology: Human Society.* Glenview, IL: Scott Foresman and Co. 1973. Joe DeGoshe, *A Content Analysis of a Nigerian TV Drama Series "Cock Crow at Dawn."* Chicago: Univ. of Chicago Press, 1984.

Dever G. E. Allan *Public Health and Policy in Community Health Analysis: Global Awareness at the Local Level*, 2nd ed., Gaithersburg, MD: Aspen Pub. 1991.

Dolan, J. A. *History of Nursing*, 12th ed. Philadelphia: W. B. Saunders Co., 1965.

Donabedian, A. et al.: *Medical Chart Book.* Ann Arbor, MT: Health Administration Press, 1986.

Dowie, Jonathan, and Arthur Eistein: *Professional Judgment: A Reader in Clinical Decision—Making.* New York: Univ. Cambridge Press, 1988.

Dorland's Pocket Medical Dictionary, 24th ed. Philadelphia: W. B. Saunders Co., 1982.

Dunning John J. : *The Multinational Enterprises.* London: Longman, 1971.

Eastaugh, S. R. *Health Economics: Efficiency, Quality, and Equity.* Westport, CT: Auburn House, 1992.

Ephross, Paul H. *Groups That Work:: A Structure and Process.* New York: Columbia University Press, 1988.

* *Epidemiology and Health.* London: Kingdom, 1977.*

Estimates of Kaduna State Government of Nigeria, Kaduna: Printing Services, Kaduna, 1995.

Emergency Handbook: The Science of Caring St. Joseph's Hospital. Asheville, NC: The Bridge Publication, 1984.

Ewing, A. C. *Ethics.* New York: The Free Press, 1853.

Falola, Toyin et al: *History of Nigeria.* New York: African Pub. Corp., 1968.

Fayol, Henry: *General Industrial Management.* New York: Pitman, 1942.

Federal Office of Statistics: The Health of Nigerians. Lagos, September 1985.

__Federal Research Division Library of Congress. *Nigeria: A Country Study.* Washington, D.C.: U.S. Government. Printing Office, 1992,

Fink, Arlene: *An Evaluation Primer.* Washington, D.C.: Admin. Resources Division, Capital Pub., 1978.

Flexner, Jay W. *Industrial Dynamics.* Cambridge, MA: MIT Press, 1961.

Flexner, A. L. *Remember.* New York: Simon & Schuster, 1940.

Freeman, John M., and Kevin McDonnel: *Tough Decisions: A Casebook in Medical Ethics.* New York: Oxford Univ. Press, 1987.

French, Ruth M. *Dynamics of Health Care.* New York: McGraw-Hill Book Co., 1979.

Fried, John: *Cultural Anthropology.* New York: Heaper's College Press, 1976.

Friedman, Gray D. *Primer of Epidemiology*, 4th ed. New York: McGraw-Hill Inc., 1994.

Frohlick, E. D., ed. *Rypins Medical Licensure Examination: Topical Summaries and Questions.* Philadelphia: J. B. Lippincott Co., 1981.

* Galli, Nicholas: *Foundations and Principles of Health Education,* Santa Barbara: John Willey and Sons, 1969.*

* Galli, Nicholas: *Foundations and Principles of Health Education,* Santa Barbara: John Willey and Sons, 1978.*

Gardner, John W. *Self-Renewal: The Individual and the Innovative Society.* New York: Harper and Row, 1964.

Garrison, F. H. : *An Introduction to the History of Medicine*, 4th ed., 1929.

Gentry J. T. *Introduction to Health Services and Community Health Systems: A Primer for Health Planners and Board Members.* Berkley, CA: McCutcan Pub. Corporation, 1978.

* George, D. M., Walkley, R. P., and L. S. Goerke. *Introduction to Public Health*, 6th ed. New York: MacMillan Pub., 1973.*

Ginzberg, E. ed. *Health Services Research: Key to Health Policy.* Cambridge, MA: Harvard Univ. Press, 1991.

Gish, Oscar: *Planning the Health Sector—The Tanzanian Experience.* London: Croom Helm, 1975.

Glorfeld, L. E., Laureman, D. A., and N. C. Strageberg, 3rd edition, New York: Holt, Rinehart and Winston Inc., 1974.

Gould, Stephen I.: *The Measurement of Man.* New York: W. W. Norton & Co. Inc., 1981.

Graham-Brown, R., and Tony Burns: *Lecture Notes: Dermatology*, 7th ed. London: Blackwell Sciences, 1996.

Grassian, Victor. *Moral Reasoning: Ethical Theory and Some Contemporary Moral Problems.* Englewood Cliffs, NJ: Prentice-Hall Inc., 1981.

Griffin, G. J., and J. K. Griffin: *Jenden's History and Trends of Professional Nursing*, 6th ed. St. Louis: The C. V. Mosby Co., 1981.

Guild, W. R., Fruisz, R. E., and S. Bojar: *The Science of Health.* Englewood Cliff, NJ: Prentice-Hall Inc., 1969.

Guilick, Luther, and Lyndall Urwick, editors: *Papers on the Service of Administration.* New York: Institute of Public Administration, 1987.

Guth, William. *Organizational Strategy: Analysis Commitment, Implementation.* Homewood, IL: Irwir, 1964.

Halley's Bible Handbook. Grand Rapids, Michigan: London Pub. House, 1965.

Hanlon, John J. *Public Health Administration and Practice*, 6th ed. St. Louis: The C. V. Mosby Co., 1974.

Hardcastle, Lena LaNelle. *By the Rule: Parliamentary Law: Motions Make Easy.* Gasland, Texas: Stuart Books, 1974.

Harold, H. *Hospital Management: A Guide to the Improvement of Hospital Management System.* Englewood Cliffs, NJ: Prentice-Hall Inc., 1982,

Haruna, Musa: *Addinin Krista a Kasar Jaba da Makwabtanta. Zaria.* Nigeria: Joe Talalur, Associates (Nig.) Ltd., 1993.

Harvey, A. M. et al., editors: *The Principles and Practice of Medicine.* New York: Appleton Century-Crofts, 1976.

Hatch, John. *Nigeria: The Seeds of Disaster.* Chicago: Henry Regnery Co., 1970.

Hazlitt, Henry: *The Foundations of Morality.* Lanham, MD: Univ. Press of America, 1989.

"Health and Development in Africa, June 2-4,1982." Internationales, Interdisciplinares Symposium, Universitat Bayreuth, 1983.

Heidgerken, E. E. *Teaching and Learning in Schools of Nursing: Principle and Methods.* Philadelphia: J.B Lippincott Co., 1965.

Heimann, Theo. *Supervisory Management for Health Care International.* St. Louis, Missouri: The Catholic Hospital Association, 1993.

Herter. Frederick P. et al., eds. *Human and Ethnical Issues in Surgical Care of Patients with Life-Threatening Diseases.* Springfield, IL: Charles C. Thomas Pub., 1986.

Hickman G. *Health for College Students*, 3rd ed., Englewood Cliffs, NJ: Prentice-Hall Inc., 1969.

Hickman, Cleveland, P. *Health for College Students*, 3rd ed. Englewood Cliffs, NJ: Prentice-Hall Inc., 1968.

Hodgetts, R. M., and D. M. Cascio: *Modern Health Care Administration*, 2nd ed. Madison, WI: W. S. Web Brown & Bench Work Pub., 1995.

Holy Bible (KJV), New York: Collin Clear-Typed Press, 1984.

Horwitz, Abraham: *New Dimensions in Health,* Washington, D.C.: Pan Am. Health Organization, 1964.

Jacobs, M., and B. T. Stern. *General Anthropology.* New York: Barnes and Nobles, 1955.

Jamieson, E. M., Sewall, M. F., and E. B. Suhrie: *Trends in Nursing History: Their Social, International and Ethical Relationships.* Philadelphia: W. B. Saunders Co. 1966.

Jawetz, F., Melnick, J. L. and E. A. Adelberg: *Review of Medical Microbiology,* Norwalk, CT: Appleton & Lange, 1987.

Johnson, D. G. *Physician in the Making.* San Francisco: Jessey Bass Pub., 1983.

Johnson, Phillip E. *Darwin on Trial.* Downers Grove, IL: Intervarsity Press, 1993.

Jonas, Steven: *Health Care Delivery in United States*, 2nd ed. New York: Springer Pub, Co., 1981.

Jonsen, A. R, Siegler, M., and William J. Winsland: *Clinical Ethics, A Practical Approach to Ethical Decisions in Clinical Medicine*, 2nd ed. New York: MacMillan Pub. Co., 1986.

Janqueira, L. Carlos, and Jose Carnairo: *Basic Histology*, 3rd ed. Drawer L. Los Altos, CA: Lange Medical Publications, 1980

Junqueira, L., Carlos, Carneiro, Jose, and Robert O. Kelley: *Basic Histology*, 8th ed. Standford, CT: Appleton & Lange, 1995.

Kaluzny, A. et al. *Management of Health Services.* Englewood Cliffs, NJ: Prentice-Hall Inc., 1982.

Karr, Snehendu B., editor: *Health Promotion Indicators and Actions.* New York: Springer Pub. Co., 1989.

King, M. A. *Medical Laboratory for Developing Countries.* London: Oxford Press, 1975.

Kobayashi, Shigeru. *Creative Management,* New York: Am. Management Association, 1971.

Kohn, R., and K. L. White: *Health Care: An International Study.* London: Oxford Univ. Press, 1976.

Kolnai, Aurel: *Kolnai Ethics, Values and Reality,.* Indianapolis: Hackett Pub. Co., 1978.

Koop, C. Everett and Florence Comite: *Dr. Koop's Self Care Advisor: The Essential Home Health Guide for You and Your Family.* Health Publication Group, 1996.

Krupp, Marcus A. et al: *Physician Handbook*, 21st ed. Los Angeles, CA: Lange Medical Pub., 1985.

F. Ransome Kuti, "Doctors Attitude to Health Care," *Concord*, October 11, 1986.

Knopke, H. J. and N. I. Dickelman, editors: *Approaches to Teaching Primary Health Care,.* St. Louis: The C. V. Mosby Co., 1981.

Lamberson, E. C. *Education for Nursing Leadership.* Philadelphia: J. B. Lippincott Co., 1958.

Lasch, Christopher: *The Culture of Narcism,.* New York: Warner Communication Co., 1979.

Lasse, Stanley. *The Future of Health Services: Anticipating Tomorrow.* New York: Irvington Pub., 1978.

Last, J. M. *Public Health and Human Ecology.* Ottawa: Prentice-Hall, Appleton & Lange, 1987.

Lee, P., and C. L. Estes, eds. *The Nation's Health.* Preston: Jones and Bartlett Pub., 1990.

Lehman, Edwards W.: *Coordinating Health Care Explorations in International Relations.* Vol. 17, Beverly Hills: Sage Pub. Inc., 1995.

Levey, S. and N. P. Loomba: *Health Care Administration: A Managerial Perspective,* 2nd ed. Philadelphia: J. B. Lippincott Co., 1990.

Levey, Samuel:. *Health Care Administration: Managerial Perspective.* Philadelphia: Lippincott, 1984.

Lewis, Michael: *The Culture of Inequality,.* New Year: New Am. Library, 1978.

Lewis, Naphtali, and Meyer Reinhold, eds. *Roman Civilization: Sourcebook II: The Empire.* New York, NY: Harper and Row Pub. 1966.

Loewy, Erichtt. *The Textbook of Medical Ethics,* 2nd ed. New York: Plenum Pub. Corp., 1989.

Longest, Beaufort B. *Management: Practice for the Health Professional,* 3rd ed. Reston, VA: Reston Pub., Co., 1984.

Mackintosh, D. R.: *System of Health Care,* Boulder, Colorado: Westview Press, 1978.

Malff, John: *Management: A Study Guide to A/C Company Koonts, O'Donnell and Welbrich.* New York: McGraw-Hill Book Co., 1989.

__Management Information Systems for Public Health Community Health Agencies, Conference Report, 1972.

Managle, John F., and David C. Thomasma: *Health Care Ethics: Critical Issues.* Rockville, MD: Aspen Pub., Inc., 1994.

__—. *Medical Ethics : A Guide for Health Performance.* Rockville, MD: Aspen Pub. Inc., 1988.

Mappes, Thomas A. and Jane S. Zematy: : *Biomedical Ethics,* 2nd ed., New York: McGraw-Hill Book Co., 1986.

Marshall, C. L. and D. Person: *Dynamics of Health and Disease,.* New York: Appleton-Century-Crofts, 1972.

Massier, J. L., and J. Douglas: *Managing: A Contemporary Introduction,* 2nd ed. Englewood Cliffs, NJ: Prentice-Hall Inc., 1977,

Mayo, Elton: *The Human Problems of an Industrial Civilization,* Boston, MA: Harvard Business School, 1946.

McClain. M. E., and S. H. Gregg: *Scientific Principles on Nursing,* 5th ed. St. Louis: The C. V. Mosby Co., 1996.

McGibony, John R: *Principle of Hospital Administration.* New York: G. P. Putnam & Sons, 1969.

McGregor, Douglas: *The Human Side of Enterprise,* New York: McGraw-Hill Book Co., 1960.

Meisenheimer, C. G: *Improving Quality: A Guide to Effective Programs.* Gailtersberg, MD: Aspen Pub. Inc.,1992.

Merton, R. K., et al, eds. *A Reader in Bureaucracy,* Glance, IL: The Free Press, 1952.

Metz, Helen. *Nigeria: A Country Study.* Washington, D.C.: Library of Congress Pub., 1997.

Metzge, Norman, ed.: *Handbook of Health Care for Human Resource Management.* Rockville, MD: Aspen Pub., 1981.

Miller, D. F. *Dimensions of Community Health*, 3rd ed. Dubuque, IA.: William C. Brown Pub., 1979.

Milner, Rosalind S. *Primary Health Care More than Medicine.* Englewood Cliffs, NJ: Prentice-Hall Inc., 1983.

Mish, Fredrick C.: *Webster's 9th New Collegiate Dictionary,* Spring field, MA; Merriam—Webster's Inc. Pub., 1991.

Mobabinije, Alvin R.: *Urbanization in Nigeria.* New York: African Pub. Corp., 1968.

—. *Urbanization in Nigeria II and Nigeria in the 19th Century.* Lagos: Longman, 1991.

Morgan, M. T. *Environmental Health.* Madison, WI: WCB Brown and Benchmark Pub., 1993.

Nagy, Doreen E. Venden: *Popular Medicine in 17th Century England.* Bowling Green, Ohio: Bowling Green Univ. Press, 1988.

Nanguang, D. M.: *Causes of Problems for Nursing Administration in Nigeria.* New Orleans, Louisiana: South Western Univ. Press, 1989.

Nehane, Chie: *Japanese Society,.* Berkeley, CA: Univ. of California Press, 1970.

Nelson, Eugene C,. et al: *Medical and Health Guide for People over Fifty,.* Glenview, IL: AARP Books, Washington, D.C., 1986.

Ojiako, James O. *Thirteen Years of Military Rule, 1966-79.* Lagos, Nigeria: Daily Times of Nigeria Ltd., 1979.

Okpokowuruk, H. A. "Journey Home, Health Care in Nigeria: My Personal Experience," *African News Weekly*, Vol. 5. No. 37, October 28, 1997.

Omolewa, Michael: *Certificate History of Nigeria,.* Lagos, Nigeria: Longman, 1990.

Orem, O. E. and K. S. Parker, eds. *Nursing Content: Interservice Nursing Curriculums.* Washington, D.C.: The Catholic Univ. of Am Press, 1964.

Orwell, George:. *Animal Farm,.* New York: New American Library, 1996.

Penrose, Edith T.: *The Theory of the Growth of the Firm,.* London: Oxford Univ. Press, 1959.

Perls, Frederick, Hefferline, Ralph F. and Paul Goodman: *Gestalt Therapy: Excitement and Growths in the Human Personality.* New York: Dell Publishing Co. Inc., 1951.

Pfeiffer, Carl J. A. *Disquisition on the Art and Practice of Medicine and Electric Review Physiology Principle as Espoused in Europe, Britain and the New United State of America, 1500-1825.* Jefferson, NC: Farland & Co. Inc., Pub., 1985.

Phillips, J. B. *Your God Is Too Small.* New York: Touchstone Books, 1997.

*_Puschmann, A. *History of Medical Education.* 1994.*

Rakich, J. S., Longest, B. B. and J. D. Kurt Darr: *Managing Health Services Organizations*, 2nd ed., Philadelphia: W. B. Saunders Co., 1985.

Reader, W. J. *Imperial Chemical Industries: A History*, Vol. 1870-1926. New York: Oxford Univ. Press, 1970.

Richardson, B. W.: *The Health of Nations: A Review of the Works of Edwin Chadwick*, Vol. II. London: Longmans, Green and Co., 1887.

Rights in Conflict, Violence in Chicago. New York: Putman Books, 1968.

Roemer, Milton I.: *National Health Systems of the World,* New York: Oxford Univ. Press, 1991.

Rogers, E. M. and Lyon Svenring:. *Modernization among Peasants Impact of Communication,.* New York: Holt Rinechart and Winston Inc., 1969.

Rogers, James: *The Dictionary of Clichés,* New York: Ballantine Books, 1985.

Rosen, G. A.: *A History of Public Health,.* New York: MD Pub. Inc., 1958.

Rosenthal, M.M., and M. Frankel. *Health Care Systems and Their Patients: An International Perspective.* Boulder, Colorado: Westview Press, 1992.

Ross, Austin: *Cornerstone of Leadership of Health Services Executives,.* Ann Arbor, Michigan: Health Admin. Press, 1992.

Rowland, H. S. and B. L. Rowland: *Hospital Administration Handbook.* Rockville, MD: Aspen Pub., 1984.

Robinson, L. and A. F. Wesley:. *Health Education: Foundations for the Future,*. St. Louis: Times Mirror/Mosby College Pub., 1984.

Samph, T. and B. Templeton: *Evaluation in Medical Education: Past, Present, Future.* Cambridge, MA: Ballinger Co., 1979.

Schram, Ralph: *A History of the Nigerian Health Services,* Ibadan: Ibadan Univ. Press, 1971.

Schwartz, H. and C. S. Kat: *Dominant Issues in Medical Sociology,* Addison: Wesley Pub. Co., 1978.

Shorter, Edward: *The Health Century,* New York: Doubleday, 1987.

Sheldom, Oliver. *The Philosophy in Management,* London: Sir Isaac Pitman and Sons, Ltd., 1930.

Shortell, Steven and Arnold Kalunzy: *Health Management: A Text in Organization, Theory and Behavior,* New York: John Willey & Sons, 1993.

Shaltuck, L. et al. *Report of the Sundry Commission of Massachusetts.* Borton: Bulton and Wentwork State Printers, 1850.

Sloan, Alfred P. Jr.: *My Years with General Motors,* Garden City, New York: Doubleday, 1941.

Sloan, Ruth et al: *The Educated African,* New York: Frederick A. Praeger Pub., 1967.

Smalley, Harold B. *Hospital Management: Guide to the Improvement of Management System.* Englewood Cliffs, NJ: Prentice-Hall Inc., 1982.

Snell, George D. *Search for a Rational Ethics.* New York: Springer-Verlag New York Inc., 1988.

Smillie, W. G.: "The National Board of Health, 1979-1983," *American Journals of Pub. Health* 33.925, August 1943.

Sounder, J. B. de C.: *Transition from Ancient Egyptian to Greek Medicine,*. Lawrence, Kansas: Univ. of Kansa Press, 1963.

Soran, Kango K. *Nursing in the World: The Needs of Individual Countries and Their Programmes,* BINF, 1977.

Spalding, E. K., and I. E. Notter. *Professional Nursing,* 8th ed., Philadelphia: J. B. Lippincott Co., 1970.

Spartan Health Sciences University, School of Medicine Brochure, 1990.

Specter, Raphael E. *Cultural Diversity in Health and Illness,* 2nd ed. Norwalk, CT: Appleton-Century-Crofts, 1985.

Summer, Wm. Graham: *Folkways,* New York. The American Library Inc., 1960.

* __AUPHA Manual of Health Services Management, The Gaithersberg, MD: Aspen Pub., 1994.
* __The Century Dictionary: An Encyclopedia Lexicon of the English Language, Vol. VI. New York: The Century Co., 1995.*
* The Democrat, September 29, 1988.*
* The Democrat, Vol. 1, December 24, 1988.*
* The Effective Health Care Executive: A Guide in a Winning Management Style. Rockville, MD: Aspen Pub., 1986.*
* The Europa World Year Book World Survey, vol. 2. London: The Europa Pub. Ltd., 1985.*
* The Europa World Year Book. London: Europe Pub. Ltd., 1994.*
* The Holy Bible (NIV). Grand Rapids, Michigan: Zondervan Bible Pub., 1984.*
* The Merck Manual, 5th ed., Railway, NJ: Merck Sharp & Dohme Research Laboratories, 1987.*
* The Nigerian Household. Federal Office of Statistics 1983/84. Lagos, Nigeria, 1985.*
* The Random House Dictionary. New York: Random House, 1980.
* Richardson, B. W.: The Health of Nations Review of the Works of Edwin Chadwick, Vol. II. London: Longmans, Green and Co., 1887.
Thompson, J. S., and M. W. Thomson: Genetics in Medicine, 4th ed. Philadelphia: W. B. Saunders Co., 1986.
Today, August, 1986.
Tripp, Rhoda T.: The Thesaurus of International Quotations,. New York: Harper-Row Pub., 1970.
Troyer, Glenn T. and Steven L. Salman, editors: Handbook of Health Care Risk Management, Rockville, MD: Aspen Pub., 1986,
Turaki, Y. An Introduction to the History of SIM/ECWA in Nigeria, 1893-1993. Jos, Nigeria: Challenge Press, 1993.
—. The British Colonial Legacy in Northern Nigeria: A Social Ethnical Analysis of the Colonial and Post Colonial Society and Politics in Nigeria. Jos: Challenge Press, 1993.
Veatch, Robert. Cross Cultural Perspective in Medical Ethics Reading. Boston, MA: James Barlett Pub., 1989.
Vency, James E.: Evaluation and Decision Making for Health Services Programs, Englewood Cliffs, NJ: Prentice-Hall, 1984.
Vivas, Elisco: The Moral Life and Ethical Life, New York: Univ. Press of American, 1965.

Waters, W. E. and K. S. Clift: *Community Medicine: A Textbook for Nurses and Visitors.* London: Groom Helm, 1983.

Wear, A., French, R. K., and I. M. Lonie, editors, *The Medical Renaissance of the Sixteenth Century.* London: Cambridge Univ. Press, 1995.

Williams, David: *President and Power in Nigeria: The Life of Shehu Shagari.* London: Prank Cass and Co., Ltd., 1982.

Williams, Roberts B., editor: *Hospital Pharmacy Management Primer,* Bethesda, MD: America Society of Hospital Pharmacist, 1985.

Wilner, D. M., Walkley, R. P. and L. S. Georke: *Introduction to Public Health*, 6th editor. New York: MacMillan Pub., 1973.

Wilson and D. Neuhauser: *Health Services in the United States*, 2nd ed. Cambridge, MA: Ballinger Pub. Co., 1985.

Winslow, C. E. A. : *The Conquest of Epidemic Diseases,* Princeton, NJ: Princeton Univ. Press, 1943.

Whitaker's Almanac, 12th ed. London: J. Whitaker & Sons., 1993.

Wolf, Thomas. *The Nonprofit Organization: An Operating Manual.* New York: Prentice-Hall, 1984.

Wright, Richard A. *Human Values in Health Care: The Practice of Ethics.* New York: McGraw-Hill Book Co., 1989.

Yoshino, M. *Japan's Managerial System: Tradition and Innovation.* Cambridge, MA: MIT Press, 1968.

APPENDIX

COMMON TERMS, SHORTHAND, ACRONYMS, AND CODING SYSTEM USED

HIV/AIDS	. . .	AIDS
Univ.	. . .	University
Sync.	. . .	Synchrony
Sml.	. . .	Small/tiny
Orgn.	. . .	Organization
Behv.	. . .	Behavior
Dev't.	. . .	Development
Dep't.	. . .	Department
Supvs./Supvrs.	. . .	Supervisor
OC	. . .	Chief or Office in Charge
Oga Kpatakpata	. . .	Overall boss
Prodox	. . .	Production/Productive
lntn'l.	. . .	International
WHO	. . .	World Health Organization
UNESCO	. . .	United Nations Education
		Cultural
Ed.	. . .	& Scientific Organization
Nrsg.	. . .	Education
Supot.	. . .	Nurse
Hosp.	. . .	Support
Ctr.	. . .	Hospital
Regres.	. . .	Center
Prog.	. . .	Regression
Admin.	. . .	Programs
Minim.	. . .	Administration
Ecol.	. . .	Minimum
Exec.	. . .	Ecology
		Executive

Eval.	...	Evaluation
Strt./Stract.	...	Structure
Pt.	...	Patient
Pub.	...	Public
Promo.	...	Promotion
Medi.	...	Medicine
Med'l.	...	Medical
>	...	Over/more than
<	...	Less/less than
->	...	Leading to
NA	...	Nurse Attendant
Ns A	...	Needs addition
TC	...	To continue
FRR	...	Further Research Required
FFR	...	For Further Research
Situ.		Situation
Info.	...	Information
Intro./Introdox.	...	Introduction
Ds	...	Disease
Hx	...	History
C'mon	...	Common
Rxn.	...	Reaction
Max.	...	Maximum
Supres.	...	Suppression
CEO.	...	Chief Executive Officer
Magt.	...	Management
PE	...	Physical Examination
Econ.	...	Economy
Epidem.		Epidemiology
Serv.		Service(s)
Grp./group		Group

ABOUT THE AUTHOR

Dr. Daniel M. N. McDikkoh was born in 1945 in Jzheik Town or Kurmin Musa in the current Kachia local government of Kaduna State, Nigeria. He was born into a large family and is the sixth child of eleven children.

His education started at the then Sudan Interior Mission (SIM) Elementary School through then the Senior Primary School from 1951-1962 in Kurmin Musa, his birthplace, after spending four years (1951-1954) in the first grade and two years (1956-1957) in the third grade. In 1959, he did not attend any school, but helped his father in the farm because there were no "qualified grade two teachers" who could teach a fifth-grade class that Dr. McDikkoh had then reached.

From 1960 through 1962, he attended and completed the senior primary education and obtained his First School Leaving Certificate, then went to the Kagoro Bible College, about fifty miles east of Jzheik Town, his birthplace, where he spent the next two years. In 1964, he was admitted to study to become a nurse at the Vom Christian Hospital, Sudan United Mission Nurse Training School. He then left the Kagoro Bible College and started the nurse training in Vom, Plateau Province, Nigeria, from 1965 through 1968, by the end of which he finished and passed the Nigerian Registered Nurse certification. He was then deployed and worked for Sudan United Mission at Gindiri and for one year (1969).

At the end of 1969, he left being the school nurse for the Gindiri and Schools complex to work with the new Ahmadu Bello University Teaching Hospital in Zaria in the then North Central State of Nigeria. Dr. McDikkoh worked as the nurse in charge of the Casualty Theater or Unit (an emergency unit) for two years (1970-1971) and was later transferred to the A. B. University—Main Campus Sick Bay at the end of 1971, where he worked for another year (1972) before leaving for the United State in January 1973.

He started work as nurse at the Saint Barnabas Medical Center, Livingston, New Jersey, in January 1973 and was then admitted to the baccalaureate nursing program at Rutgers State University of New Jersey in September 1974 and graduated with BSN degree in 1978. Prior to attending Rutgers University, he had spent the spring semester of 1974 taking courses at the Essex County Community College in Newark, New Jersey.

After his graduation at the College of Nursing, Rutgers University, he attended Teachers College Columbia University, New York City, from 1978 through 1980, where he earned masters in nursing administration and masters in nursing education. He then was admitted to study sociology of education and spent the next two years (1983-1985) at the Rutgers University, New Brunswick, New Jersey. Dr. McDikkoh then transferred to study at the Southwestern University, New Orleans, Louisiana, where he earned a his PhD in health care management and administration in 1990. He finally completed his medical education in 1994 that he had enrolled and started at the Spartan Health Sciences University in the Caribbean Island of Saint Lucia in 1989.

Dr. Daniel McDikkoh now lives in El Paso, Texas, after moving there from New Jersey to Johnson City, East Tennessee, in the spring of 1991 and from there to El Paso in November that same year. He is a professor in mental health nursing in the Division of Nursing at El Paso Community College. He is married to former Miss Leticia Corona Garibay and has four girls: two (Danielle Gimbia and Epiphany Seim) with her and the other two (Diana Celestia and Cynthia "Cinda" Gimbiya) who were bought from Nigeria in 2007.

He has traveled far and wide in West Africa, North America, Europe, the Caribbean, and parts of the Middle East and loves some of the outdoor sports like tennis, soccer, bicycle riding, hiking, and fishing.

Lightning Source UK Ltd.
Milton Keynes UK
UKHW040354270419
341665UK00014B/247/P

9 781450 021043